D1029529

INTEGRATION IN THE NERVOUS SYSTEM

A Symposium in Honor of
DAVID P.C. LLOYD and RAFAEL LORENTE DE NÓ

The Rockefeller University
May 4–5, 1978

Edited by

HIROSHI ASANUMA, M.D. and VICTOR J. WILSON, Ph.D.
The Rockefeller University, New York, NY

IGAKU-SHOIN   Tokyo · New York

Published and distributed by

IGAKU-SHOIN Ltd.,
  5-24-3 Hongo, Bunkyo-ku, Tokyo.
IGAKU-SHOIN Medical Publishers, Inc.,
  50 Rockefeller Plaza, New York, N.Y. 10020

ISBN: 0-89640-033-6
Library of Congress Catalog Card Number: 79-84783

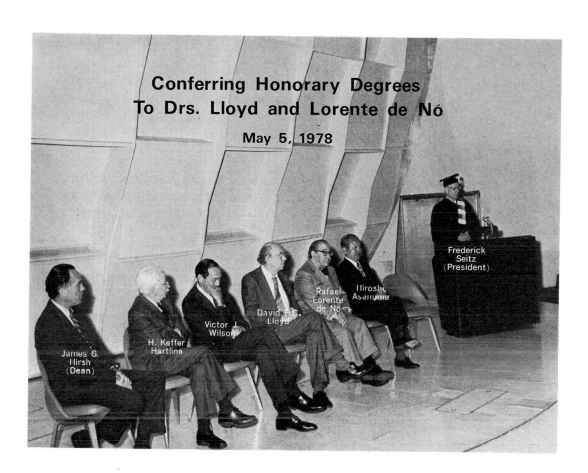

**Conferring Honorary Degrees
To Drs. Lloyd and Lorente de Nó**

May 5, 1978

James G. Hirsh (Dean)

H. Keffer Hartline

Victor J. Wilson

David P.C. Lloyd

Rafael Lorente de Nó

Hiroshi Asanuma

Frederick Seitz (President)

PREFACE

All of us who study the nervous system are greatly indebted to David P.C. LLOYD and Rafael LORENTE DE NÓ, both of whom were towering figures in Neurophysiology and spent many years at the Rockefeller. It seemed to us who followed them that an appropriate way to acknowledge this debt was to hold a symposium in their honor, at which some of the neurophysiologists who studied with them, or were influenced by them, could present some data and some thoughts about the current state of three topics on which LLOYD and LORENTE DE NÓ had a particular impact: the spinal cord, the vestibular system and cortical and subcortical organization.

There should be little need to point out the numerous fundamental contributions that LLOYD and LORENTE DE NÓ made to our understanding of the functioning of the central nervous system, directly by their own research and less directly through the work of the many investigators who spent part of their formative years working in the Rockefeller laboratories. Suffice it to say that LLOYD used newly-developed electrophysiological methods to unravel some of the intricacies of synaptic transmission and of reflex organization. In so doing, he produced the first truly important advance from SHERRINGTON's pioneering work on the reflex organization of the spinal cord. LORENTE DE NÓ opened a new field by combining the study of structure and function in the central nervous system. His discoveries of reverberating circuits in the vestibular system and of the radial arrangement of neurons in the cerebral cortex, and his analysis of field potentials in relation to structure, laid the foundations for many succeeding studies.

We are pleased that the symposium, which was held at Rockefeller University on May 4–5, 1978, was such a success and want to present this book as a tribute to our great predecessors.

VICTOR J. WILSON
HIROSHI ASANUMA

LIST OF PARTICIPANTS

Dr. VAHÉ E. AMASSIAN
Department of Physiology
SUNY-Downstate Medical Center
450 Clarkson Avenue
Brooklyn, NY 11203

Dr. HIROSHI ASANUMA
The Rockefeller University
1230 York Avenue
New York, NY 10021

Dr. ROBERT BAKER
Department of Physiology and Biophysics
New York University Medical School
550 First Avenue
New York, NY 10016

Dr. VERNON B. BROOKS
Department of Physiology
University of Western Ontario
London, Ontario
CANADA N6A 3K7

Dr. ROBERT E. BURKE
Laboratory of Neural Control
Bldg. 36, Rm. 5A29
National Institutes of Health
Bethesda, MD 20014

Dr. CLAUDE GHEZ
The Rockefeller University
1230 York Avenue
New York, NY 10021

Dr. ANN M. GRAYBIEL
Department of Psychology and Brain Science
Massachusetts Institute of Technology
Cambridge, MA 02139

Dr. HARRY GRUNDFEST
Columbia University
College of Physicians and Surgeons
New York, NY 10032

Dr. H. KEFFER HARTLINE
The Rockefeller University
1239 York Avenue
New York, NY 10021

Dr. ELWOOD HENNEMAN
Department of Physiology
Harvard Medical School
25 Shattuck Street
Boston, MA 02115

Dr. CARLTON C. HUNT
Department of Physiology and Biophysics
Washington University School of Medicine
St. Louis, MO 63110

Dr. YVES LAPORTE
Laboratoire de Neurophysiologie
Collège de France
11, place Marcelin Berthelot
75231 Paris Cedex 05
FRANCE

Dr. RODOLFO LLINÁS
Department of Physiology
New York University Medical School
550 First Avenue
New York, NY 10016

Dr. ANDERS LUNDBERG
Department of Physiology
University of Göteborg
Fack
S-400 33 Göteborg 33
SWEDEN

Dr. JEAN MASSION
Département de Neurophysiologie Générale
I.N.P.-C.N.R.S.
31, chemin Joseph Aiguier
13274 Marseille, Cedex 2
FRANCE

Dr. VERNON B. MOUNTCASTLE
Department of Physiology
The Johns Hopkins University
School of Medicine
Baltimore, MD 21205

Dr. BARRY W. PETERSON
Department of Neurophysiology
The Rockefeller University
1230 York Avenue
New York, NY 10021

Dr. CHARLES G. PHILLIPS
Department of Anatomy
University of Oxford Medical School
43 Woodstock Road
Oxford, OX2 6HG
ENGLAND

Dr. DOMINICK P. PURPURA
Rose F. Kennedy Center for Research in
Mental Retardation and Human
Development
Albert Einstein College of Medicine
1410 Pelham Perkway South
Bronx, NY 10461

Dr. HIROSHI SHIMAZU
Department of Neurophysiology
Institute of Brain Research
School of Medicine, University of Tokyo
7–3–1 Hongo, Bunkyo-ku, Tokyo
JAPAN

Dr. PETER L. STRICK
Research Service (151)
Veterans Administration Hospital
800 Irving Avenue
Syracuse, NY   13210

Dr. VICTOR J. WILSON
The Rockefeller University
1230 York Avenue
New York, NY   10021

CONTENTS

SPINAL CORD

VESTIBULAR SYSTEM

CORTICAL AND SUBCORTICAL INTEGRATION (1)

CORTICAL AND SUBCORTICAL INTEGRATION (2)

SPINAL CORD

Chairman: CARLTON C. HUNT

INNERVATION OF CAT MUSCLE SPINDLES BY FAST CONDUCTING SKELETO-FUSIMOTOR AXONS*

Yves LAPORTE

Laboratorie de Neurophysiologie, Collège de France
Paris, France

Skeleto-fusimotor axons are axons which supply both extrafusal and intrafusal muscle fibres. In lower vertebrates, they constitute the whole motor supply to muscle spindles whereas in mammals the intrafusal muscle fibres are mostly but not exclusively innervated by a specific set of axons, the fusimotor or γ axons. In cat spindles, skeleto-fusimotor axons, which regardless of their conduction velocities are conveniently referred to as β axons, were first demonstrated in a small distal muscle of the hind-limb, the first deep lumbrical muscle (BESSOU et al., 1963b, 1965; ADAL and BARKER, 1965) but recently β axons were also found in large muscles such as the flexor hallucis longus, the peroneus brevis, the tibialis anterior and the soleus (EMONET-DÉNAND et al., 1975). In the peroneus brevis muscle, 70 per cent of the spindles have a skeleto-fusimotor innervation and 18 per cent of the motor axons are β axons (EMONET-DÉNAND and LAPORTE, 1975). In this muscle there is a high incidence of spindles innervated by p_1 plates which are considered to be the endings of β axons (BARKER et al., 1970). In the tenuissimus and the abductor digiti quinti muscles, McWILLIAM (1975) has found that 30 to 40 per cent of the spindles are β innervated.

In the above-mentioned physiological studies the identification of β axons rested on the observation that repetitive stimulation of some single motor axons supplying extrafusal muscle fibres also excited muscle spindles; these axons were considered as β only if the increase in rate of discharge of primary endings elicited by their stimulation persisted after selective elimination of extrafusal contraction by curarization (BESSOU et al., 1965) or by stimulation at high frequency (EMONET-DÉNAND and LAPORTE, 1974). Nearly all the β axons identified in this way had conduction velocities in the 40–85 m/s range and exerted a dynamic action on the responses of primary endings (EMONET-DÉNAND et al., 1975). Dynamic β axons, as shown by the glycogen depletion method of EDSTRÖM and KUGELBERG (1968), supply intrafusal muscle fibres of the bag$_1$ type and extrafusal muscle fibres of the slow oxidative type (BARKER et al., 1977).

In the present paper, it will be reported that cat muscle spindles may be supplied by another kind of β axon, which differ from the previously known β axons by their conduction velocities as well as by the muscle fibres they supply and their action on spindle sensory endings. The demonstration of the existence of very fast conducting skeleto-fusimotor axons was obtained in a series of experiments designed to answer a question which arose from the observation that nearly all the β axons that had been identified in previous investigations by physiological testing had conduction velocities slower than 85 m/s. Was it because there are no skeleto-fusimotor axons among the fastest motor axons or because the techniques used were inappropriate to detect them? The size of motor units increase with the diameter and conduction velocities of their motor axons (BESSOU et al., 1963a;

* This work was supported by grants from INSERM (ATP 76–61) and the Foundation pour la Recherche Médicale Française.

McPHEDRAN et al., 1965; WUERKER et al., 1965; OLSON and SWETT, 1966; APPELBERG and EMONET-DÉNAND, 1967; BURKE, 1967; JAMI and PETIT, 1975). It is therefore conceivable that the contraction of a large number of extrafusal muscle fibres might conceal a weak excitatory effect of an intrafusal contraction by its unloading effect on primary ending discharge. Furthermore, it could not be taken for granted that all β axons had intrafusal neuromuscular junctions relatively more resistant to curare and/or repetitive stimulation than their extrafusal junctions.

The glycogen-depletion method has hitherto been used to determine the type, number and situation of muscle fibres supplied by single motor axons of *known* function: *skeletomotor* (EDSTRÖM and KUGELBERG, 1968; KUGELBERG, 1973; BURKE et al., 1973, 1974); *fusimotor* (BROWN and BUTLER, 1973, 1975; BARKER et al., 1976); *skeleto-fusimotor* (BARKER et al., 1977; BURKE and TSAIRIS, 1977). But actually this method can also serve to find out whether certain motor axons of a given muscle participate in spindle innervation, the evidence being the glycogen depletion observed in some intrafusal muscle fibres after appropriate stimulation of the axons. Such technique necessitates that as many as possible of the muscle spindles be examined for glycogen depletion and requires a great amount of histological work which explains why these experiments were carried out on a relatively small muscle of the leg, the peroneus tertius (also called peroneus digiti quinti) muscle (HARKER et al., 1977).

In each experiment single motor axons to the peroneus tertius were prepared by splitting ventral roots and only the ventral root filaments containing axons with a conduction velocity faster than 85–90 m/s were preserved (Fig. 1). All the fast conducting motor axons were then simultaneously stimulated following a pattern of stimulation (see HARKER et al., 1977 for details) known to produce glycogen depletion in intrafusal as well as in extrafusal muscle fibres. Histological examination was made on transverse sections of fresh-frozen muscle stained to demonstrate glycogen with the periodic acid-Schiff (PAS) method. The number of axons stimulated in each experiment ranged from 12 to 23 and the number of examined spindles from 12 to 21 (Table 1). It was found that of 99 examined spindles 27 presented zones of glycogen depletion. These zones were almost exclusively located in one or two of the longest chain fibres in any spindle pole, as illustrated by Figure 2; the lengths of the depleted zones ranged from 165 μm to 1700 μm. In terms of the 31 spindle

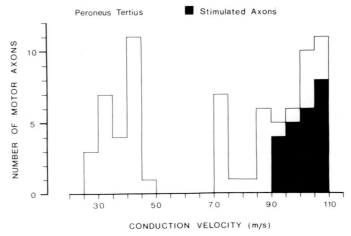

Fig. 1 Conduction velocities of single peroneus tertius motor axons which were prepared during the same experiment. The filled squares correspond to the 23 axons with a conduction velocity faster than 90 m/s which were simultaneously stimulated (from HARKER et al., 1977)

Table 1 Number of peroneus tertius spindles supplied by very fast conducting skeleto-fusimotor axons (from HARKER et al., 1977).

Expt	No. of Stimulated motor axons	No. of examined spindles	No. of spindles with zones of glycogen depletion
1	15 (85–100)	12	4
2	12 (95–105)	18	4
3	19 (92–105)	15	7
4	17 (92–105)	21	3
5	15 (97–102)	16	4
6	23 (90–109)	17	5
Total		99	27

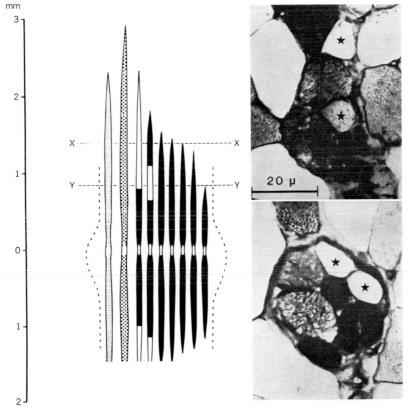

Fig. 2 Schematic reconstruction of a peroneus tertius spindle showing zones of glycogen depletion elicited by the simultaneous stimulation of 23 motor axons whose conduction velocities were higher than 90 m/s (same experiment as in Fig. 1). Bag_1 fibre, light shading (medium glycogen); bag_2 fibre, coarse shading (medium/high glycogen) chain fibre, filled (high glycogen). The depletion is exclusively located in the two longest chain fibres. The chain fibre, which in this spindle is as long as the bag_1 fibre, is the so-called long chain fibre (see BARKER et al., 1976a). In the right part of the figure, photomicrographs of transverse sections taken through levels X and Y shown in the diagram. Asterisks indicate depleted fibres (from HARKER et al., 1977).

poles with zones of glycogen depletion, chain fibres were involved in 30 (46 chain fibres), bag_2 fibres in none and bag_1 fibres in 3 (3 bag_1 fibres). In two poles, the depletion of the bag_1 fibres was accompanied by chain fibre depletion. The third instance of bag_1 depletion was observed in isolation in one pole of a spindle the other pole of which could not be histologically examined.

Figure 3 gives a summary of the glycogen depletion elicited in some spindles of a peroneus tertius muscle after stimulating 19 fast conducting motor axons. In this experiment (experiment 3 of Figure 2) out of 15 examined spindles 7 had zones of depletion; they were exclusively found in chain fibres and without exception in the longest ones.

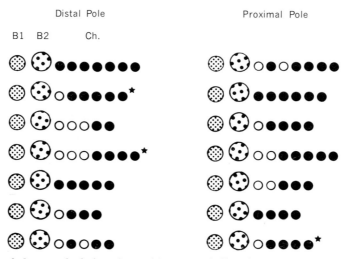

Fig. 3 Pattern of glycogen depletion observed in some spindles of a peroneus tertius muscle after stimulation of a group of fast conducting motor axons (experiment 3 of Table 1). Medium-diameter circles with light shading represent non depleted poles of bag_1 fibres; large circles with with coarse shading, those of bag_2 fibres; and small filled circles, those of chain fibres. Fibres that contained one or more zones depleted of glycogen are open circles. Asterisks indicate poles that could not be examined over their entire length (from HARKER et al., 1977).

It was checked that there are no exclusively fusimotor axons with conduction velocity faster than 50 m/s in the peroneus tertius motor supply. As in other muscles similarly tested (KUFFLER et al., 1951; ELLAWAY et al., 1972) stimulation of single motor axons in the 50–100 m/s conduction velocity range always elicited the contraction of extrafusal muscle fibres. Consequently, the glycogen depletion observed in about 25 per cent of the spindles after prolonged stimulation of several very fast conducting motor axons means that some of them (or more precisely at least one of them) must have collaterals supplying spindles, i.e. that skeleto-fusimotor axons are present in the upper conduction velocity range. Unlike the dynamic β axons, these fast skeleto-fusimotor axons almost exclusively innervate intrafusal chain fibres.

Using the same technique, fast conducting β axons supplying chain fibres were also found in tenuissimus muscles (JAMI et al., 1978). It was further observed in this study that when the group of stimulated motor axons was not limited to the fastest ones (above 85 m/s) but also included axons with conduction velocity as slow as 60 m/s, glycogen depletion was found in 40 per cent of the examined spindles with chain fibres being affected in about half of the instances and bag_1 fibres in the others. As this latter location is characteristic of slow dynamic β axons, these results show that fast and slow innervation can coexist in the same muscle. The fact that a significant number of spindles with depletion in

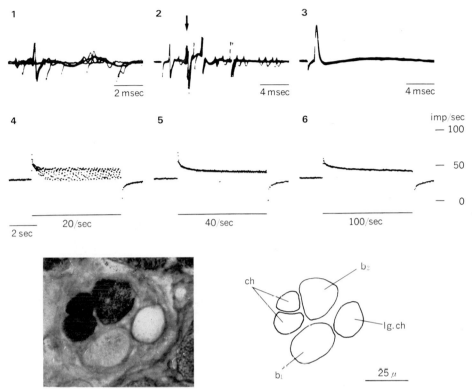

Fig. 1 Activation of a secondary ending of a tenuissimus spindle by a fast β axon.
Record 1. all-or-none behaviour of nerve and muscle action potentials elicited by threshold stimulation of a motor axon in a ventral root filament. The tenuissimus nerve was placed over the first recording electrode while the second electrode was at some distance from the muscle in order that the size of the muscle action potential be small. Superimposed traces.
Record 2: Supra maximal stimulation of the axon. Note the slower sweep speed. Conduction velocity of the axon: 103 m/s. The arrow indicates an early occurring discharge of a single afferent fibre.
Record 3: Action potential of the axon led from the cut end of the tenuissimus nerve after the muscle was excised for histological examination; this record was taken to check that the ventral root filament (stimulated in this case with a very strong stimulus) contained no other axon.
Records 4, 5, 6: Discharges of a secondary ending recorded with an instantaneous frequency meter from a group II fibre (conduction velocity: 34 m/s) in a dorsal root filament. The bars indicate the periods of repetitive stimulation of the axon at 20, 40 and 100/sec.
In the lower part of the figure, photomicrograph of a transverse section of the spindle, stained for glycogen, showing that a chain fibre was depleted (JAMI et al., unpublished data).

bag$_1$ fibres was found only when slow axons (60–85 m/s) were stimulated fits well with previous observations on the conduction velocity of dynamic β axons (EMONET-DÉNAND et al., 1975).

The centers of the zones of depletion in both bag and chain fibres were found to occur within half millimeter either proximal or distal to the extremity of the capsule; p$_1$ plates (BARKER et al., 1970) have a similar location.

In the course of a recent histophysiological study on the motor innervation of tenuissimus spindles, JAMI, LAN-COUTON, MALMGREN and PETIT (unpublished data) had the opportunity of collection several observations on single fast β axons.   These experiments were carried out on tenuissimus muscles because in this muscle it is possible to locate with precision

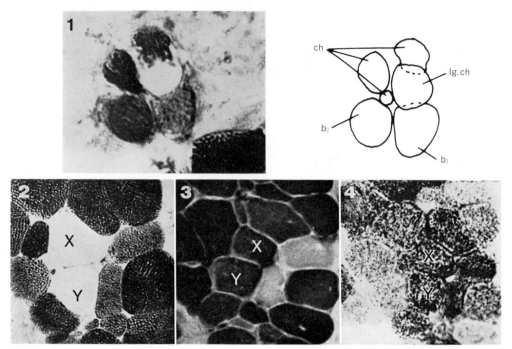

Fig. 5 Identification of the type of extrafusal muscle fibre supplied by a fast-conducting β axon.
1. Transverse section, stained with the P.A.S. method, of a tenuissimus spindle whose sensory
endings (primary and secondary) were excited by the axon. One chain fibre is blanched.
2. Transverse section stained with the P.A.S. method, showing that two large diameter extrafusal
muscle fibres (marked X and Y) are blanched.
3, 4. Transverse sections of the same muscle fibres respectively stained for alcaline ATPase (3)
and succinate dehydrogenase (4). Note the high ATPase and SDH activities of the two muscles
fibres innervated by the β axon (JAMI et al., unpublished data).

spindles whose sensory activity has been previously recorded and subsequently to examine
them for glycogen depletion.

i)   Fast β axons activate secondary endings: An example of this action is illustrated
by Figure 4 which shows that the rate of discharge of a secondary ending was increased
after repetitive stimulation of a single fast-conducting axon (conduction velocity: 103
m/s).   The spindle in which lay the secondary ending was located by the technique of
BESSOU and LAPORTE (1965) and the motor axon was then repetitively stimulated with a
pattern of stimulation adequate for glycogen depletion.   Histological examination of the
spindle revealed a zone of glycogen depletion in the longest chain fibre (see the photomicrograph of a transverse section of the spindle) thus providing 'direct evidence that in
addition to extrafusal muscle fibres this axon also supplied the spindle, in other words that
this fast-conducting axon was a skeleto-fusimotor one.

ii)   In one experiment in which the discharges of two endings belonging to the same
spindle (the primary and one secondary) were simultaneously recorded, the action of a
fast β axon on the response of the primary ending to a ramp stretch could be tested.   Repetitive stimulation of this axon which in static conditions activated both endings reduced
the dynamic index of the response of the primary ending.   This axon was shown by the
glycogen depletion method to supply the longest chain of the spindle.

iii) The extrafusal muscle fibres supplied by β axons belong to the fast oxidative-glycolytic type (classification of ARIANO et al., 1973):   An example of this identification is

illustrated by Figure 5 which shows four microphotographs of transverse sections of a tenuissimus muscle, one of them involving a spindle pole. A single motor axon activating a secondary ending had been stimulated for glycogen depletion and the spindle to which belonged this ending was histologically examined. As can be seen on transverse section 1 a chain fibre was blanched. Another PAS stained transverse section (microphotograph 2) shows two large size extrafusal muscle fibres which belonged to the β motor unit since they had been depleted of their glycogen content after stimulation of the axon. These two fibres could be traced in other transverse sections (about 100 μm distant from the PAS stained sections) that were stained for alcaline ATPase (microphotograph 3) or succinate dehydrogenase (microphotograph 4). The high ATPase and SDH activities of the two fibres (marked by X and Y) show they are fast oxidative-glycolytic fibres.

The functional role of fast β axons cannot yet be appreciated. It can be tentatively advanced that, whenever these axons are activated, the contraction of chain fibres they elicit may contribute to maintain the discharge of primary and secondary endings in spite of the presumably strong unloading effect resulting from the contraction of the extra-fusal muscle fibres they supply.

In summary, some cat spindles may be supplied by skeleto-fusimotor axons with conduction velocities faster than 85 m/s. These β axons are very predominantly distributed to the longest intrafusal chain fibres; they activate secondary endings and have a static action on primary ending discharge; the extrafusal muscle fibres they supply belong to the fast oxidative-glycolytic type. They are strikingly different from the dynamic β axons whose conduction velocity is slower and which supply bag$_1$ fibres and slow oxidative extrafusal muscle fibres.

REFERENCES

ADAL, M. N. and BARKER, D.: Intramuscular branching of fusimotor fibres. *J. Physiol. London.*, *177*: 288–299 (1965)

APPELBERG, B. and EMONET-DÉNAND, F.: Motor units of the first superficial lumbrical muscle of the cat. *J. Neurophysiol.*, *30*: 154–160 (1967)

ARIANO, M. A., ARMSTRONG, R. B. and EDGERTON, V. R.: Hindlimb muscle fiber populations of five mammals. *J. Histochem. Cytochem.*, *21*: 51–55 (1973)

BARKER, D., BANKS, R., HARKER, D., MILBURN, A. and STACEY, M.: Studies on the histochemistry, ultrastructure, motor innervation and regeneration of mammalian intrafusal muscle fibres. *In* HOMA, S. (ed.): *Understanding the Stretch Reflex. Progress in Brain Research*, Elsevier, Amsterdam, Vol. 44, pp. 67–88 (1976a)

BARKER, D., EMONET-DÉNAND, F., HARKER, D., JAMI, L. and LAPORTE, Y.: Distribution of fusimotor axons to intrafusal muscle fibres in cat tenuissimus spindles as determined by the glycogen depletion method. *J. Physiol. London.*, *261*: 49–70 (1976b)

BARKER, D., EMONET-DÉNAND, F., HARKER, D., JAMI, L. and LAPORTE, Y.: Types of intra- and extrafusal muscle fibre innervated by dynamic skeleto-fusimotor axons in cat peroneus brevis and tenuissimus muscles, as determined by the glycogen-depletion method. *J. Physiol. London.*, *266*: 713–726 (1977)

BAKER, D., STACEY, M. J. and ADAL, M. N.: Fusimotor innervation in the cat. *Phil. Trans. B.*, *258*: 315–346 (1970)

BESSOU, P., EMONET-DÉNAND, F. and LAPORTE, Y.: Relation entre la vitesse de conduction des fibres nerveuses motrices et le temps de contraction de leurs unites motrices. *C. r. hebd. Seanc. Acad. Sci. Paris.*, *256*: 5625–5627 (1963a)

BESSOU, P., EMONET-DÉNAND, F. and LAPORTE, Y.: Occurrence of intrafusal muscle fibres innervation by branches of slow motor fibres in the cat. *Nature. London.*, *198*: 594–595 (1963b)

BESSOU, P., EMONET-DENAND, F. and LAPORTE, Y.: Motor fibres innervating extrafusal and intrafusal muscle fibres in the cat. *J. Physiol. London.*, *180*: 649–672 (1965)

Bessou, P. and Laporte, Y.: Technique de preparation d'une fibre afferente I et d'une fibre afférente II innervant le même fuseau meuro-musculaire, chez le Chat. *J. Physiol. Paris.*, *57*: 511–520 (1965)

Brown, M. C. and Butler, R. G.: Studies on the site of termination of static and dynamic fusimotor fibres within muscle spindles of the tenuissimus muscle of the cat. *J. Physiol. London.*, *233*: 553–573 (1973)

Brown, M. C. and Butler, R. G.: An investigation into the site of termination of static gamma fibres within muscle spindles of the cat peroneus longus muscle. *J. Physiol. London.*, *247*: 131–143 (1975)

Burke, R. E.: Motor unit types of cat triceps surae muscle. *J. Physiol. London.*, *193*: 141–160 (1967)

Burke, R. Levine, M., Salcman, M. and Tsairis, P.: Motor units in cat soleus muscle: physiological, histochemical and morphological characteristics. *J. Physiol. London.*, *238*: 503–514 (1974)

Burke, R. E., Levine, D. N., Tsairis, P. and Zajac, F. E.: Physiological types and histochemical profiles in motor units of the cat gastrocnemius. *J. Physiol. London*, *234*: 723–748 (1973)

Burke, R. E. and Tsairis, P.: Histochemical and physiological profile of a skeletofusimotor (beta) unit in cat soleus muscle. *Brain. Res.*, *129*: 341–345 (1977)

Edström, L. and Kugelberg, E.: Histochemical composition, distribution of fibres and fatiguability of single motor units. *J. Neurol. Neurosurg. Psychiat.*, *31*: 424–433 (1968)

Ellaway, P., Emonet-Dénand, F., Joffroy, M. and Laporte, Y.: Lack of exclusively fusimotor α-axons in flexor and extensor leg muscles of the cat. *J. Neurophysiol.*, *35*: 149–153 (1972)

Emonet-Dénand, F., Jami, L. and Laporte, Y.: Skeleto-fusimotor axons in hind-limb muscles of the cat. *J. Physiol. London*, *249*: 153–166 (1975)

Emonet-Dénand, F. and Laporte, Y.: Blocage neuromusculaire sélectif des jonctions extrafusales des axones squeletto-fusimoteurs produit par leur stimulation repetitive a frequence elevee. *C. r. hebd. Séanc. Acad. Sci. Paris*, *279*, serie D: 2083–2085 (1974)

Emonet-Dénand, F. and Laporte, Y.: The proportion of muscle spindles supplied by skeletofusimotor axons (β axons) in the peroneus brevis muscle of the cat. *J. Neurophysiol.*, *38*: 1390–1394 (1975)

Harker, D., Jami, L., Laporte, Y. and Petit, J.: Fast-conducting skeletofusimotor axons supplying intrafusal chain fibres in the cat peroneus tertius muscle. *J. Neurophysiol.*, *40*: 791–799 (1977)

Jami, L., Lan-Couton, D., Malmgren, K. and Petit, J.: "Fast" and "slow" skeleto-fusimotor innervation in cat tenuissimus spindles; a study with the glycogen depletion method. *Acta Physiol. scand.*, *103*: 284–298 (1978)

Jami, L. and Petit, J.: Correlation between axonal conduction velocity and tetanic tension of motor units in four muscles of the cat hind limb. *Brain Res.*, *96*: 114–118 (1975)

Kuffler, S. W., Hunt, C. C. and Quilliam, J. P.: Function of medullated small nerve fibers in mammalian ventral roots: efferent muscle spindle innervation. *J. Neurophysiol.*, *14*: 29–54 (1951)

Kugelberg, E.: Properties of the rat hind-limb motor units. *In* Desmedt, J. E. (ed.): *New Developments in Electromyography and Clinical Neurophysiology*, Karger, Basel. Vol. 1, pp. 2–13 (1973)

McPhedran, A., Wuerker, R. B. and Henneman, E.: Properties of motor units in a homogeneous red muscle (soleus) of the cat. *J. Neurophysiol.*, *28*: 71–84 (1965)

McWilliam, P. N.: The incidence and properties of β axons to muscle spindles in the cat hind-limb. *Quart. J. Exptl. Physiol.*, *60*: 25–36 (1975)

Olson, C. B. and Swett, C. P.: A functional and histochemical characterization of motor units in a heterogeneous muscle (flexor digitorum longus) of the cat. *J. comp. Neurol.*, *128*: 475–498 (1966)

Wuerker, R. B., McPhedran, A. and Henneman, E.: Properties of motor units in a heterogeneous pale muscle (m. gastrocnemius) of the cat. *J. Neurophysiol.*, *28*: 85–99 (1965)

DISCUSSION PERIOD

HUNT: Is anything known of the nature of motor terminals supplied by fast-conducting betas on the chain type of fibre?

LAPORTE: Nothing with certainty.   There is however some indirect evidence (BARKER et al., 1970) suggesting these terminals are the p_1 plates, which are those intrafusal motor endings that very much resemble the extrafusal plates.   We are presently, David BARKER's group and mine, starting a series of experiments which might give an answer to that question.   They consist in preparing muscles in which all motor axons have degenerated but a few ones with conduction velocities faster than 50–60 m/sec.   If there are some β axons among them and if silver impregnation is satisfactory, we might be able to identify these intrafusal motor terminals.

LUNDBERG: Since only about 25 per cent of the spindles received innervation, and you dissected the majority of the alphas, would you say that it is likely that there are some spindles which don't receive innervation from fast axons?

LAPORTE: I think this is probably the correct conclusion.

LUNDBERG: That is extremely interesting.   Because this indicates that Ia afferents are not functionally homogeneous.   And then we can ask the question: What significance has that for the central nervous system and how should we go about investigating this functional difference?   We know that each motoneuron receives innervation from virtually all homonymous Ia afferents.   There is no evidence of a difference there.   I suggest that it would be interesting to look at the dorsal-spino-cerebellar tract, and see if there some neurons innervated specifically from those spindles which receive fast beta innervation.

LAPORTE: Well, that's something to try.

BURKE: I'd like to make a comment and then ask a question.   We know very well that Group Ia axons do not project back on the gamma motor neurons, so there is no feedback loop there.   But some alpha motor neurons apparently have the beta pattern of innervation, and that is in the slow twitch units.   And now we know that the fast betas are among the type FR, or fast fatigue-resistant units.   Both of those units types are projected to very heavily by Ia afferents.   So this represents an embarrassing positive feedback loop for the motor system physiologist.   The question I would like to ask is, is there any anatomical relation between the spindle in which there is a depleted intrafusal fibre and the position of depleted extrafusal motor units?

LAPORTE: No.   There is no particular relation.   We hoped there would be one but found nothing of that kind.   About the first point, Dr. BURKE, I'm not so embarassed by positive feedback.   Because after all, the frogs, the snakes, millions of animals have worked only with skeleto-fusimotor systems and so far they have done well.   You see, if the tension developed by the extrafusal fibres of a muscle is such that in spite of its load the muscle markedly shortens there should be a reduction in spindle firing and consequently the effectiveness of the positive feedback should be reduced.

Apparently, what the very-fast conducting beta axons do is to add their action to that of the predominant static gammas.   I think that whenever a fast-fatigue-resistant β motor unit is active, its contraction will not necessarily slow down the discharge of the spindle supplied by the β axon because the unloading action of the extrafusal muscle fibres, provided it is not too strong, will be opposed by the contraction of some intrafusal muscle fibres. It seems to me that the function of many excitatory collateral branches found in the central and peripheral nervous system might be to prevent some structures from being completely silenced.

FUNCTIONAL ORGANIZATION OF MOTONEURON POOLS: THE SIZE-PRINCIPLE

Elwood HENNEMAN

Department of Physiology, Harvard Medical School
Boston, MA

A relatively small population of neurons has exclusive control over a particular skeletal muscle. Each of these motoneuron "pools" receives a large number of excitatory and inhibitory impulses from many parts of the nervous system. It translates this large and varied input into a much smaller output that follows simple, logical rules. This paper reviews some recent evidence concerning the organization of these cell populations. In order to understand the collective function of such a group of cells, it is necessary to understand how various types of input are distributed to it, what the properties of the individual motoneurons are and how they react to these inputs, and finally to appreciate the individual and collective roles of the output signals in controlling muscles.

Figure 1 illustrates the location and spatial arrangement of the motoneurons comprising two closely related pools in the cat's spinal cord. In this figure from studies of BURKE et al. (1977), each motoneuron in the soleus and medial gastrocnemius pools was labelled by injecting its muscle with horseradish peroxidase (HRP). This HRP was taken up by the terminals of the motoneurons and carried rapidly by retrograde flow within the axons to their cells of origin.

In this paper I will discuss particularly the significance of the dimensions of the motoneurons making up a pool. As HODES et al. (1949) demonstrated, there are a great many small motoneurons in the spinal cord and decreasing numbers of larger and larger cells. This highly skewed distribution of sizes has been found in all pools examined to date.

At the outset it should be emphasized that a motoneuron pool is designed as it is for mechanical purposes. By means of its discharges it must combine the contractions of many individual motor units to produce precise mechanical effects in muscle at exactly the right time in a movement.

In order to understand the operations of a pool it was necessary to measure the output very precisely. Figure 2 illustrates the technique which was used. The combined nerves to the triceps surae muscles were stimulated once a second. A single, antidromic volley was set up in all the motor fibers of this muscle group. It was recorded in the distal half of the 7th lumbar or first sacral ventral root and displayed on one trace of an oscilloscope. A dromic volley set up by the same shock was conducted up the dorsal roots and elicited a monosynaptic reflex in the proximal half of the same ventral root.

The baselines of these 2 traces are superimposed in Figure 3. In each pair of responses the left one is the antidromic volley. Its amplitude indicates discharge of all the triceps motor fibers in this root. Note that it does not change in size. The right potential in each pair is the monosynaptic reflex recorded with the same gain. Its amplitude is determined by the number of triceps motoneurons discharged in the reflex. Note that before a 500 per second tetanus for ten seconds to the muscles nerves the size of the reflex was less than half that of the antidromic volley in the upper row. After the tetanus (TET) the reflex

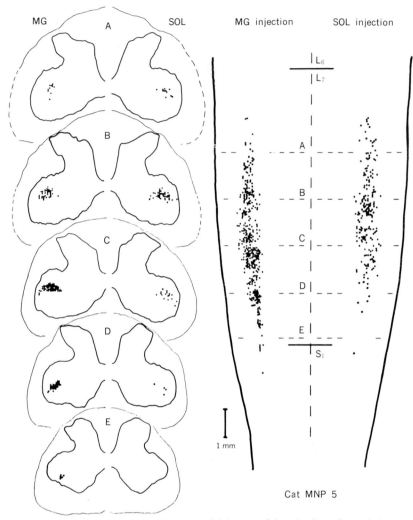

Fig. 1 Reconstructions of the MG and SOL nuclei from serial sagittal sections of the cat's spinal cord. *Right diagram*: dorsal view of the spinal cord outline (white matter-pia boundary in heavy lines) in which are superimposed positions (dots) of MG left hemicord) and SOL moto-neuron cell bodies (right hemicord). Boundaries between L_6, L_7, and S_1 segments (identified by dorsal root entry zones) are indicated by heavy lines; midline denoted by the longitudinal dashed line. Dashed lines across the cord denote levels (labeled A-E) at which reconstructions were made. *Left-hand diagrams*: reconstructions at levels A-E showing white matter-pia boundary in light lines and gray-white matter boundary in heavier lines. Neurons indicated at each level are cells located within 300-μm rostral or caudal to that cross-section. (from BURKE et al., 1977.)

was potentiated (post-tetanic potentiation) (LLOYD, 1949). In the second row at the left the reflex became as large as the antidromic volley. In later experiments the reflexes were integrated electronically to give a quantitative measure of their size.

In Figure 4 this quantitative technique was employed. The vertical lines in the upper tracing are the *time-integrals* of the monosynaptic reflexes recorded once a second. The height of each line indicates the percent discharge of the pool. The lower trace shows the simultaneous responses of a single triceps motoneuron from the same pool. As long as the response of the pool exceeded a certain level, the single unit below discharged every

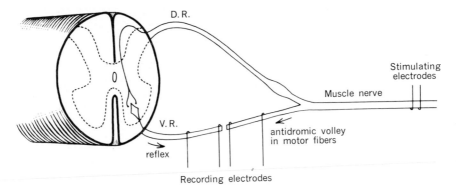

Fig. 2 Scheme of experiment used to measure maximal monosynaptic discharge of a motoneuron pool. See text. (from CLAMANN et al., 1974a.)

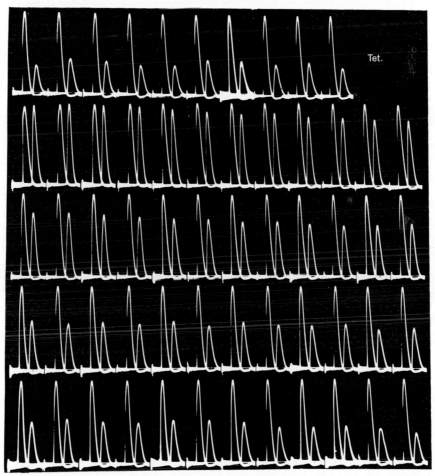

Fig. 3 Pairs of responses recorded as in Fig. 2 from proximal and distal halves of S_1VR in response to single-shock stimulation of combined nerves to MG and LG-SOL. The left and right deflectins of each pair are the antidromic and reflex responses, respectively, displayed on super-imposed traces of a two-beam oscilloscope at equal gains. First 10 pairs in upper row recorded before 12-sec tetanus (500/sec) to MG and LG-SOL nerves. Subsequent pairs recorded at 2-sec intervals after tetanus. See text. (from CLAMANN et al., 1974a.)

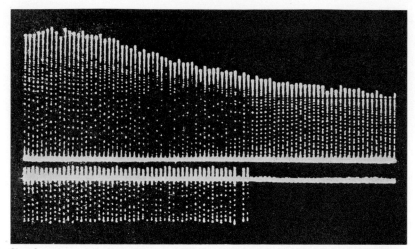

Fig. 4 Simultaneous recordings of a series of monosynaptic reflexes of the triceps surae pool (above) and a single triceps motoneuron (below), showing critical firing level of the latter. *Upper trace*: time integrals of monosynaptic reflexes recorded at 1/sec from proximal half of S_1VR. The height of each vertical line measures the size of the population response. *Lower trace*: monosynaptic reflexes of a single triceps motoneuron recorded from a small filament of L_7VR. Records were made during the decline in PTP following a brief train of conditioning shocks which were applied to the combined MG and LG-SOL nerves at 500/sec. (from Henneman et al., 1974.)

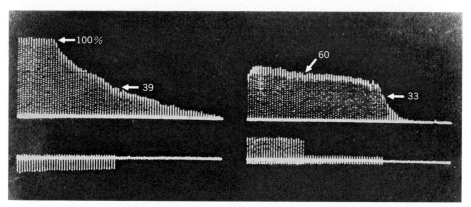

Fig. 5 Critical firing levels of three triceps motoneurons. The single unit in the lower-left tracing had a sharp threshold at 39 per cent. The two units in the lower-right tracing had thresholds of 60 and 33 per cent. The plateau in the upper-left record indicates the 100 per cent discharge level of the triceps pool. (from Henneman et al., 1974.)

time. When the responses of the pool declined below a certain level, the unit ceased to respond.

In Figure 5 the records at the upper left indicate the 100 per cent level of pool discharge. The critical firing levels of 3 units are shown. Each is sharply defined. Above a certain level each of the three motoneurons respond to every afferent volley. Below a certain level each of these units never responded again. 203 triceps units were examined and behaved in this fashion.

The critical firing level of a unit is a good predictor of its susceptibility to repetitive discharge. Figure 6 reproduces simultaneously recorded repetitive discharges from two different pairs of plantaris motoneurons. Trace "a" shows the excitatory input first increasing in intensity then decreasing. The critical firing levels for each trace are shown. In

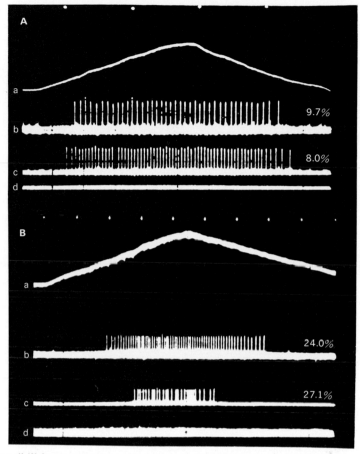

Fig. 6 Susceptibilities to repetitive discharge of two different pairs of plantaris motoneurons with known critical firing levels as indicated. Electrical stimulation of plantaris nerve at 300/sec in both cases Stimulus intensity indicated by level of trace a with reference to baseline d. Responses of plantaris units recorded on traces b and c. Time marks at 1-sec intervals for both upper and lower sets of records. (from HENNEMAN et al., 1974.)

both experiments the unit with the lower critical firing level commenced firing sooner and ceased firing later. Experiments of this type have shown that the relative excitabilities of motoneurons are the same in repetitive firing as in monosynaptic reflexes. This is an important point because the input responsible for monosynaptic reflexes is limited chiefly to impulses in Iᴀ fibers, whereas the input responsible for repetitive discharge probably includes impulses in a variety of primary afferent fibers and descending activity from brainstem centers (spino-bulbo-spinal reflexes). Thus, the rank order of motoneurons is not dependent on the distribution of input in Iᴀ fibers alone, but remains unchanged when other inputs are also involved in eliciting the discharges.

Defining the critical firing levels (CFLs) and rank orders of motoneurons more precisely and over a wider range than ever before as in Figures 4, 5 and 6 made it important to relate them to their axonal diameters and cell sizes by direct methods. An electrical technique was devised to do this, which is fully described in CLAMANN and HENNEMAN, (1976). Three procedures were carried out. (1) Reflex responses of single motor fibers were recorded monophasically from ventral root filaments. A resistor was placed in shunt across the recording electrodes and its value was varied until the action potentials

were reduced by one half.   The resistance of the nerve filament was then equal to that of
the shunt.   Dividing the voltage of the action potentials by the resistance of the filament
gave the axonal action current.   (2)   In experiments in which impulses were conducted
antidromically over long distances to yield accurate measurements of conduction velocity,
it was shown that the axonal current of an impulse varied as the square of its conduction
velocity.   (3) After the sizes of the impulses had been normalized in accordance with the
resistances of their ventral root filaments, a direct correlation was found between impulse
size and CFL.   Since both CFL and axon diameter were related to impulse size, they were
related to each other as illustrated in Figure 7.   The linearity of the data points in Figure
7 indicates that CFL is a function of a single, continuous variable, which is probably cell
size.   If CFL is very precisely and linearly related to cell size, it must be concluded that
the distribution of input to the pool and any other factors that contribute to the relationship
are also size-dependent. It is appropriate, therefore, to ask whether the scatter in the data
points of Figure 7 indicates a degree of variability or nonlinearity in this relationship.   It
does not necessarily have this implication, because the variations observed when a series
of observations was repeated several times were quite sufficient to account for all of the scatter.   Thus, the relationship between CFL and axonal diameter is probably more linear
than the data in Figure 7 indicate.   A little scatter might be anticipated since variability
in recruitment order has been observed in direct comparisons of motoneurons whose CFLs
differed by less than 2.5 per cent (HENNEMAN et al., 1974).   BARRETT and CRILL (1971)
have demonstrated a close but not perfect relationship between input impedance and conduction velocity, which might allow for some scatter.   Their methods and assumptions,
however, are probably not free of error either.

    Figure 8 adds further and more direct evidence that the distribution of input to moto-
neurons must be correlated with their size.   In this experiment a strong inhibitory input,
applied during alternate monosynaptic reflexes, caused a 20 per cent reduction in their
total response.   The horizontal line in Figure 8 shows the CFL when there was no inhibition applied (larger responses).   Extension of this line to the left also defines the critical
firing level that was found during inhibition.   It was concluded that the several types of
inhibition utilized in these experiments had no significant effect on CFL.

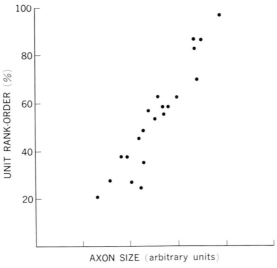

Fig. 7 Relation between axon size and CFL (rank order) of 21 plantaris motoneurons isolated
    in a single experiment. See text. (from CLAMANN and HENNEMAN, 1976.)

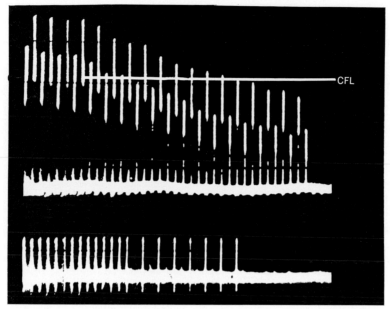

Fig. 8 Critical firing level (CFL) of a plantaris motoneuron with and without inhibitory input from the lateral popliteal nerve.
Upper tracing: time integrals of the monosynaptic reflexes of the plantaris population elicited at 2-sec intervals during the declining phase of a PTP.
Lower tracing: simultaneous responses of a plantaris unit with a critical firing level of 61 per cent Alternate reflexes preceded by a 200 msec train of pulses to lateral popliteal n. Horizontal line indicating critical firing level drawn as described in text. (from CLAMANN et al., 1974b.)

Figure 9 compares the effects of inhibition on the repetitive firing of 2 plantaris moto-neurons. 4 pairs of discharges are shown. In each pair the upper unit had a slightly higher CFL. A_1 and A_2 show the effects of recurrent inhibition on monosynaptic responses. During the period of applied inhibition (underlined) 9 of the 18 reflexes in trace 1 were silenced, but only one was silenced in trace 2. In A_3 and A_4 recurrent inhibition was produced by stimulating the proximal portion of the ventral root repetitively during the period indicated by the thickening of the baseline. In response to this form of inhibition the upper unit ceased firing entirely, but the lower unit only slowed to one half of its original rate. In part B the same pair of units was inhibited by stimulating the lateral popliteal nerve at 100/sec. In B_1 15 monosynaptic reflexes were silenced but only 4 in B_2. In B_3 and B_4 the intensity of the inhibition was gradually increased as the traces moved across the oscilloscope. Firing in the upper unit was eventually suppressed completely, whereas the lower unit was only slowed in rate. Thus, in all 4 comparisons the lower unit, with a slightly lower CFL was more resistant to inhibition.

Table 1 indicates the effects of inhibition on 133 pairs of plantaris motoneurons. In 92 per cent of these pairs, the rank order observed with simple monosynaptic reflexes was not altered during inhibition. Six different inhibitory inputs were used in these experiments, as indicated in column 1 of the table. Monosynaptic reflexes were compared in 170 tests and repetitive firing in 196 tests. Inhibition reversed the rank order in only 3 of the 170 tests. In two of these the differences in CFLs were 1.0 and 0.4 per cent, values which are probably below the accuracy of the technique. Inhibition reversed the rank order in only 4 of 196 tests with repetitive firing. In these 4 cases the average difference in CFL was 0.8 per cent.

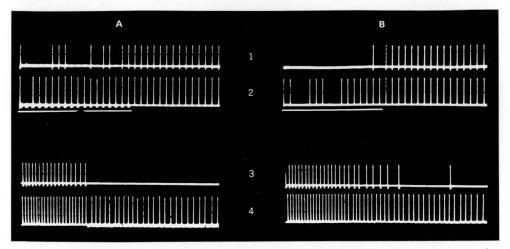

Fig. 9 Effects of recurrent inhibition (A) and lateral popliteal inhibition (B) on monosynaptic reflexes (traces 1 and 2) and repetitive firing (traces 3 and 4) of a pair of plantaris motoneurons with critical firing levels of 18.6 per cent (upper) and 18.4 per cent (lower). In traces 1 and 2 the underlined reflexes were preceded and accompanied by (A) a 100-msec train of shocks (100/ sec) to the proximal portion of L_7VR and by (B) similar stimulation of the lateral popliteal n. In traces 3 and 4 repetitive discharge of the same units was inhibited (A) by means of recurrent inhibition, indicated by thickened base line in A4 and (B) by a progressive increase in the intensity of the 100/sec shocks to the lateral popliteal n. (from CLAMANN et al., 1974b.)

Table 1 Effects of inhibition on recruitment order in motoneurons (from CLAMANN et al., 1974b).

1	2	3	4	5
	Monosynaptic reflexes		Repetitive discharge	
Source of inhibitory input	No. of tests	No. of reversals	No. of tests	No. of reversals
lat. peroneal n.	36	0	38	1
post. biceps-semitendinosus n.	36	1	37	0
sural n.	7	0	8	0
L7 ventral root	29	1	49	0
contralat. S1 dorsal root	32	1	34	2
brainstem	30	0	30	1
Totals	170	3	191	4

The six inputs used in these experiments were selected to provide contrasting types of inhibition for testing:

>   postsynaptic and presynaptic
>   spinal and supraspinal
>   unilateral and contralateral
>   recurrent and non-recurrent
>   cutaneous and muscular
>   mixed and pure

Although these inhibitory systems and the effects they exert differ from one another in many respects, none of them appeared to influence the rank order of motoneurons within a pool.   In summary, these results with inhibitory inputs strongly suggest that the location, density and distribution of active endings on motoneurons in correlated with the CFL and size of the individual cells on which they are located.

Most of the early work in this field was done on animals.   Recordings of single motor units in man agree almost completely with results in animals.   MILNER-BROWN et al. (1973) have used an averaging technique to record the twitch contractions of single units in the first dorsal interosseous muscle of man.   The twitch tensions of the motor units in this muscle varied nearly linearly with the total muscle force at which they were recruited, as illustrated in Figure 10.   Larger motor units tended to contract more rapidly than smaller units.   In short, human motor units are recruited in orderly progression according to the size of the contractions they produce as animal studies have indicated.

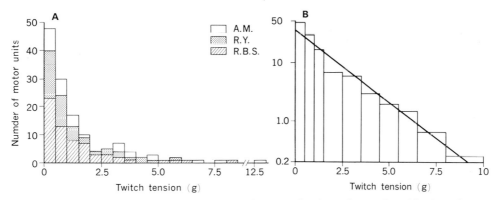

Fig. 10 Number of motor units, plotted on a linear scale (A) and on a logarithmic scale (B), having the twitch tensions indicated. The numbers from each of the three subjects are indicated on the figure. The distributions are similar for all three subjects. The computed best-fitting line on the semi-log plot of (B) indicates an approximately exponential relation between number of motor units and twitch tension. (from MILNER-BROWN et al., 1973)

Some investigators have stated that the central nervous system must have the capacity to activate units selectively, so that large or small, fast or slow units can be utilized as the occasion dictates.   In a very important paper BÜDINGEN and FREUND (1976) studied recruitment of motor units in the forearm of man to determine whether small and large units were preferentially activated by slow (50 gr/sec) and fast (2000 gr/sec) contractions.   They concluded that, when all neural and mechanical factors are taken into consideration, *mechanical recruitment occurs at approximately the same force regardless of the rate of rise of tension.*

It has been reported that recruitment may be modified in very fast, ballistic movements. These movements are presumably "preprogrammed," being completed before sensory feedback signals from muscle can modify them.   DESMEDT and GODAUX (1977) have studied recruitment in movements that produce 0.05 to 12 kg peak forces in less than 0.15 sec each.   After obtaining about 50 ballistic contractions, they arranged them in order from the weakest to the strongest as shown in Table 2.   Activity or nonactivity of the first 5 units is indicated by a + or a — sign in the table.   Unit 1 fired in all 52 trials.   Units 2–5 failed to respond below certain peak forces, but discharged with increasing probability in stronger contractions.   The lower part of the table gives the thresholds of the same 5 units for both ballistic and slow ramp contractions.   The same recruitment order was observed in both kinds of movement.   The correlation coefficient was 0.95.

It has been reported that human subjects can learn to activate or "isolate" any one of several different motor units within the recording range of the EMG electrodes in a muscle,

Table 2 Thresholds of motor units during ballistic movements (from DESMEDT and GODAUX, 1977).

Motor unit threshold data

Trial	Force (kg)	1	2	3	4	5	Trial	(kg)	1	2	3	4	5
1	0.07	+	−	−	−	−	27	2.27	+	+	+	−	−
2	0.08	+	−	−	−	−	28	2.42	+	+	+	−	−
3	0.15	+	−	−	−	−	29	2.72	+	+	+	+	−
4	0.30	+	−	−	−	−	30	2.75	+	+	+	−	−
5	0.30	+	−	−	−	−	31	3.18	+	+	+	+	−
6	0.31	+	−	−	−	−	32	3.20	+	+	+	−	−
7	0.31	+	−	−	−	−	33	3.33	+	+	+	+	−
8	0.37	+	−	−	−	−	34	3.48	+	+	+	+	−
9	0.38	+	−	−	−	−	35	3.51	+	+	+	+	−
10	0.45	+	+	−	−	−	36	3.78	+	+	+	+	−
11	0.46	+	+	−	−	−	37	4.54	+	+	+	+	+
12	0.53	+	−	−	−	−	38	4.84	+	+	+	+	+
13	0.75	+	+	−	−	−	39	4.99	+	+	+	+	+
14	0.90	+	+	−	−	−	40	5.15	+	+	+	+	+
15	0.90	+	+	−	−	−	41	5.30	+	+	+	+	+
16	0.91	+	+	−	−	−	42	5.45	+	+	+	+	+
17	1.06	+	+	−	−	−	43	5.75	+	+	+	+	+
18	1.06	+	+	−	−	−	44	6.96	+	+	+	+	+
19	1.06	+	+	−	−	−	45	8.03	+	+	+	+	+
20	1.14	+	+	+	−	−	46	8.10	+	+	+	+	+
21	1.21	+	+	+	−	−	47	8.18	+	+	+	+	+
22	1.36	+	+	−	−	−	48	8.63	+	+	+	+	+
23	1.38	+	+	+	−	−	49	9.54	+	+	+	+	+
24	1.51	+	+	−	−	−	50	9.69	+	+	+	+	+
25	1.81	+	+	+	−	−	51	10.90	+	+	+	+	+
26	1.82	+	+	+	−	−	52	12.70	+	+	+	+	+

Motor unit threshold

Unit	Ballistic force threshold (kg) Range	Mean	Ramp force threshold (kg) Range	Mean±s.d.
1	0–0.07	0.035	0.14–0.48	0.34±0.15
2	0.38–0.75	0.56	3.50–4.10	3.70±0.28
3	1.06–1.81	1.43	3.60–4.40	4.14±0.36
4	2.72–3.33	3.02	11.98–13.15	12.66±0.57
5	3.78–4.54	4.16	13.73–16.41	15.46±0.93

using auditory and visual feedback from an oscilloscope. We have not been able to confirm this selective action in human subjects (HENNEMAN et al., 1976). By dorsi-flexing the index finger our subjects were asked to recruit 2 motor units in their natural order. After establishing the normal order of recruitment by repeated testing of these units in the extensor indicis proprius muscle, the subjects were asked to reverse the normal order or to silence the first unit without silencing the second one. These were considered crucial tests of selective control.

All 9 subjects were able to isolate single units without difficulty. In 6 of the 9 subjects no changes in recruitment order were ever observed even after 2 hours of training with feedback and tests on hundreds of units. The 2 units were generally very close together in threshold.   In the other three subjects, the results were similar at most recording sites. In each of these three subjects, however, there was one site at which some variability in recruitment order was observed.   These changes seemed to occur randomly.   There was never any evidence of voluntary or conscious control over the order of recruitment.   These results demonstrate that the rank order within a pool is relatively fixed.

Recruitment of motoneurons in order of increasing size has been observed in many species.   Since its first description in the cat, it has been reported in

crab leg muscles
crab eyestalk muscles
cockroaches
locusts
dragonflies
mantids
water bugs
newts
toads
fish
and man.

There is, moreover, suggestive evidence that the size-principle may apply to other neurons in the central nervous system such as internuncial cells and pacemaker cells.

Functional Implications

Certain general principles that are of functional utility are apparent in these experiments.   They can be summarized as follows:

The neural energy required to discharge a motoneuron, the energy it transmits and releases in the muscle, its mean rate of firing and even its rate of protein synthesis, are all correlated with its size.

A pool is a hierarchy of cells of different sizes.   It also functions hierarchically.   It is designed to work incrementally by adding progressively larger or subtracting progressively smaller units from the active goup.

Human studies show that the pool controls the recruitment process in accordance with the mechanical properties of the motor units, regardless of the speed of contraction.   The critical firing level of each cell, which depends on its size, determines its susceptibility to discharge.

Whenever a particular motoneuron fires monosynaptically, all the smaller cells discharge with it.   There is, then, *a basic law of combination* that specifies how the activities of motoneurons are combined.

To appreciate the degree of simplification a rank-ordered pool represents, consider an alternative arrangement in which all possible combinations, N, of active units might occur. For a pool containing 300 cells, N is calculated as shown:

$$N = \sum_{k=1}^{300} \frac{300!}{k!(300-k)!}$$

In this example, $N > 10^{90}$.

Imagine, for example, that no rank order exists.   The central nervous system has at its disposal motor units that are large or small, fast or slow.   How should it select those it needs for a particular task and how should it combine them to produce the required tension?

It is conceivable that the nervous system might use the 300 motoneurons like the keys of a large adding mahine, picking any combination to give the proper total tension.   This would require great flexibility in the design of input to the pool so that each motoneuron could be activated selectively.   This would also require circuits to do something much more difficult: to ensure that the separate contributions of the various motor units would add up to the proper total output.

Nature's solution to these problems is the rank ordered pool, which relieves the central nervous system of selective activation of motoneurons and provides a simple rule for their combination.

REFERENCES

BARRETT, J. N., and CRILL, W. E.:   Specific membrane resistivity of dye-injected cat motoneurons. *Brain Res., 28*: 556 (1971)

BÜDINGEN, H. J., and FREUND, H.-J.:   The relationship between the rate of rise of isometric tension and motor unit recruitment in a human forearm muscle.   *Pflugers Arch., 362*: 61 (1976)

BURKE, R. E., STRICK, P. L., KANDA, K., KIM, C. C., and WALMSLE:, B.:   Anatomy of medial gastrocnemius and soleus motor nuclei in cat spinal cord.   *J. Neurophysiol., 40*: 667 (1977)

CLAMANN, H. P., GILLIES, J. D.' SKINNER, R. D., and HENNEMAN, E.:   Quantitative measures of output of a motoneuron pool during monosynaptic reflexes.   *J. Neurophysiol., 37*: 1328 (1974a)

CLAMANN, H. P., GILLIES, J. D., and HENNEMAN, E.:   Effects of inhibitory inputs on ciritcal firing level and rank order of motoneurons.   *J. Neurophysiol., 37*: 1350 (1974b)

CLAMANN, H. P., and HENNEMAN, E.:   Electrical measurement of axon diameter and its use in relating motoneuron size to critical firing level.   *J. Neurophysiol., 39*: 844 (1976)

DESMEDT, J. E., and GODAUX, E.:   Ballistic contractions in man: characteristic recruitment pattern of single motor units of the tibialis anterior muscle.   *J. Physiol., 264*: 673–693 (1977)

HENNEMAN, E., CLAMANN, H. P., GILLIES, J. D., and SKINNER, R. D.:   Rank-order of motoneurons within a pool: law of combination.   *J. Neurophysiol., 37*: 1338 (1974)

HENNEMAN, E., SHAHANI, B. T., and YOUNG, R. R.:   Voluntary control of human motor units.   *In* SHAHANI, M. (ed.):   *The motor System: Neurophysiology and Muscle Mechanisms*, Elsevier, Amsterdam, (1976)

HODES, R., PEACOCK, S. M., Jr., and BODIAN, D.:   Selective destruction of large motoneurons by poliomyelitis virus. II.   Size of motoneurons in the spinal cord of rhesus monkeys.   *Neuropathology and Experimental Neurology, 8*: 400, (1949)

LLOYD, D. P. C.:   Post-tetanic potentiation of response in monosynaptic reflex pathways of the spinal cord.   *J. General Physiol., 33*: 47 (1949)

MILNER-BROWN, H. S., STEIN, R. B., and YEMM, R.:   The orderly recruitment of human motor units during voluntary isometric contractions.   *J. Physiol., 230*: 359 (1973)

DISCUSSION PERIOD

HUNT: May I ask about the recording technique from the ventral root? How did you abolish impulse activity to record only synaptic potential?

HENNEMAN: The ventral root was sucked up into a plastic tube through which isotonic sucrose was perfused. The normal conducting medium around the initial portion of the ventral root was replaced by a non-conducting sucrose medium. Conducted impulses were abolished in the ventral root. The axons in the root, insulated by their membranes, served as wick electrodes which were used to record the intracellular potentials of the motoneurons in that segment.

HUNT: What about the intramedullary portion?

HENNEMAN: That, we don't know anything about yet. Presumably there is some current loss in that region and attenuation of potentials as a result. But it is possible that the sucrose, which permeates the ventral roots in a matter of two or three minutes, may have penetrated a short way into the cord as well. I really don't know.

LUNDBERG: I protest against your provocative hypothesis that the alternative to the size principle is an incredible number of random combinations of motor units. It is well known that we have three types of motor units. The alternative to your rank order should be separate control from the brain of three populations of motor units.

HENNEMAN: I think you echo the feelings of many people, and we would certainly like to do anything we could to clarify this point further. All I can say is the possibility you suggest has not been observed by us. A number of other groups have tried to devise situations to explore such possibilities. At least to date, I think that all of the experimental results seem to indicate that although different types of motor units might be activated, their rank order, according to motoneuron size and tension, seems to be relatively fixed. But I don't think other possibilities are excluded.

WILSON: Elwood, just in thinking of controlling different types of motoneurons, how do you reconcile your general formulation with results such as Bob BURKE's, where certain populations of cutaneous fibers selectively inhibit small motoneurons and excite large ones? I believe the same is true for rubrospinal fibers.

HENNEMAN: Yes. Those findings have troubled us. I think Bob would agree, however, that although his findings indicate some differences in input to motoneurons, that when you look at the firing order, not at the single EPSPs, that this order has not changed. A group from his own laboratory, as a matter of fact, recently published a paper pointing out the relative invariability of firing order in motoneurons.

STRUCTURAL-FUNCTIONAL RELATIONS IN MONOSYNAPTIC ACTION ON SPINAL MOTONEURONS

Robert E. BURKE, Bruce WALMSLEY* and John A. HODGSON**

Laboratory of Neural Control, NINCDS, NIH
Bethesda, MD

INTRODUCTION

This essay deals with the structure of functionally-identified group Ia muscle afferent arborizations in relation to the physiology of Ia synaptic action on alpha motoneurons. This topic seems appropriate to a symposium honoring Prof. R. LORENTE DE Nó and Prof. D. P. C. LLOYD. Prof. LORENTE DE Nó is a skilled neuroanatomist as well as an electro-physiologist. His combined studies of brainstem nuclei and the cerebral cortex demonstrate the necessity of considering the detailed structure of neuronal networks when trying to explain their physiology. Prof. LLOYD has played a central role in the development of spinal cord physiology. In particular, his studies of the synaptic interaction between muscle afferents and motoneurons are models of the inductive process and have resulted in conceptual formulations now thoroughly interwoven into current ideas about CNS reflex action. For a generation, these pioneering scientists made the Rockefeller Institute a pre-eminent center for research in what has now come to be called the Neurosciences.

GENERAL FEATURES OF GROUP IA SYNAPTIC ACTION

In the 1930's, LORENTE DE Nó demonstrated that motoneurons of extraocular muscles can be excited to synchronous discharge, after a brief but finite synaptic delay, by a synchronous volley in afferent fibers terminating directly (i.e., monosynaptically) on them (LORENTE DE Nó, 1938a, b, c). LLOYD, working in the cat spinal cord, later showed that the afferent fibers giving rise to the monosynaptic discharge of motoneurons were those with lowest electrical thresholds and fastest (group I) conduction velocities arising from end organs in muscle (LLOYD, 1943a). He further showed that the latency of this direct, or monosynaptic, reflex was identical with that due to sudden muscle stretch (LLOYD, 1943b). Furthermore, monosynaptic excitation was not confined to the motoneurons of the muscle giving rise to the afferents, but could be detected also in their synergists (LLOYD, 1946a, b) —the "homonymous" and "heteronymous" synaptic actions, respectively (LLOYD, HUNT and McINTYRE, 1955). Because the stretch-responsive group I afferents were considered to derive from muscle spindles (or type A receptors; HUNT and KUFFLER, 1951), the monosynaptic reflexes and their underlying synaptic potentials have since been ascribed to the direct action of the primary, or group Ia, muscle spindle afferents (see LLOYD, 1950).

In the 35 years since LLOYD's classic papers in 1943, the synaptic junction made by group Ia afferents on alpha mononeurons has become one of the most extensively studied systems in the mammalian CNS. Indeed, it is a textbook model for the operation of CNS excit-

* Present address: Department of Physiology, Monash University Clayton, Victoria, Australia
** Present address: Department of Physiology, University of Bristol Medical School, Bristol, England.

atory synapses. However, when the available evidence is examined in detail, it is clear
that many unresolved questions remain (see e.g., BURKE and RUDOMIN, 1977), including
the following:

1)   How many synaptic terminals from a given Ia afferent establish, on the average,
contact with an individual motoneuron, and where on the postsynaptic membrane are
they located?

2)   Is the basic junctional mechanism at Ia synapses one of "chemical" or "electrical"
transmission, or perhaps a combination of both?

3)   What accounts for the existence of all-or-none "unit" components in the synaptic
potentials produced by individual Ia fibers in motoneurons?

4)   What factor(s) account for the observed differences in group Ia efficacy among
motoneurons in a motor nucleus?

The conclusions that can be drawn from purely physiological data in response to the
above questions are for the most part not susceptible to validation by further physiological
experimentation. Rather, progress in their solution now depends in large measure on
consideration of the anatomy of group Ia arborizations within the spinal cord and of the
structure and spatial dispersion of the synaptic contacts made by Ia arbors upon cord neurons that can be definitely identified as alpha motoneurons.

Before addressing these unresolved issues in more detail, it seems important to review
briefly some aspects of Ia action that can be regarded as firmly established. Each muscle
spindle usually gives rise to a single group Ia afferent, so that their number in a muscle
nerve equals the number of spindles in the parent muscle (varying from tens to hundreds;
see MATTHEWS, 1972, for review). Each group Ia fiber establishes functional excitatory
contact directly with most, or possibly all, of the homonymous alpha motoneurons (LLOYD,
HUNT and McINTYRE, 1955; MENDELL and HENNEMAN, 1971; MENDELL et al., 1976), and
with a lesser proportion of heteronymous cells (MENDELL and HENNEMAN, 1971; SCOTT
and MENDELL, 1976). Synchronous activation of numbers of Ia afferents either by electrical stimulation of muscle nerves (e.g., BROCK et al., 1952) or by sudden muscle stretch
(LUNDBERG and WINSBURY, 1960), generates a purely depolarizing synaptic potential
(EPSP) at short (<1.0 msec) latency. This monosynaptic EPSP has a relatively rapid
rise and a slower, roughly logarithmic decay when recorded intracellularly at the motoneuron soma, and the decay phase corresponds to the decay of monosynaptic facilitation
demonstrated by LLOYD (1946a).

By using a variety of isolation methods, the EPSPs produced by individual group Ia
fibers can also be recorded in motoneurons (KUNO, 1964; BURKE and NELSON, 1966; BURKE,
1967; JACK et al., 1971; MENDELL and HENNEMAN, 1971). These individual afferent
EPSPs are in turn composed of smaller, all-or-none components (KUNO, 1964; BURKE,
1967; KUNO and MIYAHARA, 1969a; MENDELL and WEINER, 1976). Thus, there is a
hierarchy of Ia EPSPs, for which the following terms will be used:

1)   *Composite EPSP*—The synaptic potential produced in a motoneuron by synchronous
activation of more than one group Ia afferent.

2)   *Single-fiber EPSP*—The synaptic potential produced by an action potential in an
individual group Ia afferent fiber.

3)   *Unit EPSP*—An all-or-none component making up a single-fiber EPSP. Further
details and discussion of this hierarchy is available in a recent review (BURKE and RUDOMIN,
1977).

SOME PROBLEM ISSUES

Spatial Distribution of Group Ia Synapses

In the early years following the application of intracellular electrodes to study synaptic events in spinal motoneurons (BROCK et al., 1952), it was assumed that group Ia EPSPs were produced exclusively by synapses located on or near the cell soma (ECCLES, 1961; 1964). Using this assumption, the synaptic current necessary to generate observed EPSPs had to be rather prolonged, with significant "residual transmitter action" (CURTIS and ECCLES, 1959; ECCLES, 1961). However, subsequent studies of single fiber EPSPs disclosed a wide variety of EPSP shapes, both shorter and longer than the composite Ia EPSP (BURKE, 1967; MENDELL and HENNEMAN, 1971), that suggested wide spatial dispersion of Ia synapses over the motoneuron dendritic tree, including its most distal portions (RALL et al., 1967). Quantitative estimates of the spatial dispersion of Ia synapses have reinforced this conclusion, although the majority of Ia terminations appear to be on the proximal electrotonic half of the motoneuron dendrites (JACK et al., 1971; IANSEK and REDMAN, 1973), a distribution that may be explained by the relative amounts of motoneuron membrane available at different electrotonic distances (BARRETT and CRILL, 1974a; see BURKE and RUDOMIN, 1977).

The above conclusions are obviously framed in anatomical terms even though derived from electrophysiological observations. They depend critically on two factors: 1) the validity of mathematical models of motoneurons; and 2) the assumption that the duration of synaptic current is similarly brief at all Ia terminals (see RALL et al., 1967). The electrotonic model of the motoneuron formulated by RALL (1959; 1967) and extended by others (JACK and REDMAN, 1971; BARRETT and CRILL, 1974b) has in fact received substantial validation from the results of combined electrophysiological and anatomical analyses of actual alpha motoneurons (LUX et al., 1970; BARRETT and CRILL, 1974a). However, the assumption of Ia synaptic current duration is thus far unsupported by independent evidence. Some anatomical studies of Ia synapses on ventral horn neurons (e.g., CONRADI, 1969; McLAUGHLIN, 1972) are cited as showing that Ia terminals are mainly located on and near motoneuron somata. However, because of methodological limitations, these observations are in fact inconclusive as regards dendritic terminations. The issue can only be resolved by examination of the anatomy of functionally identified Ia afferents as they terminate on cells definitely identified as alpha motoneurons.

"Chemical" versus "Electrical" Transmission

It is generally assumed that group Ia EPSPs are produced by presynaptic liberation of a chemical transmitter substance, still unidentified, that causes a postsynaptic conductance change and consequent flow of depolarizing ionic currents (BROCK et al., 1952; CURTIS and ECCLES, 1959). Such a "chemical" or conductance change mechanism is compatible with observations that composite and single fiber Ia EPSPs sometimes add to one another in a less-than-linear manner (BURKE, 1967; KUNO and MIYAHARA, 1969b), and with reports that composite Ia EPSPs can sometimes be reversed with sufficient transmembrane depolarization (COOMBS et al., 1955; SMITH et al., 1967; KUNO and LLINÁS, 1970). The difficulty in demonstrating such EPSP reversal (SMITH et al., 1967) and the many instances of apparently linear addition of Ia EPSPs (ECCLES, 1964, BURKE, 1967) have been explained by invoking the influence of wide dendritic dispersal of Ia synapses discussed above (see RALL et al., 1967).

However, two recent studies of the effect of transmembrane polarization on Ia EPSPs have used methods that minimize the complications introduced by dendritic electrotonus (EDWARDS et al., 1976c; WERMAN and CARLEN, 1976).   Both sets of authors have reported failure to reverse group Ia EPSPs despite very large injections of depolarizing currents, sufficient in the case of WERMAN and CARLEN's study to reverse other types of EPSPs.   Considering the existing evidence, WERMAN and CARLEN (1976) have argued for a combined electrical and chemical mechanism at Ia terminals, while EDWARDS and coworkers (1976c) opt for a voltage—sensitive conductance mechanism.   The latter authors in fact suggest that it "...is difficult to suggest experiments through which a reasonable understanding of transmission at Ia synapses can be reached (EDWARDS et al., 1976c, p. 721).   It may be, however, that ultrastructural studies of definitively identified Ia synaptic terminations might be helpful, if not conclusive.

"Quantization" of Group Ia Transmission

In 1964, KUNO (1964) demonstrated that EPSPs produced by single Ia fibers (or small groups of them) are composed of discrete, all-or-none components, and that some afferent spikes fail to generate PSPs.   The resulting distributions of EPSP amplitudes (including "failures") fit predictions based on simple statistical models, notably the Poisson model. Subsequent work confirmed these observations (BURKE, 1967; KUNO and MIYAHARA, 1969a, b; MENDELL and WIENER, 1976), and showed that the average number (m) of unit EPSP components was usually rather small (<5) for any given afferent—motoneuron combination, but can occasionally be larger, in association with relatively large amplitude single-fiber EPSPs (BURKE and NELSON, 1966; BURKE, 1967).   The existence of "unit" Ia EPSPs has been assumed to imply that the process of liberation of the chemical transmitter thought to underlie the Ia EPSP must be "quantized" in the sense that the term is used to describe the events at the neuromuscular junction associated with individual "packets" of acetylcholine (e.g., see KUNO, 1971; MENDELL and WEINER, 1976).

BURKE and RUDOMIN (1977), in a review of synaptic transmission mechanisms in the spinal cord, have suggested that the unit Ia EPSPs can in fact only represent events that occur at individual Ia synapses and their existence does not necessarily imply a particular release mechanism.   Recent results of EDWARDS and associates (1976a, b) suggest that, at some Ia—motoneuron junctions, the amplitude of the unit EPSP components is not standard.   Instead, components of different amplitudes, occurring with highly unusual probability distributions, in fact make up some single fiber Ia EPSPs.   Many of their amplitude distributions do not fit any single statistical model.   The inferences that can be drawn from these studies are again generally framed in anatomical terms—numbers of synapses, spatial arrangements and organization of preterminal arborizations.   Further progress in understanding the phemonemon of unit EPSPs obviously requires detailed anatomical information.

Group Ia Synaptic Efficacy

LLOYD and McINTYRE (1955a) demonstrated that the responsiveness of individual motoneurons to group Ia input is graded, resulting in a spectrum of firing probabilities (or firing indices) from one motoneuron to another.   They further showed (1955b) that the firing index of a given motoneuron in homonymous Ia reflex action does not necessarily predict the relative excitability of that cell to heteronymous Ia volleys.   They suggested that gradations of responsiveness were due to corresponding variations in the presynaptic distribution of synaptic input, rather than to factors built into the postsynaptic motoneurons themselves.   Subsequent work has shown that the amplitude of composite homonymous Ia EPSPs varies among the motoneurons of a given motor nucleus (BURKE, 1968a), in a pattern matched with the type of muscle unit innervated (BURKE et al., 1976) and that the responsiveness of motoneurons in stretch reflexes is correlated with Ia EPSP amplitude (BURKE, 1968b). Several lines of evidence suggest that the wide spectrum of Ia EPSP amplitudes results from a corresponding gradation either of Ia synaptic density or of conductance change per synapse, or perhaps a combination of both factors (BURKE, 1968a; 1973; ZUCKER, 1973; BURKE and RUDOMIN, 1977; TRAUB, 1977). Direct counts of functionally identified and anatomically labeled Ia synapses impinging on similarly marked, physiologically identified motoneurons might be expected to resolve this issue.

Previous Anatomical Results

There is surprisingly little anatomical data about group Ia synaptic terminations on alpha motoneurons, despite the voluminous physiological data. Studies of fiber degeneration after dorsal root section (e.g., SPRAGUE, 1958) at the light microscopical level do not provide the necessary resolution, and ultrastructural studies are not in agreement as to whether (KUNO et al., 1973; BODIAN, 1975) or not (CONRADI, 1969; McLAUGHLIN, 1972) dorsal root terminations in the ventral horn exhibit typical degenerative changes to permit identification. Furthermore, ultrastructural studies have a very limited spatial view and attention has necessarily been concentrated on the juxtasomatic region of large cells presumed to motoneurons. Light microscopic studies of Golgi impregnated material (e.g., SCHEIBEL and SCHEIBEL, 1969) deal primarily with immature animals and there is evidence that synaptic remodeling takes place in postnatal development of the spinal cord (CONRADI and RONNEVI, 1975). It is now clear, in addition, that both group Ia and group II spindle afferents reach the ventrolateral motoneuron pool region (FU and SCHOMBURG, 1974) and make monosynaptic excitatory contacts with alpha motoneurons (KIRKWOOD and SEARS, 1975; STAUFFER et al., 1976). Thus ventral horn projection alone does not identify dorsal root projections as group Ia collaterals.

ILES (1976) has recently reported studies of dorsal root collaterals in adult spinal cords using iontophoretic application of cobalt ions to fill small groups of dorsal root fibers. Although the ventral horn projections thus visualized cannot be definitively identified, ILES demonstrated that terminal arborizations in ventral horn give rise to small numbers (1–6) of knobs or swellings along fine terminal branches which appear to contact the somata and proximal dendrites of large ventral horn cells. Both *en passant* and terminal boutons were seen, giving a picture very much like that found in Golgi-impregnated material by LORENTE DE Nó (1938b). Because the motoneuron dendrites were not visualized, ILES' results really permit conclusions only about juxtasomatic terminations of dorsal root collaterals.

HRP Marking of Functionally Identified Group Ia Afferents

Recently, several groups have shown that intracellular iontophoresis of horseradish peroxidase (HRP) produces reliable visualization not only of somata and dendrites, but also of cell axons, axon collaterals and some terminal arborizations (e.g., SNOW et al., 1976; JANKOWSKA et al., 1976), all of which can also be identified in electron micrographs (JANKOWSKA et al., 1976; CULLHEIM, KELLERTH and CONRADI, 1977). BROWN and co-workers (1977) successfully extended this method to include intra-axonal injection of HRP into functionally identified primary afferent axons, leading to visualization of their intraspinal arborizations in great detail.

Using this method, BROWN and FYFFE (1978) have very recently reported the detailed anatomical organization of identified group Ia afferents in the spinal cord of adult cats (i.e., muscle afferents with conduction velocities >80 m/sec). Initially unaware of this

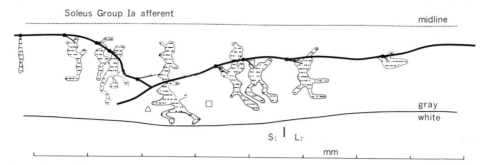

Fig. 1 Dorsal view of reconstruction (from serial sagittal sections) of the intraspinal course of a group Ia afferent from the SOL muscle, identified by conduction velocity (112 m/sec), silencing during active SOL twitch, large dynamic response to ramp stretch, and ability to follow 1:1 during 120 Hz, 100 μm vibration of the SOL tendon. The entering fiber divided into ascending and descending branches (heavy lines). The site of HRP injection was just rostral to the branch point (see Fig. 2). The descending branch gave rise to 5 rather closely spaced collaterals while the ascending branch had 4 more widely spaced collaterals. The ascending branch was about twice the diameter of the descending branch. The sets of dots enclosed by light outlines denote the projected positions of terminal arborizations of each collateral. Despite close proximity at some section levels, the adjacent arborizations did not overlap at all. The cord midline is indicated by a dashed line and the most lateral limit of the interface between gray and white matter is shown as a solid line. Most of the afferent arborizations labeled by HRP were in the rostral half of the S1 segment, as were cell bodies of 2 HRP-labeled motoneurons, a SOL type S unit (triangle) and an LG type FR unit (square). The cord was moderately post-fixed, with relatively large S1 spinal root.

work, we had begun a similar study of Ia anatomy, but our experiments also included injection of HRP into homonymous or heteronymous alpha motoneurons of known motor unit type (BURKE et al., 1973). Group Ia afferents were identified not only by conduction velocity but also by response to muscle stretch, twitch and vibration (see MATTHEWS, 1972). Our method of HRP iontophoresis was patterned on that of SNOW et al. (1976) and the animals (anesthetized with pentobarbital) survived for 8 to 15 hours after afferent injection. Following intracardiac perfusion, serial frozen sections in the sagittal plane were cut (see BURKE et al., 1977 for methods). The most successful preparations were reacted to demonstrate HRP after treatment with 0.5 per cent cobalt chloride according to the method described by ADAMS (1977).

Figure 1 shows a dorsal view reconstruction, made from 75 μm serial sagittal sections, of a soleus (SOL) group Ia afferent. The entering axon divided into descending and ascending branches (heavy lines) that ran in the dorsal column. Nine collateral branches were visualized (dots and lighter lines contacting the main branches), each (see Fig. 2) giving rise to an arborization indicated by the rows of dots within light outlines. The positions of somas of two labeled motoneurons are also indicated (triangle and square). Each collateral arborization was oriented mainly across the cord gray matter, with relatively little rostro-caudal spread. In this detail, our results differ somewhat from BROWN and FYFFE's Fig. 8 (1978) but correspond more closely to descriptions given by ILES (1976). In all, we have marked 5 group Ia fibers, 2 from SOL, 2 from medial gastrocnemius and one presumed to originate in the flexor digitorum brevis muscle. All have shown similar overall features, corresponding in most respects to descriptions given by BROWN and FYFFE (1978).

Figure 2 shows a sagittal projection of the collateral systems arising from the SOL afferent of Figure 1. The soma positions and approximate dendritic extensions (circles

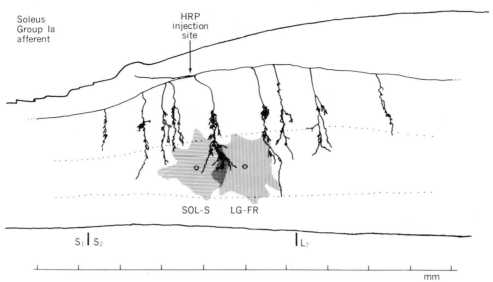

Soleus
Group Ia
afferent

HRP
injection
site

SOL-S   LG-FR

S₁ | S₂ | L₇

mm

Fig. 2 Lateral view reconstruction of the SOL Ia afferent shown in Figure 1. Because of the sagittal orientation of the serial sections, more detailed reconstruction of collateral arborizations was possible in this view. The circles and shadings denote the somata and maximum dendritic extents of the labeled SOL and LG motoneurons. Dorsal and ventral cord surfaces shown as solid lines. The dorsal and ventral limits of the ventral horn are projected as dotted lines.

and shading) of two HRP-labeled motoneurons, one SOL slow twitch (or type S) and one lateral gastrocnemius (LG) fast twitch, fatigue resistant (type FR), as defined by the innervated muscle unit (BURKE et al., 1973).   Note the slight cephelad tilt to the course of the more rostral collaterals, as described by BROWN and FYFFE (1978). Structures interpreted to be synaptic endings (Figs. 3, 5 and 6) were found in medial lamina VI, dorsolateral lamina VII and in the dorsal portions of lamina IX, as found by BROWN and FYFFE (1978). However, only 5 of the 9 labeled arborizations appeared to penetrate into the motor nuclei (compare Figs. 1 and 2); the 3 caudalmost arbors, and the most rostral one, seemed confined to more medial termination sites in laminae VI and VII.

The photomicrograph in Fig. 3 shows a fine (approx. 0.5 μm diameter) collateral from the same SOL Ia afferent (in the middle arbor of Fig. 2; see also Fig. 4).   This collateral has several swellings along its course (interpreted to be synapses *en passant*), one of which makes intimate contact with a relatively thick proximal dendrite belonging to the labeled SOL motoneuron (tailless arrow; also shown in inset A; see also Fig. 4 and 5).   There are also several terminal boutons on very fine stalks (e.g., tailed arrow).   The three boutons on the right appeared to make intimate contact with the soma of a large labeled motoneuron, clearly visualized in the original slide.   Inset B shows a terminal bouton (arrow) from the same arborization making contact with a quite distal, fine dendrite belonging to the same SOL motoneuron (see Fig. 4 and 5).   Note that the fine afferent (<0.2 μm) stalk joins that of another terminal bouton ending on an unmarked structure, presumably a neighboring dendrite of an unlabeled cell (see structure B in Fig. 5).   The HRP-labeled dendrites of this and most other motoneurons in the present study exhibited a "beaded" appearance (Fig. 3, esp. inset B; Fig. 5) particularly in their more distal regions. This phenomenon, which may be a toxic reaction to HRP (it seems to vary directly with intensity of cell label), was convenient for identification of fine dendrites but hampered attempts to reconstruct the electrotonic architecture of these motoneurons (as done by BARRETT and CRILL, (1974a).

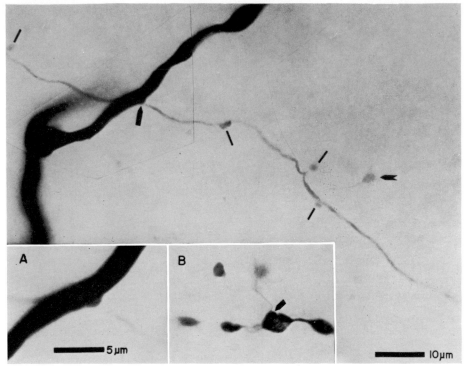

Fig. 3 Oil immersion photomicrographs of HRP-labeled collateral from the SOL Ia afferent of Figures 1 and 2. The fiber makes one *en passant* contact (tailless arrow) with a thick HRP-labeled dendrite of the SOL motoneuron (see Fig. 4 for actual position). Other presumed synaptic boutons are indicated with short lines. The tailed arrow indicates a terminal bouton on a very fine (<0.2 μm diameter) axonal twig. The section is not counterstained. Inset A shows the contact with the thick dendrite at higher magnification. Inset B shows a different contact between the same Ia arborization and a different quite distal dendritic branch of the SOL cell (structure B in Fig. 5).

Figure 4 is a sagittal projection reconstructed from 15 serial sections of two collateral arbors from the SOL Ia afferent, plus the two labeled motoneurons with which they make contact (cf. Fig. 2). The entire extent of each lamina VII and IX arborization is shown but only those motoneuron dendrites making presumed synaptic contacts are indicated (contact regions denoted by circles). The left-hand arbor made apparent contact with the SOL motoneuron (Fig. 5) but not with the LG cell, despite considerable penetration of the LG dendrites into its collateral territory. Only the right-hand arbor made contact with the LG cell (Fig. 6).

A more detailed reconstruction of the distal contact region between the Ia arbor and the SOL motoneuron (Fig. 4) is shown in Fig. 5, together with oil immersion photomicrographs of 5 of the 6 presumed synaptic contacts. Contacts A and B, also illustrated in Fig. 3, are a bouton *en passant* (A) and a terminal bouton on a fine stalk (B), respectively. Contact C has a bizarre appearance, with a relatively large (approx. 3×5 μm) *en passant* swelling (filled arrow) lying near a fine dendritic "bead" (open arrow), but connected to it by a narrow bridge filled with HRP. The bridge appeared to arise from the presynaptic swelling but its nature could not be established with light microscopy. Contact D appeared to involve no presynaptic swelling in the afferent twig, which simply lay in contact (filled arrow) with a curving portion of a SOL dendrite (open arrow). The afferent twig in D

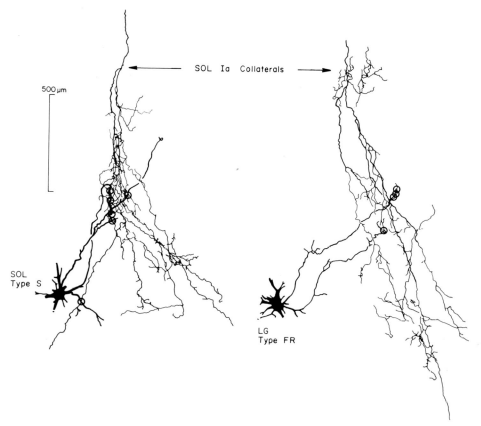

Fig. 4 Sagittal reconstruction of adjacent arborizations of the same SOL Ia afferent as Figures 1–3, which establish presumed synaptic contact with dendrites of either the SOL or the LG motoneuron at sites indicated by circles. All of the collateral fibers of each arborization in laminae VII and IX are shown, but only those dendritic branches involved in synaptic contacts are included.

branched from a thicker axon (right side of the inset) with a marked post-branching constriction. Contact E represents a bouton *en passant* (white outline; filled arrow), overlying and in contact with a dendritic "bead" (open arrow). The structure at contact F was similar to those pictured for A and E. The presumed synaptic contacts made by this SOL Ia arbor on the SOL motoneuron thus exhibited a variety of shapes and sizes.

It cannot be established from light microscopy of HRP-filled arborizations whether or not the structures shown in Figures 3 and 5 are in fact functional synaptic terminations. However, the size range and disposition of these swellings fit with the kind of structures interpreted to be synapses in electron micrographs (e.g., CONRADI, 1969; BODIAN, 1975). Synaptic specializations can also occur at nodes of Ranvier without axonal swelling (BODIAN and TAYLOR, 1963; WAXMAN, 1975), so that contact D can also be presumed to represent a functional synapse. The rest of the discussion will assume that the close contacts seen in Figure 5 are in fact functional synapses.

Figure 6 illustrates a similar reconstruction of the much simpler contact system between the more rostral Ia arbor in Figure 4 and the LG type FR motoneuron. All contacts were established on fine distal dendrites, from two presynaptic collaterals arising from the same medium-diameter parent collateral. One contact (lowermost circle) was an isolated *en passant* swelling (filled arrow in inset) and the other 3 (upper set of circles; filled arrows in

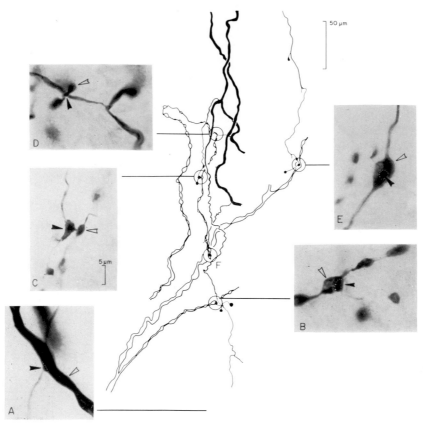

Fig. 5 Camera lucida reconstruction (sagittal view) of the distal contact region on the SOL motoneuron shown in Figure 4. The diagram includes only those afferent and dendritic branches involved in presumed synaptic contacts. Photomicrographs of 5 of the 6 contacts found are shown as insets. Contact A is the juxtasomatic structure shown in Figure 3 and indicated on Figure 4 by the circle near the SOL soma. Bouton outlines enhanced by white dots in contacts B and E. Dendrites indicated by unshaded outlines Scale in inset C applies to all insets. Further description in text.

large inset) were fusiform *en passant* swellings close together along a dendritic termination. The most distal dendritic "bead" (open arrow; large inset) was poorly labeled by HRP and was in fact the end of this dendritic branch.

Figures 4 through 6 illustrate 2 of the 3 Ia afferent—motoneuron contact systems so far reconstructed. The third system was in a different animal and involved a SOL Ia afferent making contact with an LG fast twitch (? type FF) motoneuron. Technical factors limited detailed study of 6 other possible contact systems. Simplified wiring diagrams of the 3 reconstructed systems are shown in Figure 7. Two of the patterns are relatively simple. For example, activity of the lowermost system in Figure 7 would be expected to generate single fiber EPSPs of brief duration (interpretable as juxtasomatic, or within about 0.2 space constants of the soma). The voltage change produced by synchronous action at each contact would be expected to produce less-than-linear summation (KUNO and MIYA-HARA, 1969a) since the contacts appear to be electrotonically close to one another even though one is on a different stem dendrite (see RINZEL and RALL, 1974). If all terminals are invaded by every action potential but transmission fails randomly, the amplitude fluc-tuations might be expected to indicate action of 0, 1, 2 or 3 unit EPSPs with simple statis-

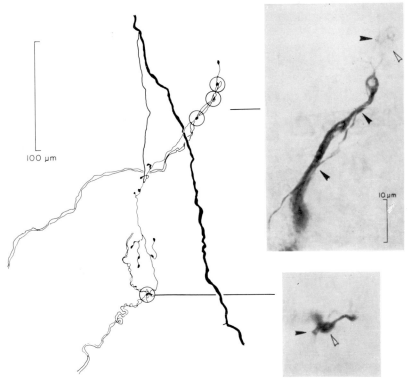

Fig. 6 Reconstruction as in Figure 5 of the contact region between the SOL Ia afferent and the LG type FR motoneuron shown in Figure 4. See text for description.

tics (KUNO, 1964). If, on the other hand, failures of transmission occur because of failure of action potential invasion into branch points (BURKE and RUDOMIN, 1977; and see below), the same number of unit components might be expected but the statistical distribution would probably be different, resembling "non-quantized" examples found by EDWARDS and coworkers (1976b). One "unit" EPSP could then involve action at the pair of *en passant* boutons while the other would reflect action at the single terminal arising from the other branch.

The contact pattern in the middle diagram of Figure 7 is equally simple although the terminations occur on dendrites at considerable electrotonic distances from the soma (Fig. 4 and 6; LG motoneuron). The voltage transient produced by such terminations would be expected to have a relatively slow rise time and long half-width (RALL, 1967), but would very likely be such that a single electrotonic locus could be assigned (JACK et al., 1971; IANSEK and REDMAN, 1973). The voltage perturbations arising at the 3 neighboring *en passant* terminals should interact quite non-linearly with one another, but the resulting net perturbation should add linearly to that produced at the single synapse on the other distal dendrite (see RALL, 1967). If the action potential invades all terminals but fails sometimes to produce conductance changes (KUNO, 1971), one would expect between 0 and 4 unit EPSPs with some simple statistical distribution. On the other hand if action potential invasion fails at the branch point giving rise to the fine preterminal axons (see Fig. 6) then the EPSP amplitude distribution might include some "unit" EPSPs more than twice the amplitude of others, representing the net action of the 3 *en passant* contacts acting as a group. The statistical distribution of EPSP amplitudes would be correspondingly complex, possibly resembling the distribution in Fig. 8 of EDWARDS et al. (1976a).

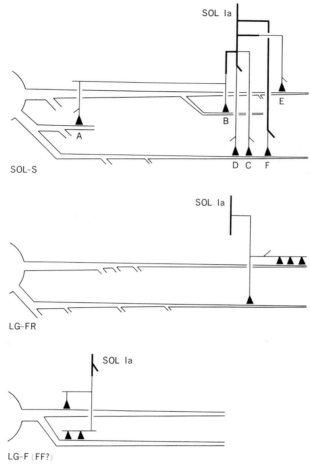

Fig. 7 "Wiring diagrams" of 3 reconstructed contact systems between group Ia afferents and alpha motoneurons. The 2 upper diagrams refer to the contact systems shown in Figure 1–6. The lowermost diagram came from a different spinal cord. The patterns of afferent branching and the approximate dendritic location of terminations are representative of the original observations. Only those afferent branches that might account for differential action of Ia terminals are included. See text for discussion.

The uppermost pattern in Figure 7 (from Fig. 5; the SOL Ia on the SOL motoneuron) is by far the most complex, involving 6 presumed synapses on 4 different dendritic branches and including terminals on both distal and proximal dendrites.   Terminals D, C, and F (see Fig. 5) would be expected to interact non-linearly (if conduction in the preterminal twigs permits synchrony of conductance changes), but otherwise, linear voltage summations would seem probable.   The existence of terminal A indicates that the waveform of the EPSP resulting from activity of this Ia arbor should have a faster rise time (due to terminal A) than expected for the long half-width contributed by the distal dendritic terminals B through F.   This kind of departure from single locus waveforms is in fact not uncommon (RALL et al., 1967; JACK et al., 1971; IANSEK and REDMAN, 1973; MENDELL and WEINER, 1976).

The different conduction paths leading to the various terminals might produce some asynchrony of synaptic action, especially in terminal A, which occurs along the course of a long but fine (approx. 0.5 μm) axon.   CNS axons with diameters <0.5 μm can be myelinated (e.g., WAXMAN, 1975) and if this branch were myelinated, its conduction velocity might be about 2–3 m/sec (WAXMAN and BENNETT, 1972). Maximum asynchrony in the network thus might be about 200 μsec, simply on the basis of different lengths of conduction paths. There is good reason to assume that axonal filling with cobalt ions or HRP permits visualization of the axis cylinders only (ILES, 1976), and it is thus impossible to determine in light microscopy where myelin sheaths end in Ia arborizations. It seems likely, however, that much of the Ia arborization is myelinated, except for the very fine terminal twigs leading to terminal boutons (e.g., Fig. 3 and 5B).

Interesting complications arise if action potentials fail to invade all branch points in this preterminal arbor. The number of possible combinations of unit EPSPs (0 to 6) might well be the same as if all terminals were invaded, with the failure process at each terminal. However, the distribution of amplitudes in the two cases would very likely be quite different, depending on which of the 6 possible branch points showed invasion failures. Furthermore, the occurrence of non-linear summation and the mixtures of juxta-somatic and dendritic components could be exected to be very complex. A presynaptic arborization of this complexity could in fact produce the kind of waveform—amplitude distribution evident in Figure 3 of EDWARDS et al. (1976b).

Whether or not action potentials sometimes fail to invade all branches of an afferent arborization remains unknown, although the possibility was suggested many years ago by BARRON and MATTHEWS (1939), with periodic revival since (McCULLOCH et al., 1950; CHIUNG et al., 1970; WAXMAN, 1975; BURKE and RUDOMIN, 1977). The phenomenon has been clearly demonstrated in branching axons of crustacea (GROSSMAN et al., 1973), but similar physiological tests in an afferent arborization (e.g., Fig. 4) would be extremely difficult. It is interesting, however, to note that branch points in Ia arborizations can be quite complex, including examples of trifurcations into daughter fibers of unequal diameter (Fig. 8A, B), bifurcations into unequal daughter branches (Fig. 5D; Fig. 8C) and simple bifurcations where, especially in finer branches, the daughter branches have diameters equal to that of the parent (Fig. 8 D). Many branch points in Ia arborizations exhibit constrictions in both parent and daughter branches (Fig. 5D; Fig. 8 A, B, C), as noted also by ILES (1976). While it is difficult to quantitate, it appears that the relative degree of constriction at many branch points is less in the parent branch than in the daughters (e.g., Fig. 5D; Fig. 8 A, B, C). From theoretical studies of GOLDSTEIN and RALL (1974) it seems possible that axonal constrictions at branch points may serve to make action potential invasion into daughter branches more secure but the pronounced residual effects of prior impulse activity, especially in fine CNS axons (e.g., SWADLOW and WAXMAN, 1976), makes prediction difficult.

ANOTHER LOOK AT UNSETTLED ISSUES

Although the information now available about Ia—motoneuron synaptic arbors is very limited, the data nevertheless permit some useful comment on the unresolved questions raised at the beginning of this essay.

The present observations clearly demonstrate that some Ia synaptic terminations occur on very distal motoneuron dendrites (Fig. 6), as well as on juxta somatic membrane regions (Fig. 7, bottom diagram). Further, some Ia contact systems clearly include terminals at different electrotonic distances from the soma (Fig. 5; Fig. 7, top diagram). This evidence strengthens inferences based on earlier anatomical results (BODIAN, 1975; BROWN and FYFFE, 1978) and suggests that the interpretation of shape differences in Ia single fiber EPSPs as due to spatial dispersion of terminals is in fact correct. It further suggests that

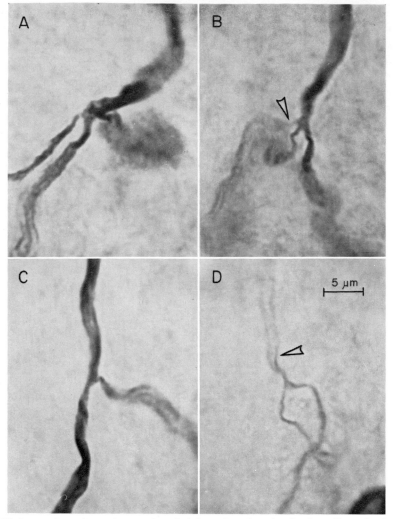

Fig. 8 Oil immersion photomicrographs of 4 branch points in the Ia collateral arborizatiton making contact with the SOL motoneuron of Figures 4 and 5. A and B show trifurcations with unequal diameter daughter branches (open arrow in B indicates fine branch leaving the plane of focus). C illustrates an example of a bifurcation that appears to be a simple side collateral (running to the right). D is an example of a fine parent branch (open arrow, leaving the plane of focus and appearing as a double image) giving rise to 2 daughter branches of the same diameter. The branch point itself seems to be a small swelling. No axonal constrictions are evident in D, but all of the other examples clearly show constrictions of all axons participating in the branch point. Constrictions seem especially pronounced in the daughter branches. Scale in D is the same for all examples.

the duration of synaptic current at Ia synapses is uniformly brief at all Ia terminals, which was a necessary assumption in the earlier physiological arguments (BURKE, 1967; RALL et al., 1967; JACK et al., 1971; IANSEK and REDMAN, 1973).

The question of how many Ia terminals occur in a given Ia—motoneuron contact system cannot be resolved by the few reconstructions now available (Fig. 7). It is a statistical question that requires a much larger sample of reconstructions done in the manner of the present work. However, the fact that all 3 synaptic systems examined had relatively few terminals on the labeled motoneurons is in keeping with estimates made on the basis of indirect evidence (KUNO, 1964; JACK et al., 1971). Only a small proportion of group Ia—motoneuron interactions (perhaps 1 per 300–500 such afferent—motoneuron contact systems) produce single fiber EPSPs with peak amplitudes and amplitude fluctuations that suggest the operation of more than 5 or 6 terminals (BURKE and NELSON, 1966; BURKE, 1967).

It is a seeming paradox that long duration single fiber EPSPs, presumably generated on distal dendrites, are not correspondingly smaller in amplitude or charge injection than the EPSPs generated closer to the soma (BURKE, 1967; JACK et al., 1971; IANSEK and REDMAN, 1973; MENDELL and WEINER, 1976). IANSEK and REDMAN (1973) have suggested that distal Ia synapses may produce larger conductance changes per terminal but the present results do not suggest that distal boutons are systematically larger, as might be consistent with such an hypothesis (see KUNO et al., 1973). Alternatively, it may be that the number of contacts formed by a given afferent arborization on distal sites may be systematically greater because of the frequency of chance encounters, even though less and less motoneuron membrane is available as electrotonic distance increases (BARRETT and CRILL, 1974a). Again, a much larger number of reconstructions must be done before this question can be settled.

With respect to the question of "chemical versus electrical" transmission, it would seem that no amount of anatomical data will permit unambiguous resolution of the problem. However, an ultrastructural study of functionally identified group Ia terminals ending on identified motoneuron dendrites would be most consistent with a "chemical" mechanism if the results confirmed existing observations of *presumed* Ia boutons (CONRADI, 1969; BODIAN, 1975). Combination of light and electron microscopy of HRP-labeled structures is now technically possible (JANKOWSKA et al., 1976; CULLHEIM et al., 1977). An additional problem, important to the transmission mechanism and not resolvable by anatomy, is the question of whether or not action potentials in fact invade Ia terminal boutons, especially those on very fine preterminal stalks (e.g., Fig. 3, Fig. 5B; see discussion in BURKE and RUDOMIN, 1977). It does seem likely, however, that action potentials must be present in boutons *en passant* (Fig. 3; Fig. 6), when these occur along the course of a collateral fiber that can travel hundreds of μm (e.g., Fig. 4).

With regard to the nature of the "unit" EPSP, BURKE and RUDOMIN (1977) have suggested in a recent review that these all-or-none synaptic potential are best considered as events associated with action at individual synaptic endings rather than as quantal packets of transmitter substance. The relatively small average number (m) of unit EPSPs in most Ia—motoneuron contacts matches the small number of anatomically demonstrable contact sites (e.g., Fig. 7). Moreover, the "non-quantized" amplitude fluctuations seen by EDWARDS et al., (1976a, b) can be explained by assuming that failure of action potential invasion can occur in presynaptic networks such as in all three examples in Figure 7. Further progress in resolving this question seems to require anatomical reconstructions of Ia—motoneuron contact systems which have also been studied physiologically. Our own attempts to do this have so far failed because of severe technical problems.

Finally, it has been suggested elsewhere (BURKE, 1968a; 1973; BURKE and RUDOMIN, 1977) that the 10-fold range in composite Ia EPSP amplitude in gastrocnemius motoneurons (BURKE, 1968a, b; BURKE, RYMER and WALSH, 1976) can be explained by a corresponding variation in the density of Ia synapses (i.e., Ia terminals per unit area of motoneuron membrane). In principle, falsification of this hypothesis should be possible using the methods of the present study, if a sufficient number of Ia contact systems can be reconstructed on motoneurons of known motor unit type. However, if it is assumed that the average m number of unit EPSP components indeed reflects numbers of contacts per afferent (see above), then currently available evidence is thus far consistent with the density variation hypothesis (see BURKE and RUDOMIN 1977).

CONCLUDING COMMENT

As Prof. LORENTE DE NÓ has amply demonstrated, analysis of the functional characteristics of synaptic interactions in the CNS must take account of the detailed structure of synaptic arborizations. This is clearly illustrated in current efforts to understand the operation of the synaptic contacts made by group Ia afferents on alpha motoneurons, which were begun with such solid grounding by the pioneering work of Prof. LLOYD.

REFERENCES

ADAMS, J. C.: Technical considerations on the use of horseradish peroxidase as a neuronal marker. *Neuroscience, 2*: 141–145 (1977)

BARRETT, J. N and CRILL, W. E.: Specific membrane properties of cat motoneurones. *J. Physiol. (Lond.), 239*: 301–324 (1974a)

BARRETT, J. N. and CRILL, W. E.: Influence of dendritic location and membrane properties on the effectiveness of synapses on cat motneurones. *J. Physiol. (Lond.), 293*: 325–345 (1974b)

BARRON, D. H. and MATTHEWS, B. H. C.: Intermittent conduction in the spinal cord. *J. Physiol. (Lond.), 85*: 73–103 (1939)

BODIAN, D.: Origin of specific synaptic types in the motoneuron neuropil of the monkey. *J. Comp. Neurol., 159*: 225–244 (1975)

BODIAN, D. and TAYLOR, N.: Synapse arising at a central node of Ranvier, and a note on fixation in the central nervous system. *Science, 139*: 330–332 (1963)

BROCK, L. G., COOMBS, J. S. and ECCLES, J. C.: The recording of potentials from motoneurones with an intracellular electrode. *J. Physiol. (Lond.), 117*: 431–460 (1952)

BROWN, A. G. and FYFFE, R. E. W.: The morphology of group Ia afferent fibre collaterals in the spinal cord of the cat. *J. Physiol. (Lond.), 274*: 111–127 (1978)

BROWN, A. G., ROSE, P. K. and SNOW, P. J.: The morphology of hair follicle afferent fibre collaterals in the spinal cord of the cat. *J. Physiol. (Lond.), 272*: 779–797 (1977)

BURKE, R. E.: Composite nature of the monosynaptic excitatory postsynaptic potential. *J. Neurophysiol., 30*: 1114–1136 (1967)

BURKE, R. E.: Group Ia synaptic input to fast and slow twitch motor units of cat triceps surae. *J. Physiol. (Lond.), 196*: 606–630 (1968a)

BURKE, R. E.: Firing patterns of gastrocnemius motor units in the decerebrate cat. *J. Physiol. (Lond.), 196*: 631–654 (1968b)

BURKE, R. E.: On the central nervous system control of fast and slow twitch motor units. *In* DESMEDT, J. E. (ed.): *New Developments in Electromyography and Clinical Neurophysiology.* Vol. 3. Karger, Basel, pp. 69–94 (1973)

BURKE, R. E., LEVINE, D. N., TSAIRIS, P. and ZAJAC, F. E.: Physiological types and histochemical profiles in motor units of the cat gastrocnemius. *J. Physiol. (Lond.), 234*: 723–748 (1973)

BURKE, R. E. and NELSON, P. G.: Synaptic activity in motoneurons during natural stimulation of muscle spindles. *Science, 151*: 1088–1091 (1966)

BURKE, R. E. and RUDOMIN, P.: Spinal neurons and synapses. *In* KANDEL, E. (ed.): *Handbook of Physiology*, Sect. 1, Vol. 1. The Nervous System: The Cellular Biology of Neurons. American Physiological Society, Washington, pp. 877–944 (1977)

BURKE, R. E., RYMER, W. Z. and WALSH, J. V.: Relative strength of synaptic input from short-latency pathways to motor units of defined type in cat medial gastrocnemius. *J. Neurophysiol., 39*: 447–458 (1976)

BURKE, R. E., STRICK, P., KANDA, K., KIM, C. C. and WALMSLEY, B.: Anatomy of medial gastrocnemius and soleus motor nuclei in cat spinal cord. *J. Neurophysiol., 40*: 667–680 (1977)

CHUNG, S., RAYMOND, S. A. and LETTVIN, J. Y.: Multiple meaning in single visual units. *Brain, Behav. Evol., 3*: 72–101 (1970)

CONRADI, S.: On motoneuron synaptology in adult cats. *Acta Physiol. Scand.* Suppl., 332 (1969)

CONRADI, S. and RONNEVI, L.-O.: Spontaneous elimination of synapses on cat spinal motoneurons after birth: do half of the synapses on the cell bodies disappear? *Brain Res.*, *92*: 505–510 (1975)

COOMBS, J. S., ECCLES, J. C. and FATT, P.: Excitatory synaptic action in motoneurones. *J. Physiol. (Lond.)*, *130*: 374–395 (1955)

CULLHEIM, S., KELLERTH, J.-O. and CONRADI, S.: Evidence for direct synaptic interconnections between cat spinal alpha-motoneurons via the recurrent collaterals: A morphological study using intracellular injection of horseradish peroxidase. *Brain Res.*, *132*: 1–10 (1977)

CURTIS, D. R. and ECCLES, J. C.: The time courses of excitatory and inhibitory synaptic actions. *J. Physiol. (Lond.)*, *154*: 529–546 (1959)

ECCLES, J. C.: Membrane time constants of cat motoneurones and time courses of synaptic actions. *Expt. Neurol.*, *4*: 1–22 (1961)

ECCLES, J. C.: *The Physiology of Synapses.* Academic Press, New York (1964)

EDWARDS, F. R., REDMAN, S. J. and WALMSLEY, B.: Statistical fluctuations in charge transfer at Ia synapses on spinal motoneurones. *J. Physiol. (Lond.)*, *259*: 665–688 (1976a)

EDWARDS, F. R., REDMAN, S. J. and WALMSLEY, B.: Non-quantal fluctuations and transmission failures in charge transfer at Ia synapses on spinal motoneurones. *J. Physiol. (Lond.)*, *259*: 689–704 (1976b)

EDWARDS, F. R., REDMAN, S. J. and WALMSLEY, B.: The effect of polarizing currents on unitary Ia excitatory postsynaptic potentials evoked in spinal motoneurones. *J. Physiol. (Lond.)*, *259*: 705–723 (1976c)

FU, T. C. and SCHOMBURG, E. D.: Electrophysiological investigation of the projection of secondary muscle spindle afferents in the cat spinal cord. *Acta physiol Scand.*, *91*: 314–329 (1974)

GOLDSTEIN, S. S. and RALL, W.: Changes of action potential shape and velocity for changing core conductor geometry. *Biophys. J.*, *14*: 731–757 (1974)

GROSSMAN, Y., SPIRA, M. E. and PARNAS, I.: Differential flow of information into branches of a single axon. *Brain Res.*, *64*: 379–386 (1973)

HUNT, C. C. and KUFFLER, S. W.: Stretch receptor discharges during muscle contraction. *J. Physiol. (Lond.)*, *113*: 298–315 (1951)

IANSEK, R. and REDMAN, S. J.: The amplitude, time course and charge of unitary excitatory postsynaptic potentials evoked in spinal motoneurone dendrites. *J. Physiol. (Lond.)*, *234*: 665–688 (1973)

ILES, J. F.: Central terminations of muscle afferents on motoneurones in the cat spinal cord. *J. Physiol. (Lond.)*, *262*: 91–117 (1976)

JACK, J. J. B., MILLER, S., PORTER, R. and REDMAN, S. J.: The time course of minimal excitatory post-synaptic potentials evoked in spinal motoneurones by group Ia afferent fibres. *J. Physiol. (Lond.)*, *15*: 353–380 (1971)

JACK, J. J. B. and REDMAN, S. J.: An electrical description of the motoneurone, and its application to the analysis of synaptic potentials. *J. Physiol. (Lond.)*, *215*: 321–352 (1971)

JANKOWSKA, E., RASTAD, J. and WESTMAN, J.: Intracellular application of horseradish peroxidase and its light and electron microscopical appearance in spinocervical tract cells. *Brain Res.*, *105*: 557–562 (1976)

KIRKWOOD, P. A. and SEARS, T. A.: Monosynaptic excitation of motoneurones from muscle spindle secondary endings of intercostal and triceps surae muscles in the cat. *J. Physiol. (Lond.)*, *245*: 64–66 (1975)

KUNO, M.: Quantal components of excitatory synaptic potentials in spinal motoneurones. *J. Physiol. (Lond.)*, *175*: 81–99 (1964)

KUNO, M.: Quantum aspects of central and ganglionic synaptic transmission in vertebrates. *Physiol. Rev.*, *51*: 647–678 (1971)

KUNO, M. and LLINÁS, R.: Alterations of synaptic action in chromatolyzed motoneurones of the cat. *J. Physiol. (Lond.)*, *210*: 823–838 (1970)

KUNO, M. and MIYAHARA, J. T.: Analysis of synaptic efficacy in spinal motoneurones from 'quantum' aspects. *J. Physiol. (Lond.)*, *210*: 479–493 (1969a)

KUNO, M. and MIYAHARA, J. T.: Non-linear summation of unit synaptic potentials in spinal motoneurones of the cat. *J. Physiol. (Lond.)*, *210*: 465–477 (1969b)

KUNO, M., MUÑOZ-MARTINEZ, E. J. and RANDIC, M.: Synaptic action on Clarke's column neurones in relation to afferent terminal size. *J. Physiol. (Lond.)*, *228*: 343–360 (1973)

LLOYD, D. P. C.: Reflex action in relation to pattern and peripheral source of afferent stimulation. *J. Neurophysiol.*, *6*: 111–120 (1943a)

LLOYD, D. P. C., Conduction and synaptic transmission of reflex response to stretch in spinal cats. *J. Neurophysiol.*, *6*: 317–326 (1943b)

LLOYD, D. P. C.: Facilitation and inhibition of spinal motoneurons. *J. Neurophysiol.*, *9*: 421–438 (1946a)

LLOYD, D. P. C.: Integrative pattern of excitation and inhibition in two-neuron reflex arcs. *J. Neurophysiol.*, *9*: 439–444 (1946b)

LLOYD, D. P. C.: On reflex actions of muscular origin. *In* BARD, P. (ed.): "*Patterns of organization in the Central Nervous System*". *Res. Publ. ARNMD*, Vol. 30; pp. 48–67, Williams & Wilkins Baltimore (1950)

LLOYD, D. P. C., HUNT, C. C. and McINTYRE, A. K.: Transmission in facilitated monosynaptic spinal reflex systems. *J. Gen. Physiol.*, *38*: 307–317 (1955)

LLOYD, D. P. C. and McINTYRE, A. K.: Monosynaptic reflex responses of individual motoneurons. *J. Gen. Physiol.*, *38*: 771–787 (1955a)

LLOYD, D. P. C. and McINTYRE, A. K.: Transmitter potentiality of homonymous and heteronymous monosynaptic reflex connections of individual motoneurones. *J. Gen. Physiol.*, *38*: 789–799 (1955b)

LORENTE DE NÓ, R.: Limits of variation of the synaptic delay of motoneurons. *J. Neurophysiol.*, *1*: 187–194 (1938a)

LORENTE DE NÓ, R.: Synaptic stimulation of motoneurons as a local process. *J. Neurophysiol.*, *1*: 195–206 (1938b)

LORENTE DE NÓ, R.: Analysis of the activity of the chains of internuncial neurons. *J. Neurophysiol.*, *1*: 207–244 (1938c)

LUNDBERG, A. and WINSBURY, G.: Selective adequate activation of large afferents from muscle spindles and Golgi tendon organs. *Acta Physiol. Scand.*, *49*: 155–164 (1960)

LUX, H. D., SCHUBERT, P. and KREUTZBERG, G. W.: Direct matching of morphological and electrophysiological data in cat spinal motoneurones. *In* ANDERSEN, P. and JANSEN, J. K. S. (eds.): "*Excitatory Synaptic Mechanisms.*" pp. 189–198, Universitetsforlaget, Oslo (1970)

MATTHEWS, P. B.: "*Mammalian Muscle Receptors and Their Central Actions*". Williams & Wilkins, Baltimore (1972)

McCULLOCH, W. S., LETTVIN J. Y., PITTS, W. H. and DELL, P. C.: An electrical hypothesis of central inhibition and facilitation. *In* BARD, P. (ed.): "*Patterns of Organization in the Central Nervous System*". *Res. Publ. ARNMD*, Vol. *30*; pp. 87–97, Williams & Wilkins, Baltimore (1950)

McLAUGHLIN, B. J.: Dorsal root projections to the motor nuclei in the cat spinal cord. *J. Comp. Neurol.*, *144*: 461–474 (1972)

MENDELL, L. M. and HENNEMAN, E.: Terminals of single Ia fibers: location, density, and terminal distribution within a pool of 300 homonymous motoneurons. *J. Neurophysiol.*, *34*: 171–187 (1971)

MENDELL, L. M., MUNSON, J. B. and SCOTT, J. G.: Alterations of synapses on axotomized motoneurones. *J. Physiol. (Lond.)*, *255*: 67–79 (1976)

MENDELL, L. M. and WEINER, R.: Analysis of pairs of individual Ia-EPSPs in single motoneurones. *J. Physiol. (Lond.)*, *255*: 81–104 (1976)

NELSON, P. G. and FRANK, K.: Anomalous rectification in cat spinal motoneurons and effects of polarizing currents on excitatory postsynaptic potentials. *J. Neurophysiol.*, *30*: 1097–1113 (1967)

RALL, W.: Branching dendritic trees and motoneuron membrane resistivity. *Expt. Neurol.*, *1*: 491–527 (1959)

RALL, W.: Distinguishing theoretical synaptic potentials computed for different soma-dendritic distributions of synaptic input. *J. Neurophysiol.*, *30*: 1138–1168 (1967)

RALL, W., BURKE, R. E., SMITH, T. G., NELSON, P. G. and FRANK, K.: Dendritic location of synapses and possible mechanisms for the monosynaptic EPSP in motoneurons. *J. Neurophysiol.*, *30*: 1169–1193 (1967)

RINZEL, J. and RALL, W.: Transient response in a dendritic neuron model for current injected at one branch. *Biophys. J.*, *14*: 759–790 (1974)

Scheibel, M. E. and Scheibel, A. B.: Terminal patterns in cat spinal cord. III. Primary afferent collaterals. *Brain Res., 13*: 417–443 (1969)

Scott, J. G. and Mendell, L. M.: Individual EPSPs produced by triceps surae Ia afferent fibers in homonymous and heteonymous motoneurons. *J. Neurophysiol., 39*: 679–692 (1976)

Smith, T. G., Wuerker, R. B. and Frank, K.: Membrane impedance changes during synaptic transmission in cat spinal motoneurons. *J. Neurophysiol., 30*: 1072–1096 (1967)

Snow, P. J., Rose, P. K. and Brown, A. G.: Tracing axons and axon collaterals of spinal neurons using intracellular injection of horseradish peroxidase. *Science, 191*: 312–313 (1976)

Sprague, J. M.: The distribution of dorsal root fibers on motor cells in the lumbosacral spinal cord of the cat, and the role of excitatory and inhibitory terminals in monosynaptic pathways. *Proc. Roy. Soc., Ser. B., 149*: 534–556 (1958)

Stauffer, E. K., Watt, D. G. D., Taylor, A., Reinking, R. M. and Stuart, D. G.: Analysis of muscle receptor connections by spiketriggered averaging. 2. Spindle group II afferents. *J. Neurophysiol., 39*: 1393–1402 (1976)

Swadlow, H. A. and Waxman, S. G.: Variations in conduction velocity and excitability following single and multiple impulses of visual callosal axons in the rabbit. *Expt. Neurol., 53*: 128–150 (1976)

Traub, R. D.: A model of a human neuromuscular system for small isometric tensions. *Biol. Cybernetics., 26*: 159–167 (1977)

Waxman, S. G.: Integrative properties and design principles of axons. *Int. Rev. of Neurobiol., 18*: 1–39 (1975)

Waxman, S. G. and Bennett, M. V. L.: Relative conduction velocities of small myelinated and non-myelinated fibres in the central nervous system. *Nature New Biol., 238*: 217–219 (1972)

Werman, R. and Carlen, P. L.: Unusual behavior of the Ia EPSP in cat spinal motoneurons. *Brain Res., 112*: 395–401 (1976)

Zucker, R. S.: Theoretical implications of the size principle of motoneurone recruitment. *J. Theoret. Biol., 38*: 587–596 (1973)

DISCUSSION PERIOD

HENNEMAN: I was fascinated by your suggestion of the possibility of a variable amount of invasion of Ia terminals, what PTP might do. We have tried the effects of PTP occasionally on EPSPs. A problem that seems to arise is that if you give a tetanus to produce a PTP and then test with a fast repetitive discharge, such as you get naturally from the stretch receptor, you can't see PTP. You can see it, if you send in a single volley. So I wonder how one should think about natural PTP, as compared with experimental PTP?

BURKE: I don't know the answer to that. However, given the data that Motoy Kuno (KUNO, 1964) has obtained, it looks very much as if PTP affects individual Ia afferents differently. In some, as you say, you can demonstrate an increase in amplitude of the single fiber EPSP. In many others, you can't demonstrate such an increased amplitude, but you do show a different probabalistic structure of the unit EPSP occurrence. And that is compatible with either model of the failure process, either a transmitter release failure or a branch point failure model, I think. I should say, in this regard, that there is no question about the existence of branch point failure in invertebrate axons. It's been demonstrated by PARNAS and coworkers (GROSSMAN, SPIRA and PARNAS, 1973) very clearly in the crayfish motor axon. And this process is a frequency filter. At certain frequencies all of the branch points of an axon will be invaded, at other frequencies only a particular branch will be invaded. It makes functional sense in the crayfish, and it's at least a solid demonstration that branch point failure does in fact occur.

GROSSMAN, Y., SPIRA, M. E. and PARNAS, I. Differential flow of information into branches of a single axon. *Brain Res., 64*: 379–386, 1973.

KUNO, M. Mechanism of facilitation and depression of the excitatory synaptic potential in spinal motoneurons. *J. Physiol. (Lond.), 175*: 100–112, 1964.

INTEGRATION IN A PROPRIOSPINAL MOTOR CENTRE CONTROLLING THE FORELIMB IN THE CAT

Anders LUNDBERG

Department of Physiology, University of Göteborg
Göteborg, Sweden

In order to exemplify integration in the spinal cord I will review recent findings regarding the control of forelimb motoneurones. It will be shown that forelimb motoneurones are excited from different higher centres via short propriospinal neurones taking origin in the C3–C4 segments and that the control of these propriospinal neurones is highly complex. Excitatory and inhibitory convergence occurs not only from different higher centres but also from forelimb afferents.

Propriospinal control of motoneurones was first investigated by LLOYD (1941). He recorded bulbospinal volleys at different segmental levels and was able to demonstrate a monosynaptic relay in neurones originating in the upper lumbar segments. The propriospinally relayed volley was correlated with the discharges in motoneurones and LLOYD postulated the existence of a disynaptic bulbomotoneuronal pathway via short propriospinal neurones. He also showed that transmission of the propriospinal volley could be facilitated by preceding stimulation of the motor cortex or of primary hindlimb afferents stimulated in the dorsal root. Further investigations of the function of short lumbar propriospinal neurones have been made by VASILENKO et al. (1967, 1972) and by KOZHANOV and SHAPOVALOV (1977 a, b).

One of our main tools in investigating interneurones in the spinal cord has been a modification of the LLOYD-RENSHAW technique of conditioning a monosynaptic test reflex. Instead of a monosynaptic test reflex recorded in the ventral roots we use a disynaptic PSP intracellularly recorded from motoneurones as test. The amplitude of test PSPs measures the number of interneurones activated by the test stimulus. An increase or decrease of the test PSP by a conditioning volley can under certain conditions (cf. LUNDBERG, 1975) be taken to indicate excitation respectively inhibition on the interneurones mediating the test PSP. This indirect technique has allowed us to investigate convergence from different sources onto cervical propriospinal neurones projecting directly to motoneurones. These results were then supplemented with recordings in the C3–C4 segments from cell bodies of propriospinal neurones.

PROPRIOSPINAL TRANSMISSION TO FORELIMB MOTONEURONES

The study of propriospinal transmission arose from an investigation of effects from the corticospinal tract on forelimb motoneurones. It appeared that corticospinal volleys evoked by stimulation of the contralateral pyramid produced disynaptic EPSPs and mainly trisynaptic IPSPs in forelimb motoneurones (ILLERT et al., 1976 a). The disynaptic EPSP was then used as test to investigate convergence on the intercalated neurones (ILLERT et al., 1976 b). Marked facilitation was produced not only by conditioning stimulation of group I muscle afferents and cutaneous afferents in the forelimb but also by volleys in the

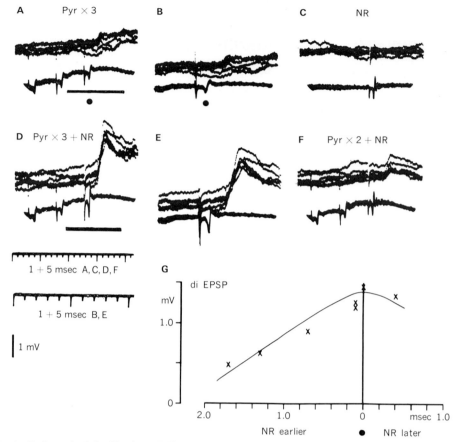

Fig. 1 Rubrospinal facilitation of disynaptic corticospinal EPSPs in a Brachialis motoneurone. Upper traces are intracellular recordings and lower traces were recorded from the C6 dorsal root entry zone. Records B and E are expanded from the corresponding left records A and D. Pyramidal stimulus strength (120 µA) was chosen to give a liminal disynaptic EPSP. A single stimulus in the red nucleus (200 µA) was without effect when given alone in C but produced a large facilitation of the pyramidal EPSP which was maximal when the rubrospinal volley was timed to arrive simultaneously with the third pyramidal volley as in D, E. The facilitation was mainly dependent on the third pyramidal volley since it decreased drastically by its withdrawal in F. The graph in G shows the effect on the pyramidal EPSP at different time intervals between the rubrospinal volley and the third pyramidal volley (ILLERT et al. 1976 b).

rubrospinal tract (Fig. 1). The time course of the rubral facilitation, obtained by changing the conditioning-test interval, strongly suggested monosynaptic excitation on the intercalated neurones both from forelimb afferents and from rubrospinal fibres (Fig. 1 G). Facilitation from forelimb afferents and from the rubrospinal tract might be exerted on different sets of intercalated neurones but interaction experiments with stimulation of all three systems together revealed that excitatory convergence from forelimb afferents, rubrospinal fibres and corticospinal fibres did indeed occur on common intercalated neurones projecting to motoneurones (Fig. 9 in ILLERT et al., 1976 b).

The finding of a convergence both from another motor centre in the brain stem and from forelimb afferents on the neurones intercalated in the fastest pathway from the motor cortex to the motoneurones seemed to merit a closer investigation of this pathway. For this purpose it was required to establish the location of the cell bodies of the intercalated neurones, which might be segmental interneurones, propriospinal neurones or bulbo-

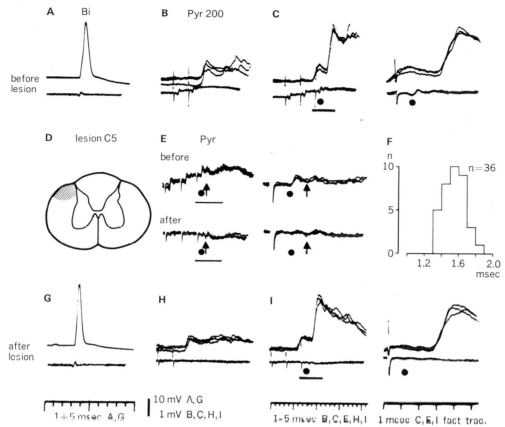

Fig. 2 Disynaptic pyramidal EPSPs recorded in a Biceps motoneurone before and after transection of the corticospinal tract in C5. Upper traces are intracellular and lower traces (all traces in E) are records from the C6 dorsal root entry zone. Stimulation of the contralateral pyramid (200 μA) in B, C, E, H and I. The left and right traces in C, E and I were taken simultaneously at different speeds. The microelectrode was withdrawn from the motoneurone before making the lesion (D) and reinserted afterwards. The transection of the corticospinal tract was monitored by recording the corticospinal volley; the discharge marked by arrow is presumably conducted in the propriospinal axons. The histogram in F gives the distribution of segmental latencies for the pyramidal EPSPs (ILLERT et al., 1977).

spinal neurones. The effect of lesions of the corticospinal tract in different cervical segments revealed that the disynaptic pyramidal EPSPs remained after a C5 lesion rostral to the forelimb segments (Fig. 2) but were entirely abolished by a corresponding C2 lesion (ILLERT et al., 1977). Accordingly it could be concluded that propriospinal neurones with cell bodies in C3 and C4, which were monosynaptically excited from the corticospinal tract, projected directly to forelimb motoneurones. C3–C4 propriospinal neurones also serve as first order intercalated neurones in a trisynaptic inhibitory pathway from corticospinal fibres to motoneurones; the last order neurones in this pathway are identical with the segmental Ia inhibitory interneurones mediating reciprocal inhibition (ILLERT and TANAKA, 1978).

Lesion experiments using the disynaptic pyramidal EPSP as test revealed that the axons of the C3–C4 propriospinal neurones which project to forelimb motoneurones are located in the lateroventral part of the lateral funiculus.

It is a great advantage that the simple procedure of transecting the corticospinal tract in C5 allows investigation of the propriospinal system in isolation from segmental neuronal pathways. It was first shown that the facilitatory interaction found in the intact cat (Fig. 1) occurred in the propriospinal neurones (ILLERT et al., 1977). Rubral facilitation of the disynaptic pyramidal EPSPs was as pronounced as before the C5 lesion with a time course showing monosynaptic rubrospinal connexions on the propriospinal neurones; the C3–C4 propriospinal neurones are in fact able to mediate large disynaptic EPSPs to moto-neurones from the rubrospinal tract. Volleys in group I muscle afferents and cutaneous afferents in the forelimb likewise facilitated the propriospinally mediated pyramidal EPSPs with a timing that was compatible with a monosynaptic linkage. The abolition of this facilitation after transection of dorsal columns in C5 showed that the primary forelimb afferents ascend to the C3–C4 propriospinal neurones in the dorsal column.

The further analysis then revealed that monosynaptic facilitation of propriospinal trans-mission to forelimb motoneurones also could be evoked by stimulation of a subtectal region in the mesencephalic tegmentum (ILLERT et al., 1977), strongly suggesting tectospinal facil-itation. This action was somewhat difficult to analyse since there was evidence of another disynaptic tectomotoneuronal pathway with a bulbar relay. However, excitation of pro-priospinal neurones from the dorsal tegmentum was proven by the finding that the facilita-tory action from the dorsal tegmentum on disynaptic pyramidal EPSPs completely dis-appeared after transection of the corticospinal tract in C2. Another complication was that the tegmental facilitation was not found in all experiments. Our interpretation was that in these cases the pyramidal EPSP used to test facilitation was transmitted by a subset of propriospinal neurones which did not receive the tectal excitatory convergence. A similar explanation was forwarded to account for the lack of facilitatory effect from primary fore-limb afferents in a few of the experiments. We then tried stimulation in the medullary reticular formation and in Deiters' nucleus. Stimulation in the medial brain stem evoked marked facilitation of pyramidal disynaptic EPSPs, again with a time course suggesting monosynaptic linkage with the propriospinal neurones (Fig. 3). The effect in Fig. 3 might be due either to stimulation of reticulospinal neurones or of vestibulospinal axons. Since in other experiments we had not found any facilitation from Deiters' nucleus we assumed that the effect was reticulospinal (BERGMANS et al., 1976; ILLERT et al., 1977). However, subsequently we have found that facilitation of disynaptic pyramidal EPSPs may be evoked also from Deiters' nucleus (ALSTERMARK, JANKOWSKA and LUNDBERG, unpublished finding). Since reticulospinal neurones have collaterals in Deiters' nucleus (ITO et al., 1970) it cannot be excluded that the facilitatory effect from Deiters' nucleus is mediated by reticulospinal neurones. Alternatively it is equally possible that the facilitation is produced by vestibulo-spinal neurones and that the facilitatory effect from the medial brain stem is due to stimu-lation of vestibulospinal fibres or their collaterals. We did obtain facilitation from regions of the reticular formation medial to that of the tracks in Figure 3 but still lateral to the medial longitudinal fasciculus where the tectospinal fibres are located. Control experi-ments showed that vestibulospinal neurones could be antidromically activated in Deiters' nucleus at weak strengths also from this more medial region. Electrical stimulation of the labyrinth (cf. ITO et al., 1969; SHIMAZU and PRECHT, 1965) did not produce facilitation of disynaptic pyramidal EPSPs, but these results cannot be taken to exclude that vestibulo-spinal fibres are responsible for the facilitation. Accordingly we are left with the conclu-sion that bulbospinal neurones excite the propriospinal neurones but cannot decide whether vestibulospinal and/or reticulospinal are responsible (cf. also next section).

It deserves to be mentioned that a similar monosynaptic facilitation of the disynaptic pyramidal EPSP can be produced from the contralateral (to the recording side) fastigial nucleus (ALSTERMARK, LINDSTRÖM and LUNDBERG, unpublished findings). It is possible

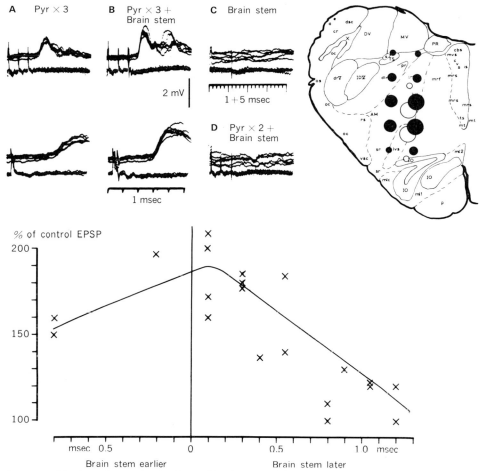

Fig. 3 Facilitation of propriospinally mediated pyramidal EPSP in a Biceps motoneurone evoked by stimulation of the medullary brain stem. Recordings were made after transection of the corticospinal tract in C5. Upper and lower traces in A and B were recorded simultaneously at different sweep speed. A single stimulus in the medullary brain stem (100 μA) was without effect alone (C) but gave a marked facilitation of the pyramidal EPSP (100 μA) in D. In the graph abscissa gives the time interval between the brain stem stimulus and effective pyramidal stimulus; ordinate gives the magnitude of the EPSP attained 0.5 msec after its onset. Diameter of circles in the histological section indicates the degree of facilitation of pyramidal EPSPs in three Biceps motoneurones (unpublished results by ILLERT, JANKOWSKA, LUNDBERG and ODUTOLA).

that this excitatory action is mediated by fastigiospinal fibres which are known to descend to the C3–C4 segments (WILSON et al., 1978) but again it cannot be excluded that the effect is due to stimulation of collaterals from neurones with cell bodies located elsewhere, which may project both to the C3–C4 propriospinal neurones and to the contralateral fastigial nucleus.

MONOSYNAPTIC EPSPs RECORDED IN C3–C4 PROPRIOSPINAL NEURONES

The indirect technique of recording from motoneurones has the advantage of proving action on neurones projecting directly to motoneurones and therefore gives a firm basis to our investigation. Many aspects of the functional organization were difficult to elucidate with this techinque and it was desirable to record directly from cell bodies of proprio-spinal neurones which might mediate the effects.   Such neurones were found in the latero-ventral part of layer VII in C3 and C4.   They were identified as propriospinal by their antidromic invasion on stimulation of the spinal cord at different segmental levels.   Many of these propriospinal neurones have axons terminating in the forelimb segments but some project beyond even to the hindlimb segments (ILLERT et al., 1978).   The long proprio-spinal neurones appear to have a similar convergence from higher centres and forelimb afferents as the short ones but their target neurones have not been identified.

Threshold mapping in the spinal cord in C5 showed that axons from propriospinal neurones were located in the ventrolateral part of the lateral funicle, i.e. in the region where a lesion interrupted the axons of the propriospinal neurones projecting to moto-neurones as was previously found with recording from motoneurones.   There is previous anatomical evidence that propriospinal neurones originating in C3–C4 project to forelimb segments (POGORELAYA and TARUSINA, 1974).   Experiments using retrograde transport of horseradish peroxidase suggest that many C3–C4 neurones with cell bodies located in layer VII project directly to motoneurones (GRANT, ILLERT and TANAKA, to be published).

With intracellular recording from cell bodies of C3–C4 propriospinal neurones it was then shown that monosynaptic EPSPs could be evoked from all the neuronal systems which influence propriospinal transmission to motoneurones (ILLERT et al., 1978).   Convergence from many sources was common and Figure 4 shows a cell with convergence from all higher motor centres tested.   With such extensive convergence the problem arises whether an effect from a particular motor centre may be due to stimulation of collaterals from other motor pathways.   This problem was discussed above in relation to the difficulty in decid-ing whether the bulbospinal effect is due to stimulation of vestibulospinal and/or reticulo-spinal neurones.   However, the independence of corticospinal, rubrospinal, tectospinal and bulbospinal effects was indicated by the linear summation of the EPSPs from all these descending tracts tested in all combinations (ILLERT, JANKOWSKA, LUNDBERG and ODUTOLA, unpublished findings).   We also found the expected monosynaptic EPSP from forelimb nerves but only in a minority of the propriospinal neurones (cf. Table 1 in ILLERT et al., 1978).   Figure 5 shows the effect of graded stimulation of the deep radial nerve in a neurone which was also monosynaptically excited from the corticospinal and rubrospinal tracts.   Note that the EPSP is evoked from very low threshold group I muscle afferents. Other propriospinal neurones were monosynaptically excited from cutaneous afferents but convergence from group I muscle afferents and cutaneous afferents was exceptional.   In most of the experiments we only investigated effects from the deep radial and superficial radial nerves but the results obtained on stimulation of the dorsal column in C4 show that about half the propriospinal neurones do not receive monosynaptic excitation from cer-vical primary afferents.   In addition to the effect from forelimb nerves we found in a few cells monosynaptic EPSPs from C2 and C3 afferents when stimulating close to the dorsal root ganglia, possibly evoked by activation of joint afferents.

The monosynaptic excitatory connexions to the C3–C4 propriospinal system are sum-marized in Fig. 6 A.   Except for the C2–C3 afferents all of them have been established with the indirect spatial facilitation technique and then confirmed and analysed with intracellular recording from the cell bodies of propriospinal neurones.   The existence of subsets of neurones with different convergence, suggested by the results obtained with the indirect technique, was confirmed with direct recording from the propriospinal neurones. Some of the connexions shown in Figure 6A may be lacking in individual neurones but extensive convergence is indeed common (cf. Table 1 in ILLERT et al., 1978).   Figure 6B shows the trisynaptic inhibitory corticomotoneuronal pathway via propriospinal neurones

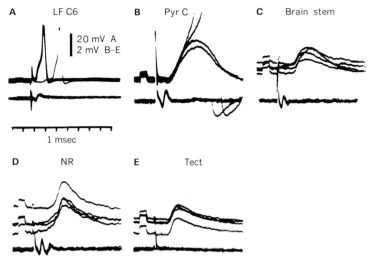

Fig. 4 Convergence of monosynaptic EPSPs from higher centres in a propriospinal neurone. Intracellular recording was made in C3 from a cell 2.7 mm from the cord dorsum which was identified as propriospinal by the antidromic invasion (A) produced by electrical stimulation of the lateral funicle in C6. 100 μA contralateral stimuli were given to pyramid (Pyr), red nucleus (NR) and superior colliculus (Tect). The ipsilateral brain stem was stimulated (100 μA) at a level 5 mm rostral to obex, 2 mm lateral to the midline at a depth of 3 mm below the floor of the fourth ventricle (unpublished results by ILLERT, JANKOWSKA, LUNDBERG and ODUTOLA).

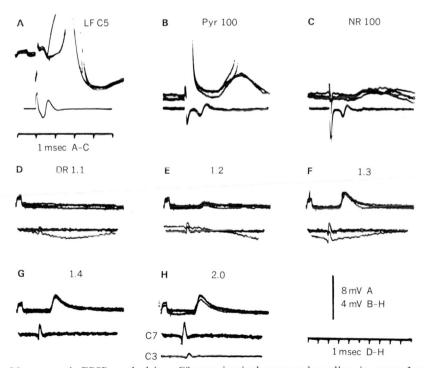

Fig. 5 Monosynaptic EPSPs evoked in a C3 propriospinal neurone by volleys in group I muscle afferents from the forelimb. Identification in A. Pyramidal and rubral monosynaptic EPSPs are shown in B and C. D–H show the effect of graded stimulation of the deep radial (DR) nerve. Stimulus strengths in D–H are given in multiples of threshold strength (ILLERT et al., 1978).

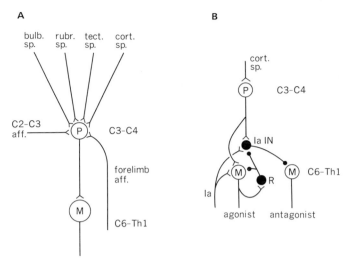

Fig. 6 *A*: Schematic representation of monosynaptic excitatory connexions to the C3–C4 pro-priospinal system (ILLERT et al., 1978). *B*: The trisynaptic inhibitory corticomotoneuronal pathway via propriospinal neurones and Ia inhibitory interneurone (ILLERT and TANAKA, 1978).

and Ia inhibitory neurones (ILLERT and TANAKA, 1978).   In view of the general paralle-lism of connexions to motoneurones and Ia inhibitory neurones (cf. HULTBORN, 1976) it is likely that the propriospinal neurones projecting to Ia inhibitory neurones have the same wide convergence as those projecting to motoneurones.   There is no evidence suggesting that some of the C3–C4 propriospinal neurones are inhibitory.

INHIBITORY PATHWAYS TO C3–C4 PROPRIOSPINAL NEURONES

The indirect technique of recording from motoneurones occasionally indicated that disy-naptic corticomotoneuronal transmission could be inhibited by volleys in forelimb nerves (ILLERT et al., 1977), but it was difficult to obtain decisive evidence since these condition-ing volleys often evoked IPSPs in the motoneurones recorded from.   With intracellular recording from the propriospinal neurones it appeared that inhibitory effects were very prominent (ILLERT et al., 1975).   In fact every system that gives monosynaptic excitation may also evoke inhibition.   Figure 7 shows the effect of three pyramidal volleys at increas-ing stimulus strength.   Superimposed on the EPSP an inhibition appears at 60 μA and increases at 100 μA (onset shown by arrow in lower trace G).   The segmental latency of 1.3 msec clearly indicates a disynaptic linkage.   A similar disynaptic inhibition was evoked by a train of volleys in the rubrospinal and tectospinal tracts.   Stimulation of forelimb afferents, both group I muscle afferents and cutaneous afferents, usually also evoked disy-naptic IPSPs with an equally brief segmental latency and in this case a single volley often sufficed.

The spatial facilitation technique was applied to investigate the connexions to the in-hibitory interneurones.   Figure 8 shows spatial facilitation of inhibitory transmission from the corticospinal and rubrospinal tracts (A–C) and between the corticospinal tract and a volley in a forelimb nerve (D–F).   Since there is no evidence for inhibitory C3–C4 proprio-spinal neurones it is unlikely that the disynaptic IPSPs are recurrent but more probable that they are mediated by special inhibitory interneurones which receive the same mono-synaptic excitatory convergence as the propriospinal neurones.   It will be shown in the

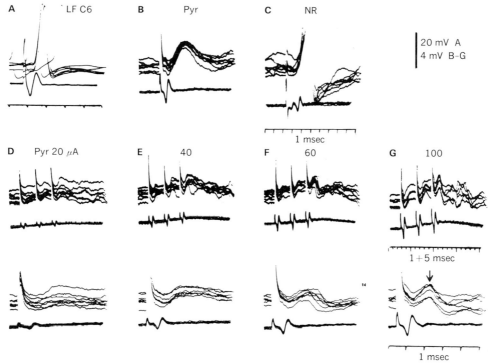

Fig. 7 Disynaptic pyramidal IPSP in a propriospinal neurone. A shows the antidromic identification and B, C the monosynaptic pyramidal and rubral EPSPs recorded immediately after impalement. D–G, obtained somewhat later when the EPSPs were smaller, show the effect of graded stimulation of the pyramid. Upper and lower traces in D, G were obtained simultaneously at different sweep speeds. The onset of the IPSP is marked with arrow in the lower trace of G (unpublished results by ALSTERMARK, ILLERT and LUNDBERG).

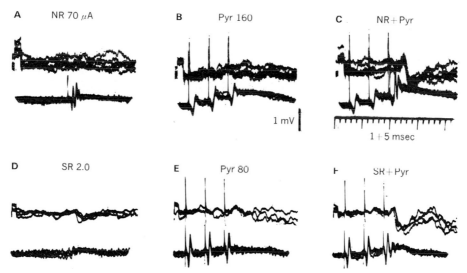

Fig. 8 Facilitatory interaction in inhibitory transmission to propriospinal neurones. Spatial facilitation between corticospinal and rubrospinal volleys is shown in A–C and between a volley in the superficial radial nerve (SR) and a corticospinal volley in D–F. Stimulus strengths in D are in multiples of threshold, all other strengths are in μA (unpublished results by ALSTERMARK, ILLERT and LUNDBERG).

end of this section that a disynaptic inhibiton from forelimb nerves can be evoked in C3–C4 propriospinal neurones via inhibitory neurones located in forelimb segments. However, the descending disynaptic IPSPs have so brief latency that they must be relayed rostral to the forelimb segments. Furthermore, the brief latency of the disynaptic IPSPs from fore-limb afferents shows that they cannot be relayed rostral to the C3–C4 segments and since they show facilitatory interaction with the descending IPSPs (Fig. 8) it is inferred that di-synaptic IPSPs are relayed also by local inhibitory interneurones in the C3–C4 segments; they are monosynaptically activated by forelimb afferents ascending in the dorsal column as evidenced by the finding that disynaptic IPSPs from forelimb nerves are evoked after complete transection of the lateral and ventral funicles (Alstermark, Lindström and Lundberg, unpublished findings) where ascending inhibitory neurones from the forelimb segments have their axons (cf. Fig. 10). Laterally in layer VII in C3 and C4 we found many cells which could not be antidromically activated from the lateral funicle in C6; these cells might be local inhibitory interneurones. It is likely that the activation of this inhibitory pathway may give feed-forward inhibition so that higher centres, when activating a population of propriospinal neurones required for a certain movement, inhibit proprio-spinal neurones to other muscles, thus providing spatial selectivity. The disynaptic in-hibition from primary afferents appears to be stronger than the descending one since usu-ally a single volley suffices, particularly when skin nerves are stimulated. It is not certain that this inhibition is evoked only by the interneurones which receive the same convergence as the propriospinal neurones. We have confirmed that volleys in group I muscle afferents and in cutaneous afferents evoke large monosynaptic focal potentials in a very medial region at the base of the ventral horn in C3–C4 (Rosén, 1969). It remains to find out a region where forelimb group I muscle afferents and cutaneous afferents evoke large mono-if the neurones in this region project to the propriospinal neurones and how they are governed from higher centres. The inhibitory effect from the forelimb nerves may not have as their sole function to assist higher centres in producing feed-forward inhibition. There is clearly also the interesting possibility of *a feed-back mechanism allowing signals from the forelimb to regulate propriospinal transmission during movements.*

Early on it became clear that the propriospinal neurones also have other inhibitory con-nexions. Stimulation of the lateral funicle in more caudal segments in order to identify the neurones antidromically produced large monosynaptic IPSPs, whether from descending or ascending fibres could not be decided. Stimulation in the medullary brain stem pro-duced IPSPs in some propriospinal neurones (Bergmans et al., 1976 and unpublished find-ings). The latency was occasionally brief enough to prove a monosynaptic inhibitory link-age (Fig. 9). In many other cells the latency was longer and might allow for one or more intercalated neurones (cf. graph Fig. 9). However, monosynaptic linkage from slow con-ducting inhibitory fibres is a more likely explanation because late unitary IPSPs were found to be evoked after a very fixed latency at threshold stimulation. Stimulation below thresh-old for the inhibitory neurones revealed pronounced temporal facilitation possibly because the weak stimuli activated presynaptic fibres and thereby lowered the threshold for direct activation by a succeeding stimulus. It is tentatively suggested that monosynaptic IPSPs evoked by stimulation of the medial reticular formation are due to stimulation of reticulo-spinal neurones and not to antidromic activation of ascending spinoreticular inhibitory neu-rones which may have collateral connexions with the propriospinal neurones (cf. below).

Many propriospinal neurones did not receive inhibition from the medullary brain stem (3–5 mm rostral to obex) but large IPSPs were nevertheless evoked by stimulation of the lateral funicle in C6. This observation suggested the existence of other inhibitory con-nexions and led us to explore effects from more caudal brain stem levels. Figure 10

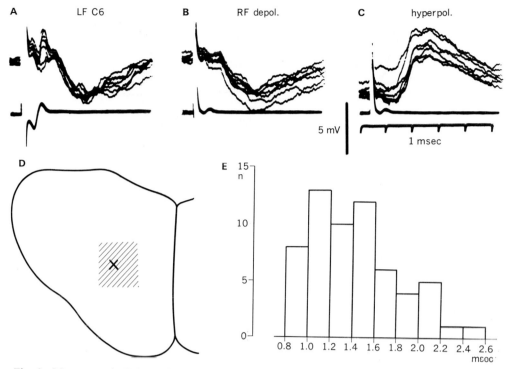

Fig. 9 Monosynaptic IPSP evoked from the reticular formation (RF) in a propriospinal neurone. Identification in A. Recording was made with a NaCl electrode but passage of depolarizing current prevented the reversal of the IPSP. C shows the reversal of the IPSP during passage of hyperpolarizing current (10^{-9}A). The IPSP was evoked by stimulation of the site marked by a cross in D and the stimulus strength was 100 μA (threshold 30 μA). The hatched area shows the region from which IPSPs usually were evoked at low strength but in some cells the region was wider including parts of the contralateral RF. The histogram in E gives the distribution of latencies for the onset of the IPSPs from the earliest descending volley evoked by the stimulus (unpublished results by ILLERT, JANKOWSKA and LUNDBERG).

illustrates the finding that very large monosynaptic IPSPs can be evoked by stimulation in the lateral reticular nucleus (LRN). There is no evidence that descending fibres originate in the LRN. For example, KUYPERS and MAISKY (1975) did not find retrograde transport of horseradish peroxidase from the spinal cord to cells in LRN and ANDERSSON and EKEROT (personal communication), who recorded from several hundred cells in LRN, did not find antidromic activation from the spinal cord in a single cell. It is therefore more likely that the monosynaptic IPSPs are produced by antidromic activation of terminals from ascending inhibitory fibres which also have inhibitory projection to the propriospinal neurones. The existence of ascending inhibitory fibres to LRN has been shown by EKEROT and OSCARSSON (1975) who in fact demonstrated the existence of two ascending systems with this action.

Our further analysis revealed that stimulation of nerves in the ipsilateral forelimb did evoke disynaptic IPSPs in propriospinal neurones after a complete transection of the dorsal column (Fig. 10). It is likely that these IPSPs are mediated by ascending inhibitory neurones which also have collateral projection to the LRN. The activation of this pathway from group I muscle afferents suggests that it is identical with the ipsilateral forelimb tract (iF tract) described by EKEROT and OSCARSSON (1975). Inhibition of the propriospinal neurones may well be the major function of these neurones and the collateral connexion

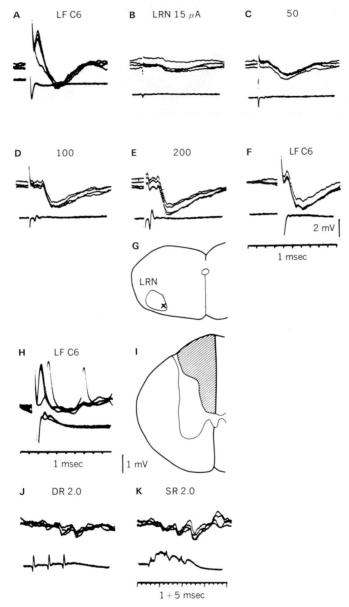

Fig. 10 A–G illustrate monosynaptic IPSPs evoked in a C3 propriospinal neurone by stimulation of the ipsilateral lateral reticular nucleus (LRN). Identification in A. B–E: Increasing strength of LRN stimulation at site shown in G. The IPSP in F was evoked by supramaximal stimulation of the lateral funicle in C6, possibly by stimulation of the fibres activated in LRN. H–K recorded in another experiment show that volleys in forelimb nerves evoke disynaptic IPSPs also after transection of the dorsal column which interrupts transmission from forelimb nerves to the C3-C4 inhibitory interneurones which also are assumed to mediate disynaptic IPSPs to propriospinal neurones (see text). It is proposed that the IPSPs from LRN are evoked by antidromic stimulation of ascending inhibitory neurones which can be monosynaptically activated from forelimb nerves and also project to C3–C4 propriospinal neurones (unpublished results by ALSTERMARK, ILLERT and LUNDBERG).

to LRN allows information of this inhibitory action to reach cerebellum. Further information regarding the organization of the iF tract is clearly required to assess its function. It remains to find out the relative role played by descending systems and the primary forelimb afferents in the activation of the tract.

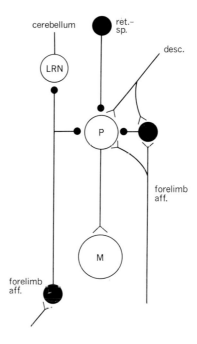

Fig. 11 Schematic representation of the proposed inhibitory pathways to C3 C4 propriospinal neurones.

Figure 11 summarizes schematically the inhibitory pathways discussed in this section. This diagram should be viewed as a working hypothesis. For example, as has appeared from the discussion above, considerable difficulties exist with respect to the evaluation of whether monosynaptic IPSPs evoked by electrical stimulation of the brain are mediated by descending or ascending neurones. Since at least three different sets of inhibitory neurones seem to project to the propriospinal neurones it is clearly difficult to analyse the pathway mediating a particular disynaptic IPSP whether evoked from higher centres or peripheral nerves. It is nevertheless important to pursue this analysis since the inhibitory control of transmission in the C3–C4 propriospinal transmission is likely to be of decisive importance for the assessment of the functional role of this system.

COLLATERAL CONNEXIONS FROM THE C3–C4 PROPRIOSPINAL NEURONES TO THE LATERAL RETICULAR NUCLEUS

It has been suggested that several ascending tracts are informing higher centres of intrinsic spinal activity (LINDSTRÖM, 1973; LUNDBERG, 1959, 1964; OSCARSSON, 1973). It is assumed that interneurones to motoneurones also project to ascending neurones which thus may carry information of the activity reaching the motoneurones. The organization of connexions to the C3–C4 propriospinal neurones described above suggests a complex integration of information from many higher centres and forelimb afferents, which presumably requires a feed-back control in order to function optimally.

ILLERT and LUNDBERG (1978) and ALSTERMARK, LINDSTRÖM, LUNDBERG and SYBIRSKA (unpublished findings) recently showed that some C3–C4 propriospinal neurones could be

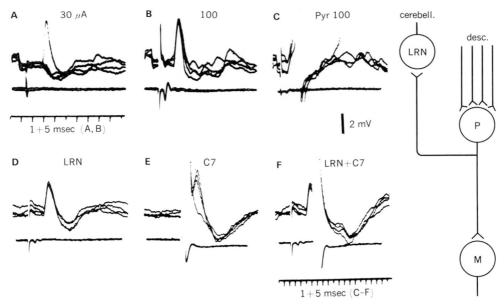

Fig. 12 Antidromic activation of a C3 propriospinal neurone from the lateral reticular nucleus (LRN). The cell was identified as a propriospinal neurone by the antidromic invasion evoked by stimulation of the lateral funicle in C7 (E). A shows antidromic stimulation of LRN at threshold for the axon. D–E show collision of antidromic spikes evoked from LRN and C7 (ILLERT and LUNDBERG, 1978).

antidromically activated also from the lateral reticular nucleus (Fig. 12) which projects to the cerebellum.   Evidently, these propriospinal neurones also function as spinoreticular neurones and continuously inform cerebellum of the activity which reaches the forelimb motoneurones.   The detailed analysis of this ascending collateral projection to LRN revealed a difference between propriospinal neurones which terminated rostral to the midthoracic segments and those projecting beyond to more caudal spinal segments, in that collaterals to LRN were found in the great majority of the former but not in any of the latter neurones (ALSTERMARK et al., unpublished findings).   These results suggest that the ascending projection occurs from virtually all the propriospinal neurones projecting to fore-limb segments but not from those projecting to hindlimb segments.   If the propriospinal neurones recorded from in C3–C4 project directly to motoneurones, as shown in the diagram in Figure 12, stimulation in LRN should give rise to monosynaptic EPSPs in fore-limb motoneurones.   Large EPSPs were indeed evoked from the LRN (which has no descending projection, cf. KUYPERS and MAISKY, 1975) in different species of forelimb motoneurones (cf. Fig. 2 in ILLERT and LUNDBERG, 1978).   There can be little doubt that these EPSPs are monosynaptically evoked and that the long latency and rise time is due to rather slow conduction velocity in the propriospinal axons and their branches (ILLERT and LUNDBERG, 1978, ALSTERMARK et al., unpublished observations).   EKEROT (1978) has shown that neurones with cell bodies in the upper lumbar segments project both to LRN and to more caudal lumbar segments.   HIRAI et al. (1978) found that some direct spino-cerebellar neurones originating in cervical segments have collaterals descending to lower lumbar segments.   Their findings make it likely that information via ascending collat-erals is conveyed also from other spinal centres than the C3–C4 propriospinal system.

Ascending collaterals from neurones projecting directly to motoneurones clearly is a very direct way of informing higher centres of the activity reaching the motoneurones.

Since several of the descending pathways exciting the C3–C4 propriospinal neurones (Fig. 6) are strongly controlled from cerebellum there is the possibility for a continuous feedback control of the activity in the propriospinal neurones. If, as a result of the highly complex integration, inappropriate activity is produced in propriospinal neurones, either with respect to the species of neurones or to the quantity of activation, then cerebellum might take corrective measures with a minimal delay by its control of rubrospinal and bulbospinal neurones projecting to the C3–C4 propriospinal neurones.

ROLE OF C3–C4 PROPRIOSPINAL NEURONES IN MOTOR BEHAVIOUR

It is important to keep in mind that the C3–C4 propriospinal system is one of several motor systems for the control of motoneurones. The forelimbs are also controlled by descending fibres which project monosynaptically to the motoneurones (cf. WILSON and YOSHIDA, 1969) and in all likelihood also by descending activity relayed by segmental interneurones. The relative role of each of these subsystems may be elucidated in behavioural experiments and investigations of the effect of different spinal cord lesions do indeed suggest that the C3–C4 propriospinal system plays an important role in motor behaviour.

ALSTERMARK et al. (1979) investigated the ability of cats to take food with the forepaw from the bottom of a cylinder (height 40 mm, diameter 30 mm) placed either vertically on the floor or horizontally 150 mm above the floor). These tests were used in a previous investigation by GORSKA and SYBIRSKA (unpublished findings) who showed severe impairment of contralateral forelimb movements after transection of the pyramid and lesions of the red nucleus. We transected the dorsal part of the lateral funicle in C2 or C5; the C2 lesion was made in order to interrupt the rubrospinal and corticospinal connexions both to the C3–C4 propriospinal system and to the forelimb segments. The C5 lesion, on the other hand, would interrupt these connexions to the forelimb segments but not to the C3–C4 propriospinal neurones and not interfer with their more ventrally located axonal projection to motoneurones. The dorsal C2 lesion gave severe motor defects similar to those found after a combined lesion of the pyramid and red nucleus (GORSKA and SYBIRSKA, unpublished findings). Cats with a dorsal C5 lesion, in contrast, were able to place the forepaw into the cylinder rapidly and accurately already 10 days after the lesion while the movements of the forepaw and digits, required to take the piece of food to the mouth, were lacking during the entire postsurgical period (3 months).

Other cats were investigated after a ventral C5 transection of the lateral funicle where the propriospinal axons are located. They could lift the forelimb in the direction of the cylinder but the movement was very atactic. Since a corresponding ventral lesion in C2 had no effect on the test movements it is unlikely that the motor defects observed after the ventral C5 lesion is caused by interruption of other descending fibres with the same transverse location as the propriospinal axons. Once having reached the food the cats with a ventral C5 lesion were able to grasp the food and take it to the mouth in the same way as normal cats.

These results suggest that the C3–C4 propriospinal system is used in precise, rapid movements of the forelimb which are so essential in feline behaviour, e.g. in catching prey (LEYHAUSEN, 1973); fine movements of the digits, on the other hand, appear to depend mainly on the control of interneuronal systems located within the forelimb segments.

COMMENTS

In all likelihood the C3–C4 propriospinal system is only one of several systems by which higher centres can control forelimb motoneurones. From an analytical point of view it has the great advantage that it can be experimentally isolated from other systems and therefore is amenable to detailed investigations including its role in motor behaviour. There can be no doubt that the main function of this system is to transmit excitation from higher centres to forelimb motoneurones and that the convergent effect from forelimb afferents, excitatory and inhibitory, has a regulatory role.

If the finding of an extensive convergence from higher centres on the propriospinal neurones appears surprising it is only because we have had preconceived ideas of how motor pathways function. The tradition has been to consider one pathway at a time and activity in a given pathway is often tacitly assumed to represent a command signal for a movement. The convergence on common propriospinal neurones suggests that several higher motor centres may participate in activation of motoneurones via these premotoneurones. In this connexion it is of interest that there is now increasing evidence for simultaneous activity in many higher motor centres during movements as was first shown in high decerebrate cats during stereotype locomotion on a treadmill (ORLOVSKY, 1970, 1972 a, b).

The results of the behavioural experiments suggest that the C3–C4 propriospinal system is indeed used in precise rapid forelimb movements. It might be possible to elucidate the contribution of individual higher centres, e.g. the superior colliculus by investigation of propriospinally mediated movements after selective higher lesions. It also seems within experimental reach to test our working hypothesis that forelimb activity provides feed-back regulation of transmission in the C3–C4 propriospinal system during movements.

It is of considerable interest that cerebellum receives information about the activity in the propriospinal neurones via their ascending collaterals to the lateral reticular nucleus. The findings suggesting that also one of the inhibitory pathways to the C3–C4 propriospinal neurones has a collateral projection to LRN provide additional evidence that cerebellum takes a great interest in the function of the propriospinal system and probably plays an essential role in the regulation of this system.

ACKNOWLEDGEMENTS

I am indebted to Drs. ALSTERMARK, ILLERT, JANKOWSKA, LINDSTRÖM, ODUTOLA and SYBIRSKA for permission to discuss unpublished results.

REFERENCES

ALSTERMARK, B., LUNDBERG, A., NORRSELL, U. and SYBIRSKA, E.: Role of C3–C4 propriospinal neurones in forelimb movements in the cat. *Acta physiol. scand.*, (1979 in press)

BERGMANS, J., ILLERT, M., JANKOWSKA, E. and LUNDBERG, A.: Reticulospinal control of propriospinal neurones mediating disynaptic corticomotoneuronal excitation in the cat. *Acta physiol. scand.*, *96*: 5A (1976)

EKEROT, C. -F.: Information mediated by the lateral reticular nucleus. Abstract, ENA Meeting, Florence (1978)

EKEROT, C. -F. and OSCARSSON, O.: Inhibitory spinal paths to the lateral reticular nucleus. *Brain Res.*, *99*: 157–161 (1975)

HIRAI, N., HONGO, T. and YAMAGUCHI, T.: Spinocerebellar tract neurones with long descending axon collaterals. *Brain Res.*, *142*: 147–151 (1978)

HULTBORN, H.: Transmission in the pathway of reciprocal Ia inhibition to motoneurones and its control during the tonic stretch reflex In HOMMA, S. (ed.): *Understanding the Stretch Reflex. Progress in Brain Research. 44*: 235–255 (1976)

ILLERT, M., and LUNDBERG, A.: Collateral connections to the lateral reticular nucleus from cervical propriospinal neurones projecting to forelimb motoneurones in the cat. *Neuroscience Letters., 7*: 167–172 (1978)

ILLERT, M., LUNDBERG, A., PADEL, Y. and TANAKA, R.: Convergence on propriospinal neurones which may mediate disynaptic corticospinal excitation to forelimb motoneurones in the cat. *Brain Res., 93*: 530–534 (1975)

ILLERT, M., LUNDBERG, A., PADEL, Y. and TANAKA, R.: Integration in descending motor pathways controlling the forelimb in the cat. 5. Properties of and monosynaptic excitatory convergence on C3–C4 propriospinal neurones. *Exp. Brain Res., 33*: 101–130 (1978)

ILLERT, M., LUNDBERG, A. and TANAKA, R.: Integration in descending motor pathways controlling the forelimb in the cat. 1. Pyramidal effects on motoneurones. *Exp. Brain Res., 26*: 509–519 (1976a)

ILLERT, M., LUNDBERG, A. and TANAKA, R.: Integration in descending motor pathways controlling the forelimb in the cat. 2. Convergence on neurones mediating disynaptic cortico-motoneuronal excitation. *Exp. Brain Res., 26*: 521–540 (1976b)

ILLERT, M., LUNDBERG, A. and TANAKA, R.: Integration in descending motor pathways controlling the forelimb in the cat. 3. Convergence on propriospinal neurones transmitting disynaptic excitation from the corticospinal tract and other descending tracts. *Exp. Brain Res., 29*: 323–346 (1977)

ILLERT, M. and TANAKA, R.: Integration in descending motor pathways controlling the forelimb in the cat. 4. Corticospinal inhibition of forelimb motoneurones mediated by short propriospinal neurones. *Exp. Brain Res., 31*: 131–141 (1978)

ITO, M., HONGO, T. and OKADA, Y.: Vestibular-evoked postsynaptic potentials in Deiters' neurones. *Exp. Brain Res., 7*: 214–230 (1969)

ITO, M., UDO, M. and MANO, N.: Long inhibitory and excitatory pathways converging onto cat reticular and Deiters' neurons and their relevance to reticulofugal axons. *J. Neurophysiol., 33*: 210–226 (1970)

KOZHANOV, V. M. and SHAPOVALOV, A. I.: Synaptic organization of the supraspinal control of propriospinal ventral horn interneurons in cat and monkey spinal cord. *Neurophysiology (Kiev), 9*: 177–184 (1977a)

KOZHANOV, V. M. and SHAPOVALOV, A. I.: Synaptic actions evoked in motoneurons by stimulation of individual propriospinal neurons. *Neurophysiology* (Kiev), *9*: 300–306 (1977b)

KUYPERS, H. G. J. M. and MAISKY, V. A.: Retrograde axonal transport of horseradish peroxidase from spinal cord to brain stem cell groups in the cat. *Neuroscience Letters, 1*: 9–14 (1975)

LEYHAUSEN, P.: *Verhaltensstudien an Katzen.* pp. 232, Verlag Paul Parey, Berlin and Hamburg (1973)

LINDSTRÖM, S.: Recurrent control from motor axon collaterals of Ia inhibitory pathways in the spinal cord of the cat. *Acta physiol. scand.*, Suppl. 392 (1973)

LLOYD, D. P.: Activity in neurons of the bulbospinal correlation system. *J Neurophysiol., 4*: 115–134 (1941)

LUNDBERG, A.: Integrative significance of patterns of connections made by muscle afferents in the spinal cord. *Symp. XXI Int. Physiol. Congr.*, Buenos Aires, 1–5 (1959)

LUNDBERG, A.: Ascending spinal hindlimb pathways in the cat. *In* ECCLES, J. C. and SCHADÉ, J. P. (eds.): *Progress in Brain Research, Physiology of Spinal Neurons.*, Elsevier, Amsterdam, *12*: 135–163 (1964)

LUNDBERG, A.: The control of spinal mechanisms from the brain. *In* TOWER, D. B. (ed.): *The Nervous System*, Vol. 1. pp. 253–265, Raven Press, New York (1975)

ORLOVSKY, G. N.: Activity of reticulospinal neurones during locomotion. *Biofizika, 15*: 728–764 (1970) (English transl. *Biophysics* p. 761–771).

ORLOVSKY, G. N.: Activity of vestibulospinal neurons during locomotion. *Brain Res., 46*: 85–98 (1972a)

ORLOVSKY, G. N.: Activity of rubrospinal neurons during locomotion. *Brain Res., 46*: 99–112 (1972b)

OSCARSSON, O.: Functional organization of spinocerebellar paths. *In* IGGO, A. (ed.): *Handbook of Physiology.* Vol. II, pp. 339–380. Springer-Verlag, Berlin, Heidelberg, New York (1973)

POGORELAYA, N. K. and TARUSINA, B. N.: Experimental-morphological study of lateral funiculus propriospinal fibre terminals in cat cervical spinal cord. *Neurophysiology (Kiev)*, *6*: 44–51 (1974)

ROSÉN, I.: Localization in caudal brain stem and cervical spinal cord of neurones activated from forelimb group I afferents in the cat. *Brain Res.*, *16*: 55–71 (1969)

SHIMAZU, H. and PRECHT, W.: Tonic and kinetic responses of cat's vestibular neurons to horizontal angular acceleration. *J. Neurophysiol.*, *28*: 991–1013 (1965)

VESILENKO, D. A., KOSTYUKOV, A. I. and PILYAVSKI, A. I.: Cortico- and rubrofugal activation of propriospinal interneurones sending axons into the dorsolateral funiculus of the cat spinal cord. *Neurophysiology (Kiev)*, *4*: 489–500 (1972)

VASILENKO, D. A., ZADOROZHNY, A. G. and KOSTYUK, P. G.: Synaptic processes in spinal neurons monosynaptically activated from the pyramidal tract. *Bull. Exp. Biol. Med. USSR.*, *64*: 20–25 (1967)

WILSON, V. J., UCHINO, Y., MAUNZ, R. A., SUSSWEIN, A. and FUKUSHIMA, K.: Properties and connections of cat fastigiospinal neurons. *Exp. Brain Res.*, *32*: 1–17 (1978)

WILSON, V. J. and YOSHIDA, M.: Comparison of effects of stimulation of Deiters' nucleus and medial longitudinal fasciculus on neck, forelimb and hindlimb motoneurones. *J. Neurophysiol.*, *32*: 743–758 (1969)

DISCUSSION PERIOD

PURPURA: Dr. LUNDBERG, in your previous formulations of hindlimb control mechanisms, you laid great stress on VSCT cells and those receiving input from descending control systems. I didn't see any consideration of that in the forelimb mechanism you're now discussing. Rather you would propose that something goes to the lateral reticular nucleus. Now, to what extent might not the RSCT system make its direct connections with a propriospinal system, and therefore, also operate in a way similar to VSCT would in the lumbar cord? You don't seem to now want to put this system into a direct pathway to the cerebellum on the way in.

LUNDBERG: The RSCT probably conveys information to cerebellum regarding segmental interneuronal pathways to forelimb motoneurones in much the same way as VSCT does for hindlimb segments. We have no evidence for a collateral projection to the cerebellar cortex or nuclei from the C3–C4 propriospinal neurones. In other words they do not seem to be identical with any of the spinocerebellar neurones originating in the upper cervical segments. It is not known whether some of the upper spino-cerebellar neurones signal activity in interneuronal pathways to the C3–C4 propriospinal system but note that there seems to exist a collateral projection to LRN from one of these interneuronal pathways. It is certainly puzzling that the lateral reticular nucleus takes care of the information from the C3–C4 propriospinal system but the results by EKEROT and OSCARSSON suggest that the lateral reticular nucleus handles information from many spinal motor centres.

PETERSON: I'd like to ask you something more about the divergence of the output of these neurons. You showed us that some go beyond the cervical enlargement. Do you have any evidence that they talk to other kinds of motoneurons than forelimb motoneurons and do they have the same input signals?

LUNDBERG; We do not know the target neurones of the long propriospinal axons but they appear to have the same convergence as those terminating in the forelimb segments, including effects from the forelimb.

HUNT: I think this morning's session points out very well how much we all owe to David LLOYD and Raphael LORENTE DE NÓ for our understanding of integrative function within the spinal cord, and I think that it also emphasizes the importance of functional organization to which they really made such important contributions. And I'd like, in closing, to add my personal comment of how much it meant to me to be able to work in DAVID's laboratory, and to have contact with Raphael and Herbert GASSER.

VESTIBULAR SYSTEM

Chairman: Dominick P. PURPURA

SOME PATTERNS OF CONNECTIVITY IN THE CENTRAL NERVOUS SYSTEM: A TRIBUTE TO RAFAEL LORENTE DE NÓ

ANN M. GRAYBIEL

Department of Psychology and Brain Science, Massachusetts Institute of Technology
Cambridge, MA

INTRODUCTION

It is no doubt true of an intellectual debt, no less than a biological debt, that one can honor it best in the prospective sense. But it is only natural to take pleasure in the direct celebration of great contributions to our field. We do so at this symposium in honor of Dr. David LLOYD and Dr. Rafael LORENTE DE NÓ.

Being asked to take part in the session on the vestibular system, I have organized these remarks around LORENTE DE NÓ's classic work on the subject, and in particular, around LORENTE's article on the vestibulo-ocular reflex arc published in 1933 (LORENTE DE NÓ, 1933 a). This paper exemplifies the enormous range of LORENTE's thinking. On the one hand, it includes detailed observations on the anatomy of the vestibulo-ocular reflex pathways, side chains in the reticular formation, and related nuclei and conduction routes. An even larger part of the paper is devoted to an account of LORENTE's ablation studies and physiological observations on vestibular nystagmus. On the other hand, the paper has a second quite different theme, carried at a more general level, that concerns the nature and complexity of organization of circuits in the brain and their relation to cerebral function.

LORENTE DE NÓ opened his 1933 *Archives* paper with a paradox: his observation that after transsecting the main bundle of the vestibulo-ocular reflex arc, the medial longitudinal fasciculus, he could still elicit vestibulo-ocular reflexes (Fig. 1). From this observation, and from related studies by GRAHAM BROWN and by HERRICK and COGHILL, LORENTE DE NÓ was forced to the conclusion that the so-called elementary reflex arcs do not represent the functional units of the nervous system.

With this fundamental conclusion in mind, LORENTE began an extensive series of experiments aimed at finding a satisfactory alternative. Almost immediately, in his ablation studies, LORENTE hit upon a second riddle; for when he left the medial longitudinal fasciculi intact, and instead made lesions in the reticular formation, he could abolish the rhythm of vestibular nystagmus (or as he put it, he could turn the nystagmus into a pseudo-postural reflex). Even slender knife cuts in the midline of the caudal pons and rostral medulla oblongata had similar effects; an example from his paper is given in Figure 2. LORENTE concluded from these experiments that the direct reflex pathway (the medial longitudinal fasciculus) could indeed carry excitation to the motoneurons but that side chains of neurons in the reticular formation were necessary for the production of the reflex rhythm. LORENTE's classic summary of these experiments is shown in Figure 3. His diagram indicates that the peripheral vestibular apparatus sets up the slow phase of the nystagmus but

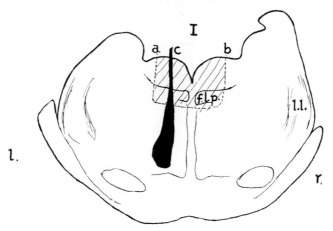

Fig. 1 Drawing from Lorente de Nó's paper illustrating a bilateral section (a–b) of the medial longitudinal fasciculus (f.l.p.) and (c) a thin longitudinal lesion of the tegmentum of the pons. (from Lorente de Nó 1933a).

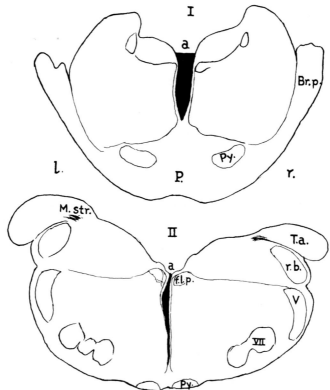

Fig. 2 Drawings illustrating the rostral (I) and caudal (II) limits of a sagittal lesion made in the ponto-medullary tegmentum. (from Lorente de Nó, 1933a rabbit 6, Figure 19).

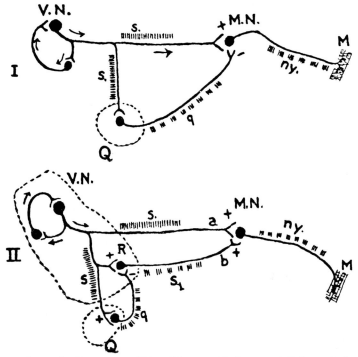

Fig. 3 Diagram drawn by LORENTE DE NÓ to illustrate his "system Q," the reticular mechanism involved in generating the reflex rhythm of vestibular nystagmus. In I, systemQ sets up a train of inhibitory bursts that are sent directly to the motoneuron (M.N.). The alternative drawn in II was favored by LORENTE because it incorporates internuncial neurons in the vestibular nuclei (V.N., enclosed in dotted outline). The theory illustrated was attributed by LORENTE to BÁRÁNY, in whose laboratory LORENTE studied. (from LORENTE DE NÓ, 1933a, Fig. 27).

that the quick phase depends on auxilliary conduction routes in the rostral medullary reticular formation, a region which he named System Q.

In these conclusions, LORENTE DE NÓ was anticipating by some thirty or forty years modern views on the organization of the reticular formation; for he stressed that connections in the reticular formation are not diffuse but highly specific as to their targets and essential to the functioning of particular sensory-motor circuits. He also was anticipating what has become a dominant theme of modern theoretical work on the oculomotor system by emphasizing reticular side chains as crucial elements in the vestibulo-ocular reflex arc and other oculomotor circuits (see, for example, ROBINSON, 1975).

In parallel with these ablation experiments LORENTE amassed a large number of observations on the anatomy of brain stem circuits related to the vestibular mechanism. Using the GOLGI method, he tried to define the nature of vestibular side paths in the reticular formation and, in his 1933 *Archives* paper, made a major effort to stress that complex circuits are not just confined to the cerebral cortex or cerebellum, but occur in the brain stem as well. From this work LORENTE DE NÓ was led to general conclusions about the organization of fiber connections in the central nervous system which he stated as two *laws of nerve circuits* in his 1933 paper on the vestibulo-ocular reflex arc. These theoretical formulations were later amplified in his paper on internuncial chains, published in the first volume of the *Journal of Neurophysiology* in 1938 (LORENTE DE NÓ, 1938 a). They also provided a major theoretical foundation for his remarkable chapter on the cerebral cortex, published in the same year in FULTON's textbook of physiology (LORENTE DE NÓ, 1938 b).

Lorente's laws will be considered in some detail in the second part of this paper. The first part deals briefly with findings on brain stem oculomotor pathways that are directly related to Lorente's own observations.

BRAIN STEM PATHWAYS OF THE OCULOMOTOR SYSTEM

Figure 4 reproduces the summary drawings by which Lorente de Nó illustrated the main vestibulo-oculomotor connections in the medulla oblongata (I) and (in II) the principal fiber connections associated with the medial longitudinal fasciculus (f. l. p. in the diagram). In diagram I Lorente emphasizes the role of the medullary reticular formation (R) both as a link in vestibulo-reticulo-oculomotor circuits and as a source of input to the vestibular nuclei. The second drawing specifically includes the pontine reticular formation (r. n. p.) within this dual plan of organization. This region was already well known to clinicians as the pontine gaze center and was of special interest to Bárány, under whom Lorente studied. Lorente's diagrams are all the more remarkable for being based on the Golgi method, for as Lorente de Nó pointed out in his 1933 paper on the Anatomy of the Eighth Nerve (Lorente de Nó, 1933 b), analysis by the Golgi method is certainly not the ideal way to study connections among neurons. But the lesion method

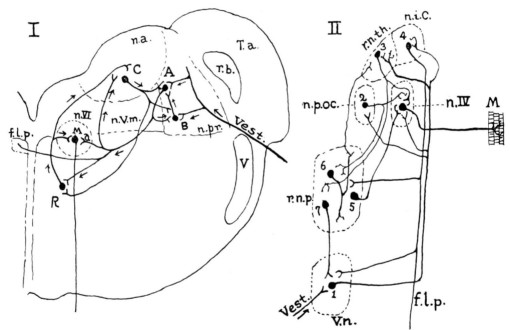

Fig. 4 Schematic diagrams from Lorente's paper illustrating, in I, what Lorente called "the smallest part of the medulla oblongata, which still is sufficient to set up the slow phase of the nystagmus in the external rectus muscle" and, in II, fiber connections associated with the medial longitudinal fasciculus (f.l.p.). Vestibular nuclei (V.n.), pontine reticular formation (r.n.p.), and regions near the oculomotor and trochlear nuclei (including the interstitial nucleus of Cajal) are indicated by broken outlines. Lorente considered n.p.o.c., nucleus para-ocularis, a "hitherto apparently undescribed part of the vestibular system;" its equivalent in modern nomenclature is uncertain. Lorente indicated r.n.th. (reticular nuclei in the thalamus) as receiving input carried over the medial longitudinal fasciculus and sending a direct projection to ocular motor neurons. This region could be interpreted as reticular formation at the meso-diencephalic border, rather than dorsal thalamus proper, in which case it could correspond to the region recently described in Büttner et al., 1977 and Graybiel, 1977b. (from Lorente de Nó, 1933a, Fig. 8)

(then the MARCHI technique) was simply not reliable because degeneration of passing fibers was produced by any lesion in the brain stem.

It is only very recently, with the development of the axon transport techniques, that it has been possible to study pathways in the reticular formation by methods designed to circumvent technical problems. In our own laboratory, we first began work on the brain stem oculomotor pathways by using the then still very new retrograde horseradish peroxidase method (GRAYBIEL and HARTWIEG, 1974). The findings corroborated previous evidence that direct fiber projections to the oculomotor complex arise in the so-called accessory oculomotor nuclei of the midbrain, regions illustrated in LORENTE's drawing II. The greatest density of labelling, however, appeared at levels corresponding to that illustrated in part I of LORENTE's summary diagram: not only in the vestibular nuclei but also in the rostral medullary tegmentum, in the nuclei of the perihypoglossal complex (most prominently the nucleus prepositus hypoglossi) and in the abducens nucleus itself (Fig. 5).

These findings had two main implications. First, the organization of the nuclei of the extraocular muscles appeared much more like that of the ventral horn of the spinal cord than one would have guessed before, for there apparently were interneurons in and around

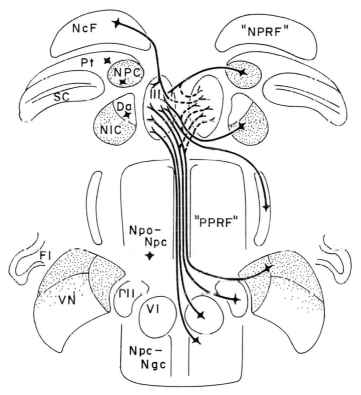

Fig. 5 Summary of afferent connections of the oculomotor complex observed in anterograde and retrograde tracer experiments in cat and monkey. Main ascending connections arise from parts of the vestibular nuclei (VN), nucleus prepositus hypoglossi (PH), ponto-medullary tegmentum (Npc-Ngc), and abducens nucleus (VI). Local connections arise in Cajal's interstitial nucleus (NIC) and the nucleus of the posterior commissure. Slightly anterior to the latter regions, in the caudal part of the subthalamus at its point of continuity with the mesencephalic reticular formation, a descending connection originates. This is considered to play an important role in the control of vertical gaze. The laterality of many of the connections is not known or cannot be illustrated in so schematic a diagram. (modified from Fig. 5 of GRAYBIEL, 1977b)

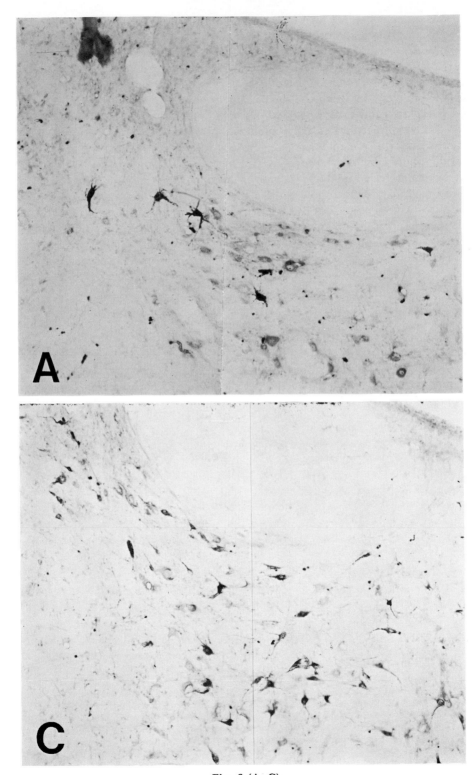

Fig. 6 (A, C)

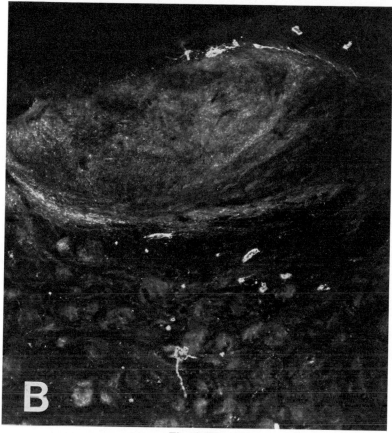

Fig. 6 (B)

Fig. 6 (A–C) Photomicrographs illustrating neurons of the abducens nucleus that are labelled by retrograde transport after injections of horseradish peroxidase (HRP) into the cerebellar flocculus of the cat. A) shows the side ipsilateral to the flocculus injections, B) the contralateral side. Somewhat lateral location of the RHP-labelled neurons in (A) was typical of cases of flocculus injection; so was the supragenual position illustrated in (B). For comparison, (C) shows a photomicrograph of HRP-labelled neurons in the abducens nucleus contralateral to an injection site in the oculomotor nucleus. Flocculus experiments carried out with Dr. B. B. GOULD.

the motoneuronal pools, at least in the abducens nucleus. We now know that some neurons (presumably interneurons) in the abducens nucleus project directly to the cerebellar flocculus (GRAYBIEL, 1977b and Fig. 6) and that neurons in or immediately alongside the oculomotor nucleus give rise to an indirect pre-cerebellar pathway (GRAYBIEL, 1977 a; MACIEWICZ, 1977 b). These pathways recall propriospinal and spinocerebellar connections and, at the behavioral level, bring to mind LORENTE's analogy between nystagmus and rhythmic spinal reflexes such as the scratch reflex (LORENTE DE NÓ, 1933 a).

A second and related implication was that a fiber system involved in the control of horizontal gaze would not necessarily need to synapse in both the IIIrd and VIth nerve nuclei but instead could project to the abducens-periabducens region, relying on ascending pathways from this region to the oculomotor complex for the coordination of conjugate gaze. Such an arrangement could account for the failure of the HRP experiments to demonstrate a fiber projection from the pontine tegmentum to the oculomotor complex (GRAYBIEL and HARTWIEG, 1974).

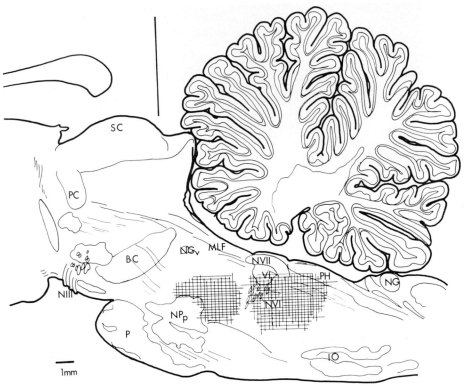

Fig. 7 Drawing of a parasagittal section through the brain stem in the cat to illustrate the approximate locations of the pontine and pontomedullary zones considered to play a role in the control of horizontal gaze. (Modified from Figure 15 of GRAYBIEL, 1977a.)

It has become clear from autoradiographic experiments we and others have since carried out that the so-called paramedian pontine reticular formation, while apparently not projecting in volume directly to the IIIrd nerve nucleus, does in fact send a direct ipsilateral fiber projection to the abducens-periabducens region (BÜTTNER-ENNEVER and HENN, 1976; GRAYBIEL, 1977 a).   The autoradiographic experiments also suggested, however, that the densest direct projection from the reticular formation to the abducens nucleus may arise just caudal to the pontine zone, in the rostrodorsal part of the medullary reticular formation of the contralateral side (Fig. 7).   This finding is in close accord with the conclusions of HIKOSAKA and KAWAKAMI (1977) and has been confirmed both in HRP experiments (GRAYBIEL, 1977 b; MACIEWICZ et al., 1977 a) and in a more recent series of autoradiographic experiments (unpublished; see Fig. 8).   All available evidence suggests that this zone corresponds to the region LORENTE DE NÓ described in his 1933 *Archives* paper as the "smallest part of the medulla oblongata which still is sufficient to set up the slow phase of nystagmus in the external rectus muscle."   Other districts related to eye movements clearly are present in the reticular formation of the brain stem, for example the so-called pauser region near the midline of the rostral medulla oblongata (KELLER, 1974), and the dorsomedial part of the prerubral field (BÜTTNER et al., 1977; GRAYBIEL, 1977 b; KING, 1976) which projects to the oculomotor complex (see Fig. 5).   There can be little doubt, however, that LORENTE DE NÓ outlined in his *Archives* paper the main pre-oculomotor pathways of the horizontal gaze mechanism of the pontomedullary tegmentum as we recognize them today.

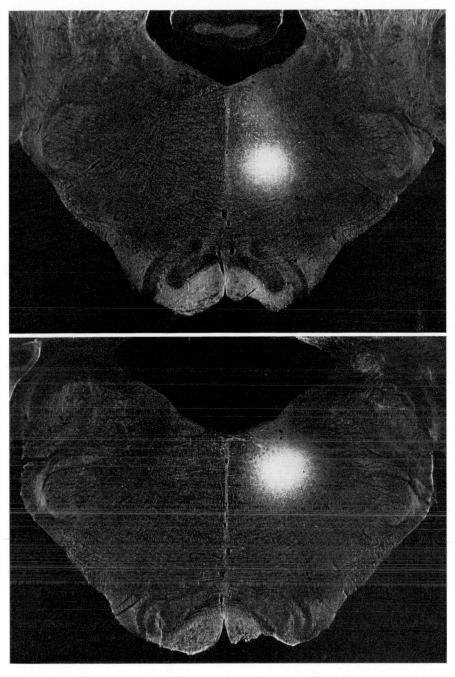

Fig. 8 Examples from autoradiographic experiments in progress illustrating locations of tritiated amino-acid deposits in the medullary reticular formation in the cat. These injections led to anterograde labelling of the contralateral abducens nucleus, perihypoglossal complex and parts of the contralateral vestibular complex. Their location corresponds closely to that of LORENTE DE Nó's system Q.

RULES OF CONNECTIVITY IN THE BRAIN STEM AND FOREBRAIN

Lorente's laws of nerve circuits

Even in a brief survey of brain stem pre-oculomotor connections, one is struck repeatedly by a characteristic plan of organization: for every direct pathway to the motoneuronal nuclei there are indirect paths paralleling and interacting with the direct ones. In the limit, of course, the notion of "indirect" pathways loses its meaning and recalls mainly the medical student's complaint that everything is connected to everything else. In a more restricted sense the distinction is useful, for the existence of a direct (or nearly direct) pathway — say, to motoneurons — means that sufficient preprocessing has occurred to produce a meaningful message or instruction. Conversely, the presence of intercalated nuclei (or synapses) along a pathway implies that corresponding modifications in the information line are necessary to produce the appropriate final effect. The particular balance between direct and indirect conduction lines, in fact, may serve as an important signature of the individual conduction routes within a system of related fiber pathways. For example, *direct* reticular paths to the abducens nucleus seem to predominate in the case of the more caudal of the reticular zones shown in Figure 7, *indirect* paths in the case of the pontine zone.

This highly characteristic plan of organization of direct and indirect pre-oculomotor pathways made a strong impression on LORENTE DE NÓ. Even though he could not trace out these brainstem paths with techniques designed to study long-axon connections, a similar pattern could be detected at the level of single-fiber analysis by the GOLGI method. LORENTE's insight was to see the generality of the pattern's underlying principles and to formulate them explicitly in laws describing fiber connections in the central nervous system. In his 1933 *Archives* paper he called the first the *law of plurality of connections*. It stated that for every through pathway there are one or more parallel pathways derived from the first and involving at least one and often more than one internuncial neuron. Some years later LORENTE returned to this principle, calling these circuits *multiple chains* (LORENTE DE NÓ, 1938 a). The second law, the *law of reciprocity of connections* stated that

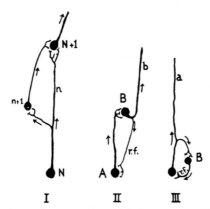

Fig. 9 This figure reproduces diagrams by which LORENTE DE NÓ illustrated his two laws of nervous connections (Figure 3 of the 1933 *Archives* paper). I depicts the law of plurality of connections. This states that "If the cells in the spinal or cranial ganglia are called cells of the 'first order' and the following ones in the transmission system cells of the second, third to...nth order, it can be said that each nucleus in the nervous system always receives fibers of at least n and n+1 order, and often of n, n+1 and n+2 order." II and III illustrate LORENTE's law of reciprocity of connections, in which he stated that "If cell complex A sends fibers to cell or cell complex B, B also sends fibers to A, either direct or by means of one internuncial neuron." (LORENTE DE NÓ, 1933a).

for each pathway there is a return, or reciprocal, pathway closing the loop either directly or by means of one or more internuncials (later called closed chains, LORENTE DE NÓ, 1938 a). He depicted these generalizations in the diagrams that are shown in Figures 9 and 10.

It is clear, in retrospect, that LORENTE DE NÓ embodied in these laws the concepts of feedforward and feedback now used by control engineers. What is remarkable is that LORENTE did this so many years before these concepts were formally incorporated into the field of cybernetics, so many years before these concepts were applied generally to the study of central nervous organization. In choosing observations to support and illustrate these principles (including some observations by his former teacher, RAMÓN Y CAJAL) LORENTE was careful to distinguish between large systems of interconnected neurons and individual fiber connections. LORENTE was, for the most part, speaking of the individual, not the col-

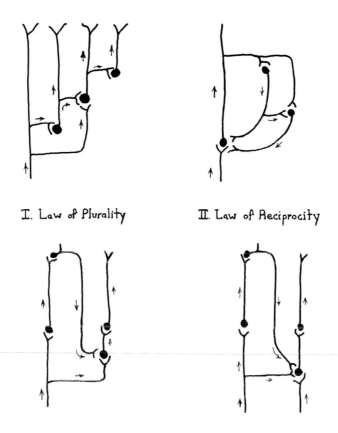

I. Law of Plurality   II. Law of Reciprocity

III. Law of indirect recursion

Fig. 10 The diagrams in I and II show LORENTE's two laws as he modified them for his 1938 paper on internuncial chains (adapted from his Figure 2), in which he used the term, *multiple chain,* to denote the first law (I), and *closed chain* to denote the law of reciprocity (II). In these diagrams, the "level" in the through-conduction increases as one moves toward the top of the diagram. The diagrams in III illustrate a third law, incorporating features of each of LORENTE's laws. The diagrams indicate characteristic patterns in which a later stage in a pathway (up in the diagram) can play back upon an earlier stage in the system without closing a loop. This *indirect reciprocity* prevents alteration of the original message likely in the case of direct reciprocity; it incorporates the notion of plurality, but suggests different functions for the multiple pathways. The diagram to the left shows indirect recursion in its simplest form. In the diagrams to the right, an independent input has been added to illustrate one likely circuit plan based on the law. The diagrams in III are not meant to be restricted to the single-fiber level of analysis.

lective case. This strategy was virtually a necessity because the analyses were largely by the GOLGI method. It was important also to the logic: multiple chains "must be thought of as being used by the impulses at the same time and for the same function." It is unclear whether this point can be carried over to studies of long tracts and available techniques are hardly adequate to decide. Even if identity of function is not assumed in the strict sense, however, LORENTE's principles nevertheless apply to these complex "long circuiting arcs," as I hope to show below, and can be extended in ways that may be useful in understanding some of the great families of related fiber connections typical of the forebrain.*

Plurality and reciprocity in long-circuiting arcs

Figure 11 shows an example of LORENTE's law of plurality extended to long-circuiting pathways of the visual system. The diagram at the top shows the more or less direct pathways leading from the optic tract to the cerebellum. The diversity of these pathways is remarkable. They range from a nearly direct pathway, recently discovered by KARTEN and his co-workers in the bird (BRAUTH and KARTEN, 1977) to indirect paths involving the midbrain, mesodiencephalic border zones and thalamocortical loops feeding back to the precerebellar nuclei which in turn give rise either to climbing fibers or to mossy fibers. Nine such pathways are depicted in Figure 11, but the number surely is not so small as this. Many have been collapsed in the diagram; for example, all descending vision-related pathways from the cerebral cortex are indicated by a single line.

The multiplicity is not limited to the visuocerebellar mechanism. The second panel in Figure 11 illustrates the relatively direct routes leading from the optic tract toward the neocortex. These play over the lateral geniculate body, the pulvinar and LP and include a curious transthalamic route from cortex to thalamus and back to cortex. Here again, the relative simplicity of the diagram should not mislead: in the retino-geniculo-striate path alone, there now are thought to be a number of separable and therefore, by implication, presumably functionally distinct channels, and within the lateral thalamic group at least four or five can be distinguished even at the relatively crude level of analysis by thalamic subdivision or cortical area (BERSON and GRAYBIEL, 1978; GRAYBIEL 1972 c). Finally, as a counterpoint to the cerebellar access routes, the third panel in Figure 11 shows the most direct paths from the visual mechanism into the basal ganglia. Here one is farthest from understanding the form of information processing, least sure of the eventual targets of the paths; yet even so, there already is evidence for some regional topographic organization within the striatum, the substantia nigra, and their outflow pathways (FAULL and MEHLER, 1976; GRAYBIEL 1978; KÜNZLE, 1975 and unpublished observations).

At the level of long-circuiting arcs, there is no need to think of redundancy as the primary outcome of this pattern of multiplicity. To summarize the situation simply by saying that for every input path there are many feedforward lines also seems an impoverished view. In fact, one of the most important lessons of recent electrophysiological work on the visual system is the unequivocal demonstration that there can be multiple input channels that are not fully, and are sometimes only partly, overlapping in origin, information content, and temporal spectrum. At the outset of the sensory pathway, the spatiotemporal

---

* It is to be hoped that if a law applies at one level of analysis it will apply to others. The most reductionistic levels currently recognized in the study of the CNS are still too imperfectly understood to permit comment. Certainly, though, the laws apply to serial and reciprocal synaptic complexes known only through the use of the electron microscope; see, for example, SHEPHERD (1972) and RAKIC (1975). The present discussion is directed toward systems of fibers but this is mainly because of the incompleteness of our knowledge at the single-fiber level.

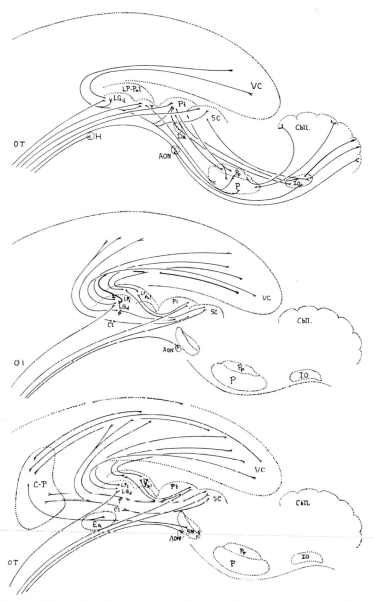

Fig. 11 Diagrams illustrating the law of plurality extended to long systems of pathways. The examples are taken from work on the visual system, and all three drawings show optic tract fibers terminating in the dorsal and ventral nuclei of the lateral geniculate body (LGd, v), pretectal region (Pt), superior colliculus (SC), accessory optic tract nuclei (AON) and suprachiasmatic nucleus of the hypothalamus (H). The top drawing depicts the relatively direct access routes by which this visual input can influence the cerebellum (Cbll.) including one representative of trans-cortical conduction pathways (heavier line). Da-nucleus of Darkschewitsch; P-pontine grey; Pp-nucleus papillioformis; IO-inferior olivary complex. The middle diagram illustrates pathways by which visual information reaches the neocortex. Lp-Pul: nucleus lateralis posterior-pulvinar complex of the thalamus; LP1-lateral part of nucleus lateralis posterior; P-posterior nuclear group; Cl-nucleus centralis lateralis. The bottom figure represents visual pathways leading toward the basal ganglia. C-P: caudoputamen; En: globus pallidus/entopeduncular nucleus; SNr, c: substantia nigra, pars reticulata, compacta. The connections drawn are meant to represent fiber systems, not single fibers.

aspects of the signals, the type of ganglion cell giving rise to the pathway, the proportional representation of various parts of the visual field, all may be different in, and even diagnostic of, groups of optic tract axons with different destinations. With the further diversification imposed at the next synaptic stations, there is added to the pattern potential flexibility, each synapse (and possibly each axonal branch point as well) representing a facultative linkage in apparently fixed lines of connectivity (see GRAYBIEL, 1972 a).

Flexibility in the processing of information is the supraordinate functional consequence of LORENTE's second law, the law of reciprocity of connections. For short of chemical modulation, only now beginning to be adequately appreciated, it is by its internal feedback pathways that the brain modifies its own functional state. In his 1933 *Archives* paper LORENTE emphasizes CAJAL's discovery of centrifugal fibers and his diagrams of complicated networks with recurrent fibers in the cerebellum. Figure 12 illustrates two other cerebellar circuits recently demonstrated by axon transport techniques: in 12.2, the cerebello-olivary pathway by which the cerebellum can modify its climbing fiber input (GRAYBIEL et al., 1973) and in 12.3, the nucleocortical pathway by which the deep cerebellar nuclei can modulate the activity of the cerebellar cortex (GOULD and GRAYBIEL, 1976). Constant modulation of the internal settings of the cerebellar circuits must be essential to the function of the cerebellum, which LORENTE epitomized in his internuncial chains paper as "a giant chain of internuncial neurons superimposed upon the reflex arcs in the spinal cord and medulla" and charged with the responsibility of "regulating the transmission of impulses through the shorter arcs." It is no exaggeration to add that an entire subfield of physiology is currently devoted to studying this regulation using exactly LORENTE's model: the vestibulo-ocular reflex arc (ITO, 1975).

The overwhelming impression LORENTE leaves us with, in discussing the implications of his laws, is one of an active central nervous system. The internal activity created in the brain by reciprocal internuncial circuits means above all that the brain can impress a pattern of activity on incoming information by virtue of its own intrinsic activity. It is this intrinsic activity, in turn, that gives the brain its flexibility. As LORENTE DE NÓ (1933 a) stressed:

"... the whole vestibular system is a physiological unit that finds itself in constant activity, and according to its functional state the afferent impulses set up reflexes of a determined pattern, because they find open only a limited number of the extremely numerous anatomic paths." (p. 279)

And again

"That the vestibular impulses really have at their disposal different anatomic paths is demonstrated by the fact that no labyrinthine excitation necessarily sets up a determined reaction ... In a similar way the state of the reticular relays modifies the function of the vestibular nuclei according to the impulses concurrent with the vestibular ones; this would explain the reflex reversal conditioned by extralabyrinthine impulses ... (p. 282, 283)

These passages constitute a remarkably accurate prediction of current work on the "plasticity" (that is, functional and/or structural modifiability) of the vestibulo-ocular reflex induced, for example, by visual inputs. More importantly, they mark a central theme of LORENTE's thinking about the brain, namely, that it is physiologically meaningless to think of circuits as having fixed numbers of synapses and hence necessary to look to complex systems of circuits for the functional units of the brain.*

---

* It is interesting that at the level of single neurons, SHEPHERD has recently made a comparable point based on electron microscopic evidence for dendrodendritic synapses and other local-circuit devices (SHEPHERD, 1972).

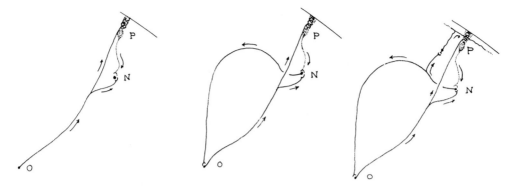

1. COLLATERALS OF THE CLIMBING FIBERS   2. CEREBELLO - OLIVARY PATHWAY   3. CEREBELLAR - NUCLEOCORTICAL PATHWAY

Fig. 12 Examples of LORENTE's law of reciprocity, drawn from experiments on the climbing fiber pathway to the cerebellum, shown in (1). (2) illustrates a conduction route by which the cerebellum can modify its climbing fiber input (GRAYBIEL et al., 1973). (3) an intrinsic circuit of the cerebellum allowing the deep cerebellar nuclei to influence the cerebellar cortex (GOULD and GRAYBIEL, 1976).

Feedback without closure: law of indirect recursion

In musicology it is common to make a distinction between monophonic music, in which a single melodic line is carried without accompaniment, and homophonic music, consisting of a main melodic line supported by harmony; these in turn are contrasted with contrapuntal or polyphonic music, in which two and sometimes several related but independent melodic lines are elaborated. It was a richness characteristic of the homophonic forms that LORENTE DE NÓ stressed in his rejection of the reflex arc (monophonic) as "only an anatomic idealization of the structure of the nervous system," and his embracing of the multiple and closed chain (homophonic) concepts of central nervous organization. It is the lines of partially independent conduction characteristic of polyphony that are emphasized in the more complex forms of connectivity that become apparent in analyzing systems of long-circuiting pathways in the brain. It is to these forms that the remainder of this paper is addressed.

The third panel in Figure 10 illustrates in simple circuit form a pattern of *indirect recursion* that appears over and over again in the study of functionally related systems of pathways in the brain: a pattern in which a through-conduction path influences a parallel path by a recurrent fiber system that does not close a loop and yet feeds back to an early stage in the system. The diagram to the left shows the simplest case, in which the relationship between two lines originating in a single source is reiterated by a recurrent fiber farther along the system. The diagram to the right shows a more complicated (and probably more typical) form in which the parallel path is driven not only by the common source and the recurrent fiber, but also by an independent afferent line. Despite the fact that they were derived from study of fiber systems, not individually recognizable fibers, the drawings in Figure 10 III have been made in the style of LORENTE's own to emphasize the point that these are recursive circuits just as are the reciprocal pathways that LORENTE discussed. The type of recursion, however, is important. First, indirect recursion allows for feedback without closure. Second, it allows for a spectrum in the degree of coupling of related lines of conduction. Third, it allows for an interlocking of lines of independent origin, an interweaving of one conduction network with another. These characteristics do not apply to direct reciprocity, leaving aside membrane fluctuations and other devices that may be used to introduce modulation of apparently hardwired connections.

Figure 13 illustrates an example of indirect recursion taken from the visual system. Both diagrams in the figure are organized around the parallel conduction routes leading from the retina to the lateral geniculate body (LG), superior colliculus (SC) and pretectal region (Pt), and the pathways leading from these three regions toward the neocortex. The geniculo-striate path to area 17 is direct, but both the tectofugal and the pretectofugal pathways require additional synaptic links in the caudal thalamus (the lateralis posterior-pulvinar complex) before reaching the extrastriate cortex. A striking feature of this group of related pathways is that the striate cortex projects back upon all three of the pathways and, in doing so, projects to the regions that receive direct projections from the retina. The descending fibers from area 17, to do this, must almost literally avoid the thalamic links in the extrageniculate paths (traveling farther to reach the retino-recipient superior colliculus and pretectum); yet, fibers from area 17 do terminate in the thalamic region

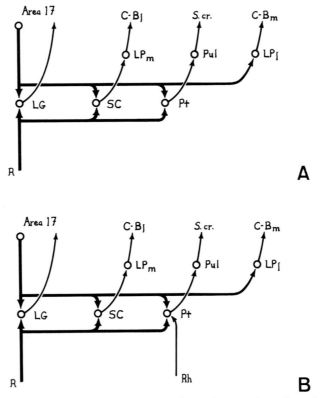

Fig. 13 (A) Example of the law of indirect recursion, drawn from work on the pulvinar-posterior system and visual association cortex in the cat (BERSON and GRAYBIEL, 1978; GRAYBIEL, 1972b, c). The diagram has been organized around fiber pathways that originate in the retina (R) and striate cortex (area 17), and lead into the extrageniculate visual mechanism. The diagram shows retinal projections to the lateral geniculate body (LG), superior colliculus (SC) and pretectum (Pt). The superior colliculus and pretectum in turn project to the pulvinar-posterior system, specifically the medial part of the nucleus lateralis posterior (LPm) and the Pulvinar (Pul). These thalamic subdivisions, together with the lateral part of the n. lateralis posterior (LPl), project to areas of visual association cortex (the medial and lateral parts of the Clare-Bishop complex, C-Bl and C-Bm, and the crown of the suprasylvian gyrus, SCr). An important point to note is that area 17 projects to regions receiving input from the retina, i.e. to the early stages of the tecto-thalamo-cortical and pretecto-thalamo-cortical channels, thus modulating them by recurrent fibers that do not close a loop. Compare with the direct, reciprocal area 17-LG path. (B) Same as A except that one example of an additional input system (rhombencephalic tegmental input to the pretecto-pulvinar channel, (see GRAYBIEL, 1977a) has been added. Compare with Figure 10-III.

physically adjacent to the tectorecipient and pretectorecipient zones, namely, in the lateral part of the nucleus lateralis posterior, LP1 (see BERSON and GRAYBIEL, 1978; GRAYBIEL, 1972 b).

In these visual feedback pathways, one can see example of the two types of recursion under discussion: *direct recursion* (reciprocity) in the striato-geniculate path, *indirect recursion* (non-reciprocal recursion) in the striato-tectal and striato-pretectal paths. The remarkable point about the arrangement is that the brain seems to recognize, in its own morphological arrangement, the type of recursion in these circuits. Two different layers in cortical area 17 participate in the two different types of circuit: pyramidal cells in layer VI provide the direct reciprocal pathway, pyramidal cells in layer V provide the pathways of indirect recursion.*

SUBDIVISIONS OF THE BRAIN: RELATION BETWEEN THEIR INTRINSIC FUNCTIONAL OPERATIONS AND PRINCIPLES OF EFFERENT INFORMATION-DISTRIBUTION

The subject of complex nerve circuits leads naturally to inquiry about the logic of individual functionally identified pathways; for almost certainly, the constraints that result in such patterns of connectivity as here discussed must have to do at least in part with the functional peculiarities of the particular pathways—that is, with the logic of the particular circuits involved. But we are far from understanding any single instance. A typical problem is illustrated in Figure 13. The thalamic LP1 region receiving input from area 17 is shown to project to its cortical receiving area, the medial part of the Clare-Bishop complex (C-B_m; BERSON and GRAYBIEL, 1978; GRAYBIEL, 1972 b, c and BERSON and GRAYBIEL, in preparation). This cortical area itself receives a fiber projection directly from area 17. Why is the trans-thalamic path: area 17-LP_1-C-B_m superimposed upon the direct area 17-C-B_m route? Part of the answer may ultimately lie in the new finding that LP1 has some source of ascending input, so that the trans-thalamic route is actually a partly autonomous circuit embedded within another main conduction line. This line of reasoning is specifically addressed to identifying functionally distinct visual pathways. Another possible approach involves noticing that the direct transcortical input to the C-B_m area arises from the supragranular layers of area 17, the trans-thalamic input indirectly from the infragranular layers. This second possibility is less strictly tied to the example of the visual cortex; it suggests that some property of the intrinsic structural arrangement of the cortex may be an observable indication of an underlying functional logic, and that the particular pathways emerging from area 17 reflect this logic. At this level, the pathway analysis has gone beyond the particularized case dealing with extrageniculate visual pathways. The design of the pathway is seen not solely as a consequence of the need for processing of visual information, but also as a functionally and perhaps also developmentally necessary consequence of a set of rules describing the operations of the subdivisions of the brain engaged by the particular pathways under discussion.

Such general constraints may play a basic role in the form of particular patterns of connectivity. Consider what is meant by the common phrase, "precerebellar nuclei"—that is, those nuclei whose efferent fibers are distributed in large part, if not entirely, within the

---

* It seems probable that with double or multiple retrograde labelling techniques, we will be able to extend the schema of classification of layer V pyramids much farther than is presently possible. Differential patterns of projection of layers V and VI were first documented in 1974–1975 (see GILBERT and KELLY, 1975). It now appears that pyramidal cells in layer V also give rise to other projection fibers (corticostriate, cortico-pontine, etc.). It may be that these are parts of one or more collateral systems originating in layer V.

cerebellum.   At first glance, the phrase simply calls to mind certain nuclei of the brain stem, for example, the inferior olivary complex or lateral reticular nucleus or the pontine nuclei.   Seen in a slightly different way, however, the phrase conveys the meaning that only a few parts of the brain are *allowed* to project to the cerebellum and, conversely, that many are not allowed to do so.

The very simple diagrams of Figure 14 are intended to illustrate how common the "pre-cerebellar" pattern is.   They are focused on the relationship between the neocortex and three great districts of the brain: the pallidum, cerebellum, and hippocampus.   The point of the figure is that the neocortex, despite its close association with all three regions, does not project directly to any of them.   It must instead, in each instance, use interme-diaries in order to reach them.   It is important to stress that this is apparently true of all neocortex, not just one or several areas of neocortex.   In other words, this pattern of con-nectivity does not seem to express a rule based solely on the modality or function of a par-ticular cortical area.   Nor does the notion need to be keyed to the neocortex alone.   In

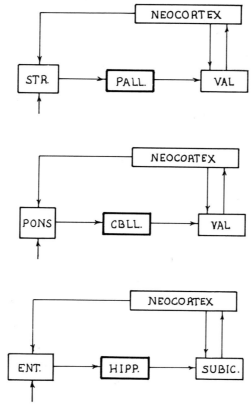

Fig. 14 Schematic diagrams illustrating characteristic pattern of the access routes by which the neocortex can exert its influence upon the pallidum (PALL.), cerebellum (CBLL.) and hippo-campus (HIPP.). In each of these examples, the neocortex must use intermediaries in order to gain access to these major target regions: to influence the pallidum, the cortex projects to the striatum (STR.); to reach the cerebellum, it projects to the pontine nuclei (PONS); to reach the hippocampus, it projects first to the entorhinal area (ENT). Note that, considered from the standpoint of the ventral anterior and lateral nuclei of the thalamus (VAL) or, for the hippo-campal example, the subiculum (SUBIC) (ROSENE and van HOESEN, 1977), these last named con-nections could be considered as side-chains of the more direct pathways shown at the righthand side of each diagram. A possibility to be considered is that directness of access is related logically, and perhaps developmentally as well, to the type of process occurring in brain-compartments such as those illustrated in the figure.

each of the three examples shown in Figure 14, the intermediary is one of a very small class of staging centers with direct access to their respective target. This plan of organization lends itself to a partial interlocking of related fiber systems because the links formed between the intermediaries do not necessarily affect the primary functional autonomy of the principal pathways involved (see Fig. 15). The main implication of the plan is that at least some circuits in the brain are based on rules that describe the connections different subdivisions of the brain are allowed and not allowed to make.

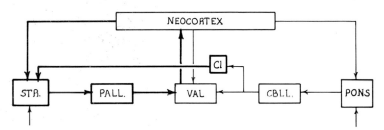

Fig. 15   Diagram illustrating one possible consequence of the schemes of restrictde access illustrated in Figure 14. The top and middle networks of Figure 14, illustrating loop systems of the motor system, are here shown interlocked by means of an additional link through the intralaminar nuclei of the thalamus (Cl-nucleus centralis lateralis).

Figure 16 expresses the concept in its more general form, namely, that each subdivision of the brain (nucleus, cortical area, embryological subdivision) can be defined by the nature of its access routes to other parts of the brain: by their type, and by the degree of multiplicity embodied in LORENTE's first law. According to this line of thinking, the neocortex can be defined as that part of the brain with the greatest access to all other subdivisions; indeed it has direct access to all other major subdivisions. This situation is shown at the top left in Figure 16, and is contrasted with the much more limited efferent domain of the non-cortical hemisphere (exemplified by the basal ganglia, BG). The other diagrams in Figure 16 illustrate the *dorsal thalamus*, whose efferents nearly all ascend to the cerebral hemisphere; the *midbrain*, which, aside from its aminergic neurons, lacks major access routes to the cerebral hemisphere (the dopaminergic nigrostriatal system is shown as the most massive and discretely organized of the midbrain-hemisphere connections); the *rhombencephalon*, with widespread brain stem connections illustrated by the cerebellofugal pathways and direct effector channels carried by cranial nerves; and finally, the *biogenic amine* and other special fiber systems, including adrenergic and dopaminergic fibers innervating the hemisphere (DESCARRIES et al., 1975; LINDRALL et al., 1974), serotonin-containing fibers innervating the ventricular ependyma (CHAN-PALAY, 1976), and hypothalamic neurons innervating blood vessels (HAYMAKER, 1969). Most of the last-named neural or neurohumoral pathways are still very poorly understood. It is not even clear whether they use the mechanisms of synaptic transmission thought to characterize most other neurons in the mammalian brain. The electron microscopic observations of DESCARRIES and his colleagues, in fact, suggest that the biogenic amine pathways may not (see DESCARRIES et al., 1975). If so, we may in time be able to learn a different set of rules, having to do with the modifying of the local or regional chemical milieu in which classic synaptically-linked chains of neurons are active.

The notion of trying to distinguish among different subdivisions of the brain is, of course, not new at all. In the present context the attempt has the advantage of emphasizing that the long connections of the major subdivisions may be as distinctive as their local patterns of connectivity. But the main point in stressing subdivisions is the possibility that we could relate the long circuits and local circuits in a rational way.   The key question here is whether there are different functional algorithms that characterize different parts of the brain by virtue of the intrinsic organization of those parts; that is, whether we can discover different subprinciples that govern the integrative activity of different parts of the brain, subprinciples that allow the individuation of Lorente's laws according to region, that let us ask how a particular pattern of connectivity works in a particular instance to bring about

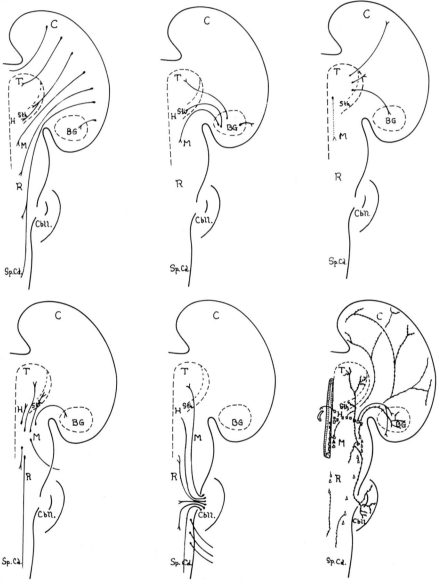

Fig. 16 Drawings designed to illustrate principle that differential access routes permitted major subdivisions of the mammalian brain in their communication with other parts of the brain may be defining characteristics of these subdivisions. Principal efferent pathways are illustrated, from upper left to lower right, for the cerebral cortex (C); the basal ganglia (BG); the thalamus, (T, as part of the diencephalon); the midbrain (M, mesencephalon); the hindbrain (R, rhomben-cephalon). The lower righthand diagram shows biogenical amine and neurohumoral pathways. Sp. Cd-spinal cord; Sth-subthalamus; H-hypothalamus.

a particular result.   For if we can accept the notion that such functional distinctions are in order, then it may be possible to view the restriction of output of a given region, or allowance of input to the region, as being at least in part developmentally and functionally related to the intrinsic organization of that part.   Accordingly, we could begin to look at the long circuits of the brain as expressing corresponding principles of routing of information.

Ordinarily something quite different is done.   We classify much of the brain according to modality or prevailing input.   We think of "the visual system"; or "the greater visual system" including all the extrageniculate paths; of the "rhinencephalon;" or the "vestibulocerebellum."   This means that a fiber system can be traced from A to B to C to Z for the reason that A, B, C...Z deal with visual (olfactory, vestibular) information.   There are obvious reasons for thinking along these lines, but we are left with extremely perplexing problems.   In the main sensory channels, for example, what accounts for the obligatory synaptic link in the specific sensory nuclei of the thalamus?   The fact that the term, relay nuclei, was for many years applied to these thalamic way stations actually expressed the query well.   The term is no longer used, but the question still remains.   It is problems such as this that point to the usefulness of thinking, in addition, of information of a particular modality or functional affiliation as being routed according to a set of distribution principles that express the functional operations of different neural compartments.   For example, in the case of central visual pathways involved in oculomotor control, one could consider a series of simultaneously active pathways such as those schematized in Fig. 17, one shunting information rapidly to the brain stem oculomotor apparatus, conveying the general directions for the eye movement; another path sending the visual information to the striatum, perhaps for modulation by the dopamine system; yet other pathways leading into limbic system or cerebellum or association cortex, each with a particular functional consequence.   At least in the case of the striatum, one has the chance of identifying a likely defining peculiarity of the compartment—the dopamine innervation.   For the cerebellum, the ideas of a clock (BRAITENBERG and ATWOOD, 1958; BRAITENBERG, 1961) and of an idiosyncratic modulation by climbing fibers (e.g. MARR, 1969) have attracted serious interest.   For the superior colliculus, a perhaps unique overlaying of spatial maps related to different modalities could be the important feature.   At best, these characteristics are only clues; in most instances we do not even have clues.   Even so, there clearly is an arbitrariness in limited definitions of such functional groups as "the visual system."   The routing itineraries in Figure 17 are intended to suggest a shift in emphasis from the input side to the effector side of the different compartments, and to stress how useful it could be to work out at least a taxonomy, if not indeed a grammar, of these circuits.

COMPARTMENTALIZATION AND GEOMETRIC ORGANIZATION

Fundamental advances in the physical and biological sciences have depended, above all, on the identification of the elements of the subject matter and the rules relating those elements.   LORENTE DE NÓ, in his emphasis on seeking the "elementary units" of function in the central nervous system, was clearly striving for a comparable advance.   It has been the purpose of this paper to demonstrate the great increase in understanding he achieved. He set aside as an "elementary unit" the two-neuron arc and in fact, any arc with a fixed number of internuncials.   He substituted, in place of these, multiple and closed chains of neurons and argued forcefully for the generality of his laws of connectivity.   This theme of LORENTE's work was carried through to his observations on the cerebral cortex (LORENTE DE NÓ, 1938b), with remarkable results:

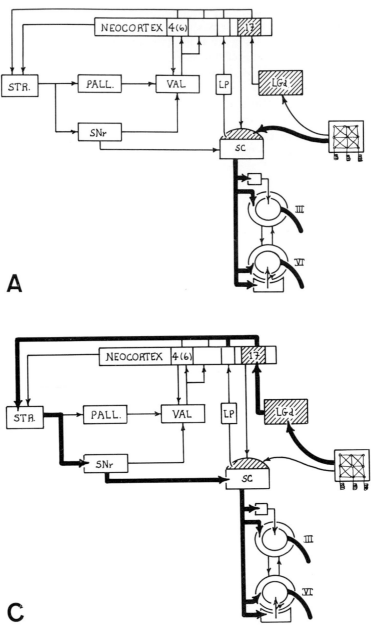

Fig. 17 Circuit diagrams illustrating different lines of communication involved in visuo-oculo-motor control especially as mediated by the superior colliculus. The basic plan of the diagram is the same in all 4 panels: the neocortex is shown at the top (only area 4, 6 and visual cortex, area 17, specified); thalamic nuclei and basal ganglia in next lower tier, superior colliculus and its variably complex linkages with the oculomotor apparatus toward the bottom (III and VI= oculomotor and abducens nerves). In each panel, retinal fibers lead in from right. In (d), cerebellar and vestibular circuits are added. Pathways considered "active" in each panel are

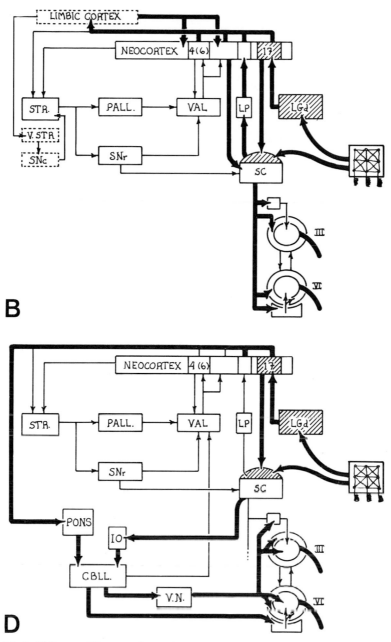

B

D

emphasized in bold lines to illustrate the notion of visual information being routed along multiple lines of conduction each one of which may have a functional peculiarity by virtue of the operations carried out along each route. The channels are viewed as being simultaneously active; they have been pulled apart as though separating the sections of an orchestra, or the themes of a fugue. In the diagrams, the superior colliculus (A), visual cortex and affiliates (B), corpus striatum (C) and cerebellum (D) are emphasized; the type of processing, not the modality, is stressed.

  a)   LORENTE recognized, many years before the celebrated microelectrode studies of
the late 1950's and 1960's (HUBEL and WIESEL, 1959, 1962; MOUNTCASTLE, 1957), the importance of vertical ordering in the neocortex.

"Studies on the fine structure of the cortex have revealed that, although in architectonic pictures
the horizontal stratification seems to be the most important factor in cortical organization, the intracortical connections are established chiefly in vertical directions so that the whole vertical section
of the cortex must be considered as a unitary system."   (p. 339)

  b)   LORENTE suggested that cylindrical volumes of tissue in the neocortex were the
likely units of cortical function (although, of course, he had no means of recognizing
discrete entities).
  [Referring to his classic figure summarizing cortical organization, p. 302]

"The small strip reproduced on the left of figure 63 is the vertical section of a cylinder having a
specific afferent fiber like *a* as axis.   All the elements of the cortex are represented in it, and therefore it may be called an *elementary unit*, in which, theoretically, the whole process of the transmission
of impulses from the afferent fibre to the efferent axon may be accomplished."   (p. 311)

  c)   LORENTE formulated the notion that the neocortex is made up of large numbers of
vertically disposed repeating units cutting across its horizontal layers.

"Thus it comes about that the area striata is composed of an enormous number of vertical
parallelopipedons with the longer horizontal axis parallel to the main system of fibers in the stria of
Gennari and related to the numerous shallow sulci detectable in the surface of the calcarine cortex.
In each parallelopipedon, which has a microscopic size, the thickness of the layers and even the relative number of cells of each type varies between considerable limits.   The drawing of Campbell
(fig. 62) happens to include different parts of two adjacent parallelopipedons."   (p. 316)

  These quotations have been included to demonstrate LORENTE's emphasis on the actual
detailed steric configuration of the neocortex and his idea that the unit of cortical processing (his parallelopipedon, with a deduced discreteness) is a unit that is repeated over and
over again.   These two points clearly lie at the basis also of modern work on the columnar
organization of the neocortex.   But it is important to stress that their implications can be
cast in a more general way.   One of the most important outcomes of anatomical work of
the past five years, attributable to the use of the new tracer techniques, is the realization
that the inherent geometrical arrangement of tissue elements is a crucial fact of central
nervous organization.   Even in noncortical tissue of the brain stem, even in regions where
at first glance the neuropil seems almost completely homogeneous, repeating units or small
compartments have been found to exist.   In some instances the tissue compartments have
been identified by virtue of a systematic fractionation of one or more input systems terminating within a region.   In other instances, the constituent neurons of a region have
been shown to be grouped into units by virtue of particular patterns of efferent fiber projection.   Finally, histochemically distinct compartments have been identified in certain
regions, including two illustrated in this paper: the superior colliculus (Fig. 18), a lay-
ered but non-cortical structure in the midbrain; and the caudate nucleus (Fig. 19), a part
of the cerebral hemisphere that long had been held in contrast to the highly structured cortex as being a more or less uniform, homogeneous collection of neurons.   In the superior
colliculus the histochemical compartmentalization may be related to the discontinuous
pattern in which afferent fibers terminate in that structure.   In the caudate nucleus, the
histochemical findings may reflect efferent compartments in the striatum.   In both instances the compartments thus appear to serve as mechanisms for selective channeling of
information; their particular role in processing of information has not yet been studied.

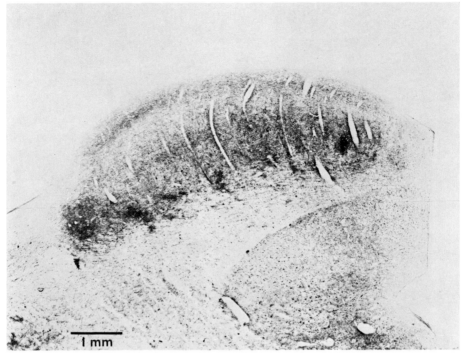

Fig. 18 Histochemically defined compartments in the superior colliculus of the human being visualized by the acetylthiocholinesterase method in a 75 μm thick transverse section. The cholinesterase-rich patches, about 200 μm wide, lie at a depth level corresponding to the intermediate gray layer. They are spaced at roughly 1 mm intervals (refer to GRAYBIEL, in press).

These examples are included here because in both colliculus and caudate nucleus, the use of histochemical techniques has given us the opportunity to extend evidence for compartmentalization to the brain of the human being (GRAYBIEL, in press; GRAYBIEL and RAGSDALE, 1978).

Much as the chemistry of the cell could not be understood without reference to the structural elements that organize the cytoplasm into units, so it seems likely that we will not understand the physiology and anatomy of the brain without taking into account its subdivision into compartments. It would be misleading to say that "columnar organization" is a general characteristic of the mammalian brain. The term has a specific meaning in reference to the structure of the neocortex. But compartmentalization of nervous tissue, observed as a clustering of fiber terminals, neurons or neurotransmitter-related molecules, is clearly not confined to the neocortex (or even to cortex in general); it is more and more appearing to be a very general organizational feature of the brain. The degree to which such compartmentalization represents the consequence of developmental constraints is not yet known. Nor is it clear how the developmental histories of the compartments relate to their role in fractionating the channeling and processing of information in the brain. The very ubiquity of some form of compartmentalization is itself important, however, and leads back to LORENTE's admonition that we must not think of complex circuits—or even circuit arrangements, such as stereometrically defined repeating units— as being limited to what seem to us to be the "complex" parts of the brain, to the cerebral or cerebellar cortex. For in fact, it is probably mainly because we find it natural to think

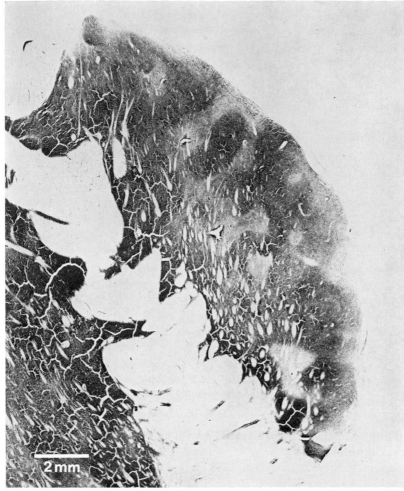

Fig. 19 Photomicrograph illustrating cholinesterase-poor compartments in a 75 μm-thick frontal section through the caudate nucleus of the human being. The enzyme poor-zones are about half a millimeter in diameter and variable in cross-sectional shape (refer to Graybiel and Ragsdale, 1978).

in hierarchies that this limitation would occur to us at all.   In fact, what Lorente de Nó achieved in his 1933 *Archives* paper was a clear demonstration that the most sophisticated connectional patterns yet known to occur in the brain, the patterns which he thought must surely represent the functional units of the nervous system, occur even in the supposedly lowly reflex centers of the brain stem.

ACKNOWLEDGMENTS

I thank the National Science Foundation for support, and Mr. Henry F. Hall and Miss Elaine Yoneoka for their valuable help.

REFERENCES

BERSON, D. M. and GRAYBIEL, A. M.:   Parallel thalamic zones in the LP-pulvinar complex of the cat identified by their afferent and efferent connections. *Brain Res., 147*: 139–148 (1978)

BRAITENBERG, V.:   Functional interpretation of cerebellar histology. *Nature, 190*: 539–540 (1961)

BRAITENBERG, V. and ATWOOD, R. P.:   Morphological observations on the cerebellar cortex. *J. Comp. Neurol., 109*: 1–27 (1958)

BRAUTH, S. and KARTEN, H. J.:   Direct accessory optic projections to the vestibulocerebellum: a possible channel for oculomotor control systems. *Exp. Br. Res., 28*: 73–84 (1977)

BÜTTNER, U., BÜTTNER-ENNEVER, J. A., and HENN, V.:   Vertical eye movement related unit activity in the rostral mesencephalic reticular formation of the alert monkey. *Brain Res., 130*: 239–252 (1977)

BÜTTNER-ENNEVER, J. A. and HENN, V.:   An autoradiographic study of the pathways from the pontine reticular formation involved in horizontal eye movements. *Brain Res., 108*: 155–164 (1976)

CHAN-PALAY, V.:   Serotonin axons in the supra- and subependymal plexuses and in the leptomeninges; their roles in local alterations of cerebrospinal fluid and vasomotor activity. *Brain Res., 102*: 103–130 (1976)

DESCARRIES, L., BEAUDET, A., and WATKINS, K. C.:   Serotonin nerve terminals in adult rat neocortex. *Brain Res., 100*: 563–588 (1975)

FAULL, R. L. M. and MEHLER, W. R.:   Studies of the fiber connections of the substantia nigra in the rat using the method of retrograde transport of horseradish peroxidase. *Neurosci. Abstr., 2*: 62 (1976)

GILBERT, C. D. and KELLY, J. P.:   The projections of cells in different layers of the cat's visual cortex. *J. Comp. Neurol., 163*: 81–106 (1975)

GOULD, B. B. and GRAYBIEL, A. M.:   Afferents to the cerebellar cortex in the cat: Evidence for an intrinsic pathway leading from the deep nuclei to the cortex. *Brain Res., 110*: 601–611 (1976)

GRAYBIEL, A.:   Contributions of the space program to our knowledge of motion sickness. *Acta Astronautica, 17*: 5–25 (1972a)

GRAYBIEL, A. M.:   Some extrageniculate visual pathways in the cat. *Invest Ophthal., 11*: 322–332 (1972b)

GRAYBIEL, A. M.:   Some fiber pathways related to the posterior thalamic region in the cat. *Brain Behav. Evol., 6*: 363–393 (1972c)

GRAYBIEL, A. M.:   Direct and indirect preoculomotor pathways of the brainstem: An autoradiographic study of the pontine reticular formation in the cat. *J. Comp. Neurol., 175*: 37–78 (1977a)

GRAYBIEL, A. M: Organization of oculomotor pathways in the cat and rhesus monkey. *In* BAKER, R. and BERTHOZ, A. (eds.):   *Control of Gaze by Brainstem Interneurons,* pp. 79–88, Elsevier, Amsterdam (1977b)

GRAYBIEL, A. M.:   Organization of the nigrotectal connection: an experimental tracer study in the cat. *Brain Res., 148*: 339–348 (1978)

GRAYBIEL, A. M.:   Periodic-compartmental distribution of acetylcholinesterase in the superior colliculus of the human brain. *Neuroscience,* (1979 in press)

GRAYBIEL, A. M. and HARTWIEG, E. A.:   Some afferent connections of the oculomotor complex in the cat: an experimental study with tracer techniques. *Brain Res., 81*: 543–551 (1974)

GRAYBIEL, A. M., NAUTA, H. J. W., LASEK, R. J. and NAUTA, W. J. H.:   A cerebello-olivary pathway in the cat: An experimental study using autoradiographic tracing techniques. *Brain Res., 58*: 205–211 (1973)

GRAYBIEL, A. M. and RAGSDALE, C. W., Jr.:   Histochemically distinct compartments in the striatum of human being, monkey and cat demonstrated by acetylthiocholinesterase staining method. *Proc. Nat. Acad. Sci., 75*: 5723–5726 (1978)

HAYMAKER, W.:   Hypothalamo-pituitary neural pathways and the circulatory system of the pituitary, *In* HAYMAKER, W., ANDERSON, E. and NAUTA, W. J. H.:   *The Hypothalamus,* pp. 219–250, Charles C Thomas, Springfield, Ill. (1969)

HIKOSAKA, O. and KAWAKAMI, T.:   Inhibitory reticular neurons related to the quick phase of vestibular nystagmus—their location and projection. *Exp. Br. Res., 27*: 377–396 (1977)

HUBEL, D. H. and WIESEL, T. N.: Receptive fields of single neurones in the cat's striate cortex. *J. Physiol., Lond., 148*: 574–591 (1959)

HUBEL, D. H. and WIESEL, T. N.: Receptive fields, binocular interaction and functional architecture in the cat's visual cortex. *J. Physiol., Lond., 160*: 106–154 (1962)

ITO, M.: The vestibulo-cerebellar relationships: vestibulo-ocular reflex arc and flocculus, *In* NAUNTON, R. F. (ed.): *The Vestibular System*, pp. 129–145, Academic Press, New York (1975)

KELLER, E. L.: Participation of medial pontine reticular formation in eye movement generation in monkey. *J. Neurophysiol., 37*: 316–332 (1974)

KING, W. M.: Quantitative analysis of the activity of neurons in the accessory oculomotor nuclei and the mesencephalic reticular formation of alert monkeys in relation to vertical eye movements induced by visual and vestibular stimulation. Doctoral dissertation, University of Washington, Seattle (1976)

KÜNZLE, H.: Bilateral projections from precentral motor cortex to the putamen and other parts of the basal ganglia. An autoradiographic study in *Macaca Fascicularis*. *Brain Res., 88*: 195–209 (1975)

LINDVALL, O., BJÖRKLUND, A., MOORE, R. Y. and STENEVI, U.: Mesencephalic dopamine neurons projecting to neocortex. *Brain Res., 81*: 325–331 (1974)

LORENTE DE NÓ, R.: Vestibulo-ocular reflex arc. *Arch. Neurol. Psychiat., 30*: 245–291 (1933a)

LORENTE DE NÓ, R.: Anatomy of the eighth nerve. The central projection of the nerve endings of the internal ear. *Laryngoscope (St. Louis), 43*: 1–33 (1933b)

LORENTE DE NÓ, R.: Analysis of the activity of the chains of internuncial neurons. *J. Neurophysiology, 1*: 207–244 (1938a)

LORENTE DE NÓ, R.: The cerebral cortex: architecture, intracortical connections and motor projections. *In* FULTON, J. F.: *Physiology of the Nervous System*, pp. 291–325, Oxford University Press, London, (1938b)

MARR, D.: A theory of cerebellar cortex. *J. Physiol., 202*: 437–470 (1969)

MACIEWICZ, R. J., EAGEN, K., KANEKO, C. R. S. and HIGHSTEIN, S. M.: Vestibular and medullary brain stem afferents to the abducens nucleus in the cat. *Brain Res., 123*: 229–240 (1977a)

MACIEWICZ, R. J., ROMAGNANO, M. A., BAKER, R. and HIGHSTEIN, S. M.: Two projections of the oculomotor internuclear neurons. *Anat. Rec., 187*: 642–643 (1977b)

MOUNTCASTLE, V. B.: Modality and topographic properties of single neurons of cat's somatic sensory cortex. *J. Neurophysiol., 20*: 408–434 (1957)

RAKIC, P.: Local circuit neurons. *Neurosci. Res. Prog. Bull., 13*: 291–446 (1975)

ROBINSON, D. A.: Oculomotor control signals. *In* LENNERSTRAND, G. and BACH-Y-RITA, B. (eds.) *Basic Mechanisms of Ocular Motility and Their Clinical Implications*, pp. 337–374, Pergamon Press, Oxford, 1975.

ROSENE, D. L. and VAN HOESEN, G. W.: Hippocampal efferents reach widespread areas of cerebral cortex and amygdala in the rhesus monkey. *Science, 198*: 315–317 (1977)

SHEPHERD, G. M.: The neuron doctrine: a revision of functional concepts. *Yale J. Biol. Med., 45*: 584–599 (1972)

THE PARABDUCENS NUCLEUS

Robert BAKER and Robert McCREA

Department of Physiology and Biophysics, New York University Medical Center
New York, NY

INTRODUCTION

The use of contemporary morphological techniques coupled with electrophysiological studies has now provided convincing evidence for the presence of neurons other than motoneurons both in and around the classically defined borders of the abducens nucleus (Graybiel and Hartwieg, 1974; Baker and Highstein, 1975; Grantyn et al., 1977; Baker and Berthoz, 1977). This paper describes eight potential subclasses of neurons in the abducens nucleus based upon differences in projection and termination sites. As such, these data stress the important role the abducens nucleus must play in the organization of horizontal eye movement. Historically, the abducens nucleus and its immediate surround have been emphasized in the oculomotor literature as being *essential for horizontal conjugate gaze*. In fact, the necessary structural, functional and theoretical organization required to ensure horizontal conjugate eye movement has been embodied by the concept of a 'parabducens nucleus'. Much to our surprise, a search of the oculomotor literature not only showed that it was difficult to determine who first used the term "parabducens nucleus", but also to decide how and on what morphological and physiological grounds it was being employed by different authors. In the first section of this paper, the origin and usage of "parabducens nucleus" is discussed.

Since one purpose of this paper is to comment on further use of the expression parabducens nucleus in oculomotor literature, we have taken into account nearly all existing morphological and physiological studies which either directly or indirectly have referred to a "parabducens nucleus". The second and third sections of this paper deal with early anatomical and physiological work which predate use of the term, but which undoubtedly are in reference to it. When the early work is viewed in perspective with our recent studies, it will be shown that it is relevant to contemporary ideas regarding organization of the abducens nucleus.

Finally, after presenting the different classes of neurons in the abducens nucleus, we discuss whether the parabducens usage should continue in view of our present understanding of the neuronal organization of horizontal gaze. In short, we will suggest that morphologically the concept of the parabducens nucleus has always been too ambiguous and therefore, probably is not meaningful on those grounds. However, conceptually, if one argues that the parabducens nucleus concept refers to a 'class of information' carried by neurons both *in and around* the abducens nucleus, then it might be useful to speak of a parabducens role in horizontal conjugate eye movement as separable from the purely motor task of the abducens nucleus. Even so, we conclude that more experimentation is required before the latter suggestion is worth further consideration.

ORIGIN OF THE TERM "PARABDUCENS NUCLEUS"

Somewhat surprisingly, the expression "parabducens nucleus" appears to have been first used in a *textbook description* of lateral gaze by Strong and Elwyn in 1943. These authors employed it because they wanted to describe the central mechanism underlying conjugate lateral eye movement in a simple fashion. It is our surmise that they adopted the expression, "parabducens" as a result of the influence of H. ALSOP RILEY who contributed heavily to their textbook.* In 1930 RILEY stated "In certain instances when the abducens nucleus was completely destroyed, there was loss of movement in the ipsilateral eye outward but retention of conjugate movement of the contralateral eye inward". Although the latter contention was erroneous, he obviously concluded that "the center for lateral eye movement" could not be situated directly in the abducens nucleus itself (see Figure 1). Even so, other evidence, mostly from pathological material, indicated that the center must be close to the abducens nucleus which led RILEY to conclude that it was not identical with, *but situated in the vicinity of*, the abducens nucleus. RILEY did not use "parabducens nucleus" either in text or in diagram, but instead labeled the area as "center for lateral gaze" (see Figure 1).

The first paper to actually show a figure clearly labeling the 'parabducens nucleus' as such, was CROSBY's in 1950. As indicated in Figure 1 (lower right) she cautiously abbreviated it "P.Ab." Although a reason was not explicitly expressed in that paper, CROSBY stated that "the abducens nucleus proper consisted of *large neurons* from which arose motor fibers of the abducens nerve and *small cells* forming the parabducens nucleus". The latter neurons were believed to send fascicles through the homolateral MLF to the nucleus of Perlia [an incorrect view from a textbook by SPIEGEL and SOMMER (1944)]. In her 1953 paper CROSBY took a more definitive stance toward localizing the parabducens nucleus. She stated that "In the reticular gray *adjacent to* the abducens nucleus and *intermingled with* the abducens neurons are *small associative cells* which constitute the parabducens nucleus". It was clear that even while doing so, the author herself did not have any new supportive experimental data and, again, referred back to the textbook of STRONG and ELWYN (1948 edition rather than the 1943 one). As has already been mentioned, their viewpoint was not apparently based upon any documented experimentation. After evaluating the paper by COGAN, KUBIK and SMITH (1950), CROSBY in the 1953 paper correctly placed the fibers related to conjugate deviation as ascending in the contralateral MLF.

In the early 1960's the notion that the parabducens nucleus was a "center for horizontal eye movement" was attacked on the grounds that it was both an anatomical and physio-

---

* Even though STRONG and ELWYN (1943) assumed RILEY's logic that cell groups in the nearby reticular formation close to the motor cells of the abducens nucleus gave rise to internuclear or interocular fibers they admitted to the reader that the course of such an ascending tract had not been determined. However, they made an interesting change in the transition between their diagram and RILEY's. Note that RILEY had connections from the center for lateral gaze passing contralaterally to the abducens nucleus, and ipsilaterally up to the internal rectus. Without explanation, RILEY stated exactly the opposite in his text! Namely, that fibers originated in the homolateral abducens nucleus and then decussated to travel to the oculomotor nucleus by the contralateral MLF. In contrast, STRONG and ELWYN showed the associative neurons to originate in ipsilateral abducens nucleus and ascend up the ipsilateral MLF to terminate on medial rectus motoneurons which then decussated to innervate the contralateral internal rectus. CROSBY in both the 1950 and 1953 paper apparently solved this pathway problem by showing medial rectus motoneurons in both the ipsi- and contralateral oculomotor complex, but she associated the internuclear fibers with the ascending contralateral MLF (see text). For inexplicable reasons, all these authors were evidently not aware of prior studies which could have supported their diagrams and statements.

Riley 1930

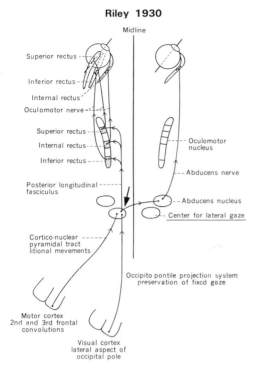

Strong and Elwyn 1943

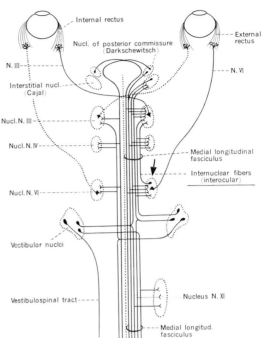

Fig. 1 Diagrams showing internuclear connections between the abducens and oculomotor nucleus. All diagrams are reproduced exactly as they appeared in the original articles. The only modifications are 1) the arrows which point out cellular origin of the internuclear connections and 2) the expression each author uses to refer to the lateral gaze center is underlined. The diagram on the upper left is Figure 4, "Mechanism for lateral deviation of gaze" reproduced from page 652 of the article by RILEY, H. A.: *Arch. Ophthalmol., 4*: 640–661. ⓒ 1930, American Medical Association. The diagram on the upper right is Figure 202, "Diagram showing some of the important components of the medial longitudinal fasciculus" obtained from the physiological textbook by STRONG, O. S. and ELWYN, A.: Human Neuroanatomy. ⓒ 1943 The Williams & Wilkins Co., Baltimore. The insert on the lower right shows, Figure 2, "Diagram of certain vestibular connections underlying conjugate deviation of the eyes in the horizontal plane" acquired from CROSBY, E. C.: *J. Neurosurg., 7*: 566–183, 1950. Also shown on the lower right, is Figure 2, "A diagram showing some connections of the vestibular system related to horizontal conjugate deviation of the eyes" reproduced from a later article by CROSBY, E. C.: *J. Comp. Neurol., 99*: 437–479, 1953. Permission to reproduce these diagrams has been obtained from the publications in which they appeared.

Crosby 1953

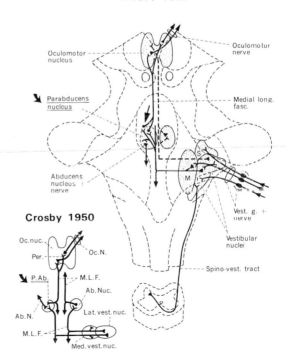

Crosby 1950

logical misconception.   In fact, BENDER and SHANZER (1964) used that precise expression. Even though they admitted that it would be a convenient structure to serve as an anatomical substrate for a complex gaze mechanism, they rightly attacked CROSBY's ambiguous description of the nucleus; (i.e. the idea that the parabducens nucleus consisted of *small cells adjacent to* the abducens nucleus and *intermingled with* the abducens motoneurons.) We believe these authors were expressing the concern of most experimental neurologists at that time which was trepidation about the rapid inclusion of the term parabducens into the neurological textbooks.   The tenuous nature of the CROSBY scheme was pointed out well in the article by BENDER and SHANZER (1964; page 134 and 135) who closely scrutinized the papers and experimental work which the hypothesis was based on.   They pointed out that in addition to the STRONG and ELWYN (1943) textbook the only other reference employed by CROSBY was to CRANMER (1951) who, in only indirect fashion, supported the postulate of a parabducens nucleus.   In a more general sense, *all* participants at the oculomotor symposium in 1964 were doubtful of the existence of a center for horizontal eye movement.   In principle, they were not against areas *near to* the abducens nucleus either rostral or ventral to it participating in some manner of integration for oculomotor function, but, at the same time, they did not want to either justify or invoke a center, i.e. an anatomic locality subserving a specific function, without evidence.

Other more tangible (i.e. experimental) reasons for not accepting a postulated parabducens nucleus surfaced following the oculomotor symposium.   The most significant was general agreement that one could distinctly separate the oculomotor disorders following either MLF or tegmental lesions (ventrally situated paramedian reticular lesions) into two classes (CARPENTER and HANNA, 1962; CARPENTER and STROMINGER, 1965).   In a sense, the BENDER (1964) denunciation of the parabducens concept was based upon his knowledge that impairment of adduction in the homolateral eye (a paresis) and associated contralateral abductor nystagmus was due to a MLF lesion and that a lesion in the paramedian pontine tegmentum produced paralysis of horizontal conjugate ocular movement (BENDER and WEINSTEIN, 1944, 1950).   As thoroughly summarized in recent years by many authors, evidence was put forward in the late 60's that the paramedian pontine reticular area provided a unique neuro-organization and function for horizontal eye movements somewhat different from that entailed by the parabducens nucleus concept (CARPENTER, 1971; COHEN, 1971; COHEN and HENN, 1972; BAKER and BERTHOZ, 1977; FUCHS, 1977).   Morphological and physiological evidence, especially neuronal correlate-data, accumulated rapidly indicating the pontine reticular area to be substantively more influential, in a hierarchial supranuclear sense, as a brainstem center (see GRAYBIEL, 1977; BÜTTNER-ENNEVER and HENN, 1976; RAPHAN and COHEN, 1978; BAKER and BERTHOZ 1977 for reviews).   In recent years the latter belief often included the necessity for postulating that reticular neurons whose axons ascended in (or juxta-to) the MLF (NAUTA and KUYPERS, 1958; BÜTTNER-ENNEVER and HENN, 1976) might explain the adductive paresis following MLF lesion.   Assuming the latter viewpoint, the MLF lesions and the subsequent eye movement deficits were viewed as only a problem of interfering with one leg, or branch, of the reticular system.   Given the absence of any new and compelling data, either morphological or physiological, concerning neurons in and around the abducens nucleus, then certainly the above authors could not be criticized for their beliefs.   On the other hand after reviewing the earlier literature, it is clear that many experimental studies concerning the abducens nucleus were overlooked, misinterpreted but, most of all, ignored!

EARLY ANATOMICAL WORK

The perspective which is to follow has used, as a stepping stone, the bibliography included in the excellent survey of the literature by M. B. CARPENTER et al. in their work concerning the MLF (1962, 1965) and disturbances of conjugate horizontal eye movements following abducens and MLF lesions (1963, 1971). Interestingly, CARPENTER et al., due to cautious interpretation of their own data, never supported the concept of parabducens nucleus even though careful review of their results indicates that their observations were compatible with the idea. Unfortunately, the physiological evidence at the time was leaning largely towards the pontine reticular formation as a preferential site for the *initiation of all* horizontal conjugate eye movements and, therefore, neurons in and around the abducens nucleus were to be largely ignored. Yet, nearly every anatomical study ever reported provided some evidence that not all neurons in the abducens motor nucleus were motoneurons!

Without a doubt, the first creditable morphological and physiological description of the parabducens nucleus as an entity dates back to over a century ago. GRAUX (1878) in his doctoral dissertation clearly pointed out for the first time *not only the theoretical but also the actual anatomical* basis for internuclear pathways between the oculomotor and abducens nucleus. Neurons, other than motoneurons, with axons projecting anterior towards the oculomotor complex were postulated on the basis of anatomical evidence. Out of necessity, these observations were based upon use of the MARCHI technique whose merit and interpretive value were already much discussed and debated at that time (CAJAL, 1909). In Van GEHUCHTEN's (1904) detailed review article concerning vestibular, reticular and oculomotor pathways GRAUX's work was not referenced; however, many other studies supportive of his findings were mentioned. Both BRUCE (1903) and FRASER (1903) contended that ascending fibers in the MLF originated from the nucleus of nerve VI and were present in the cat. Both THOMAS (1903) and Van GEHUCHTEN (1898 and 1904) disagreed with the latter contention because of the absence of retrograde chromalytic reaction in nucleus VI neurons following lesion of the MLF. Van GEHUCHTEN even made the statement that "Nous croyons en effect, avoir démontré que, après section du nerf VI, *toutes les cellules du noyaux "origine se mettent en chromolyse"* (1904). The latter was categorically a strong stance and Van GEHUCHTEN supported it at least on two separate occasions in the 1904 article (pp. 44 and 57). We cannot, of course, know how much the finding of Van GEHUCHTEN was predicated upon the work of CAJAL or if he even was aware of CAJAL's work at that time. In none of the earlier papers before 1900 or in his later collected work (1909), did CAJAL ever mention neurons other than abducens motoneurons in the abducens nucleus. His Golgi presentation of only abducens motoneurons on Page 854 (1909) reflects that opininon. However, CAJAL refers to work by STILLING, NEYVERT, CLARKE and DUVAL who, in the anterior region of the abducens nucleus, had visualized axons ascending toward the facial nerve. Although he indicated that modern histologists (referring to those of his time) could not confirm with any direct technique such conjecture his negative reasoning was actually based more on the absence of any retrograde chromatolysis in the abducens nucleus following section of the facial nerve. As is shown in Figures 4, 11 and 12, the axons of internuclear neurons were probably the ones visualized by the earlier workers because these fibers ascend dorsally toward the facial nerve to enter the MLF. CAJAL was well aware that synergistic contraction of the medial and lateral rectus was required for abduction and adduction of the ocular globe, but he chose to explain the synergy by supposing (incorrectly) that vestibular fibers gave direct collaterals to the abducens and medial rectus motoneurons.

Other morphological studies by TSUCHIDA (1906) and FUSE (1912) clearly demonstrated internuclear pathways based upon brainstem lesions which 1) severed the root fibers of the abducens nerve, 2) interrupted the MLF at the oculomotor level and 3) split the MLF slightly rostral to the abducens nucleus.   Collectively, this work showed that severence of the abducens nerve did not cause all large cells in the abducens nucleus to disappear and secondly that there was loss of cells in the abducens nucleus following interruption of the MLF thereby indicating that axons originated from cells in this area and ascended in the MLF bundle.   These two lengthy papers contain such sufficient undeniable evidence that alone they could have substantiated the parabducens concept.   Yet they did not differ much in content and conclusion from the work of GRAUX in 1878.   The early physiological work which paralleled the above anatomical studies was equally as clear and it is mentioned next in combination with later morpho-physiological studies.

EARLY PHYSIOLOGICAL WORK

One of the most remarkable papers concerning a center for lateral eye movement is that by BENNETT and SAVILL (1889) entitled "Case of Permanent Conjugate Deviation of the Eyes and Head: The Result of a Lesion Limited to the Sixth Nucleus".   The lesion in the sixth nucleus is shown as an inset in Figure 2.   These authors found that with a lesion on the left, both eyes were *firmly* and *permanently* fixed towards the right side and the strongest voluntary effort could barely bring them towards the midline.   In this regard, the left eye was especially deficient.   Both eyes converged when an object was brought close to them.   The head was firmly and permanently rotated towards the right and could not voluntarily be brought into a straight position.   It is interesting to point out that the diagnosis of a sixth nucleus lesion was made during life in the patient and afterwards proved by postmortem examination to have been correct i.e. the ocular phenomenon was due to a lesion of the sixth nucleus. The remarkable point is that these authors were not only able to recognize and describe such a lesion restricted to a minute area, but they would not even take credit for establishing that the sixth nucleus was the reflex center presiding over a "complicated automatism by which the eyes, head and neck move harmoniously in concert".   Instead, they gave the credit to other authors such as LANDOUZY 1876, GRAUX 1878, DUVAL and LABORDE 1880 and GAREL 1882.   Although BENNETT and SAVILL were not aware of FOVILLE's (1858) clinical observations*, the fashion in which they summarized

---

* According to DUVAL and LABORDE (1880), ANDRAL first noted in 1834, paralysis of conjugate deviation of the eyes.   Similar clinical observations were also reported by MILLARD (*Bulletin de la Société Anatomique* 1856) and GUBLER (*Gazette hebdomadaire* 1858).   Yet, in the opinion of HUNNIUS (1881), FOVILLE (1858) really deserves most credit for first postulating a center for lateral gaze situated near the abducens nucleus (rather than the more frequently cited LUTZ (1923) and SPILLER (1924) papers.   Notably, RILEY in 1930 refers to the syndrome of internuclear ophthalmoplegia as "The Syndrome of FOVILLE".   FOVILLE's findings on horizontal gaze paralysis were extended by DESNOS (*Bulletin de la Société médicale des hôpitaux* 1873), HALLOPEAU (Archives de physiologie 1876) and FÉRÉOL (*Bulletin de la Société médicale des hôpitaux* 1873).   FÉRÉOL (1873) was likely the first person to clearly diagnose and report a case with autopsy.   In fact, paralysis of conjugate eye movements in the subsequent experimental work of DUVAL, LABORDE and GRAUX was referred to as the "Malade de FÉRÉOL".   In 1877 DUVAL and LABORDE were already emphasizing fibers in the MLF arising from the sixth nucleus.   Later their colleague GRAUX made this topic the subject of his thesis study (1878).   DUVAL and LABORDE then published their results (1880) which completely corroborated the GRAUX work.   Notably, all of these studies included experimental production of strabismus and other conjugate eye movement disorders by central lesions.   Later, BECHTEREW (1899) distinguished between internuclear and vestibular origin of fibers in the MLF by observing that internuclear fibers were smaller and developed later than those derived from the vestibular nucleus.   Finally the much debated issue of whether internuclear fibers terminated in the oculomotor nucleus or entered the third nerve rootlets (BLOCQ and GUINON, 1891), was resolved in favor of the former hypothesis by FRASER (1901 and 1903).

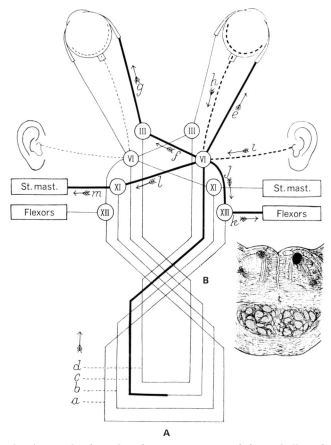

Fig. 2 Diagram showing mechanism of conjugate movements of the eyeballs and rotation of the head and neck (from BENNETT and SAVILL, 1889). "The dark lines represent the voluntary motor tract from the cortex to the sixth nucleus, as well as the efferent tracts from this centre by which conjugate movements of the eyeballs, head and neck are accomplished. The dotted lines indicate the afferent tracts from the eye and ear to the sixth nucleus. The arrows show the direction of the different nerve currents. The diagram attempts to show how various connections may take place and the relation that exists between he sixth and eleventh nuclei of opposite sides, and between the former and the cervical ganglia on the same side. An impulse, whether voluntary (c), or from sensory impressions, (h and i) acting on the sixth nucleus (VI), through its influence will cause contraction of the external rectus (e) and the flexors of the neck (k) through connections with the cervical ganglia (XIII) on the same side; and simultaneously contrtaction of the internal rectus (g), and the sternomastoid (m) through the eleventh nucleus (XI) of the opposite side. The result of this is a conjugate movement of both eyeballs, and a rotation and inclination of the head towards the side of the sixth nucleus which receives and distributes the impulse. Destruction of this centre would of course, have exactly the opposite effects. The inset on the lower right shows a transverse section of the pons at the level of the sixth nucleus showing a limited softening of that centre from which the authors based their observations. A. Cortex Cerebri: a. Voluntary tract from cortex to cervical ganglia; b. Ditto to eleventh nucleus; c. Ditto to sixth nucleus; d. Ditto to third nucleus; B. Decussation of voluntary motor trtacts in medulla and pons; III. Third nucleus; VI. Sixth nucleus; XI. Eleventh nucleus; XIII. Upper cervical ganglia; e. Motor fibres from sixth nucleuss to external rectus; f. Crossed tract between third and sixth nuclei; g. Motor fibres from third nucleus to internal rectus; h. Afferent tract from retina to sixth nucleus; i. Afferent tract from ear to sixth nucleus; j. Communicating tract between sixth nucleus and cervical ganglia on the same side; k. Motor nerve from cervical ganglia to flexors of neck; l. Crossed tract between sixth and eleventh nuclei of opposite sides; m. Motor nerve from eleventh nucleus to sterno-mastoid muscle." (This figure and its legend have been reproduced by permission of the Journal exactly as they appeared in the paper by BENNETT and SAVILL in 1889.)

the conjugate gaze mechanism as affected following a sensory flash of light or any sensory stimulus which reflexly produces conjugate gaze was insightful.

"Sensory impression is conveyed to the corresponding sixth nucleus exciting there a motor impulse which is directly carried by the sixth nerve to the external rectus, thus causing the contraction of that muscle. This eye takes a lead in the action and moves outward. Almost simultaneously the motor impulse is directed by a cross-communicating tract to the third nucleus of the opposite side and through this by fibers in the third nerve to the internal rectus muscle which also contracts. Thus both eyeballs are directed toward the light or sound, the sixth nucleus being the reflex centre by which the combined act is carried on"!

The diagram which these authors provided supports a mechanism for reflex conjugate eye movement organized as a special center in the sixth nucleus (Figure 2). Surprisingly, it even includes special cortical wiring which projects to the third nucleus so that vergence is present in the absence of paralyzed conjugate movement. Not only do the authors include the appropriate cortical decussations, but also their subsequent neurological analysis indicated that they could discern lesions at various levels of the neuroaxis with great facility. The above description of circuitry relating only to reflex and/or voluntary eye movement, was realized to be more complicated by these authors because during targeting, both the eyes and head act conjugately so the latter is rotated and inclined to look over the shoulder. Thus they added a more intricate series of connections to the mechanism already formulated. But in so doing, importantly, *insisted* that the sixth nucleus acted as a primary starting point for *all* the latter functions. Since they were well aware that head movement is effected by rotation and partly by inclination they appropriately included the rotators sterno-mastoid and trapezius and the spleenius, recti and other muscles on the same side supplied by cervical nerves and carefully depicted the relationships between the sixth and the eleventh nuclei of the opposite side and the flow of traffic which would result in a conjugate eye movement and rotation and/or inclination of the head towards the sixth nucleus which receives and distributes the impulses. Destruction of this center, would of course, have exactly the opposite effect of its stimulation. Finally, concerning the mechanism of this highly complex physiological phenomenon, these authors stated that

"Conjugate movement of the eyeballs and head, is an act which partly, by inheritance and partly by education, has become organized in the nervous centres, reflexly in the pons, by volition in the cerebral cortex. The two are intimately connected by connecting elements which decussate in the pontine region, possibly at the corpora quadrigemina. The apparently simple act of head and eyes looking in concert towards an object, is carried on by a diverse system of nerves and muscles which have no anatomical relation one with the other, but all of which, excited by a suitable stimulus, and through the agency of a common centre act harmoniously together to effect the physiological purpose desired. Any disturbance of this centre involves derangement of the conjugate phenomenon as a whole, but leaves the individual elements with the exception of the sixth nerve, to act normally for any other purpose, and any other form except that of conjugation"!

The conclusions from other early work concerning the syndrome following either the abducens nucleus or MLF lesion were essentially the same as those by BENNETT and SAVILL (FOVILLE, 1858; GAREL, 1882; BLOCQ and GIUNON, 1891; BENVENUTI, 1901; D'ESPINE and DÉMOLE, 1917). Unfortunately following the turn of the century much of the latter experimental work was forgotten and the sequence of events presented in the first part of the paper began to de-emphasize the abducens nucleus as being the origin for the increasingly well delineated symptomotology of internuclear ophthalmoplegia following either abducens nucleus or MLF lesion. Van GEHUCHTEN (1904), HOLMES (1921) MUSKENS (1913/14) and CAJAL (1909) did not utilize the parabducens nucleus concept (in the sense of CROSBY; page 3 and 4) to explain paralysis of conjugate lateral eye movement. Even so, in all of these studies, it was assumed that the abducens and oculomotor nuclei were connected by association fibers and these pathways were concerned with reflex movements and adjustment of the eye. But in response to the question of origin of these fibers, all authors opted for an anatomical hypothesis which assumed the separate existence of a supranuclear center in the neighborhood of the nucleus of the sixth nerve. Each author had individual themes on where they would place the central gaze center. HOLMES (1921) (for a reason not stated) shows a place oral and slightly ventral to the abducens nucleus (probably in the pontine reticular formation) and assumed that all impulses which excited conjugate lateral movement reached that center. MUSKENS (1913/14) in a superb article integrating his own experimental findings and the original work of others with clinical cases, presents a figure (Figure 14, p. 404) analyzing the vestibular system and the localization of fiber tracts in the MLF. If one ignores termination sites then the topographical organization he describes for the ascending and descending components in the MLF is remarkably accurate. However, he is openly critical of the possibility of axons emanating from neurons within the abducens nucleus as well as their utilizing the MLF as an internuclear pathway (pp. 413–419). The latter inferences were supported by the prior studies of Van GEHUCHTEN (1898 and 1904) and the later work of HOLMES (1921), WARWICK (1953) and CARPENTER et al. (1963), who maintained that extirpation of the sixth nerve produced nearly, if in fact not complete, retrograde chromatolysis of *all* cells in the abducens nucleus. Therefore, the constellation of signs referred to as internuclear ophthalmoplegia had to be produced by neurons located elsewhere in the brainstem. Following the work describing MLF lesions in the cat (CARPENTER and HANNA, 1962) and monkey (CARPENTER and McMASTERS, 1963; CARPENTER and STROMINGER, 1965) a strong argument was mounted that lateral gaze paralysis seen in the MLF syndrome was of vestibular origin (i.e. it was assumed that interruption of secondary vestibular fibers traversing first the abducens nucleus and then entering the opposite MLF accounted for the paresis of ocular adduction). This hypothesis was later abandoned when it became clear from work by these same authors (McMASTERS et al., 1966) as well as others (UEMURA and COHEN, 1973) that this was not the case. Subsequently, the search for a site for paralysis of lateral gaze moved to the pontine reticular formation in which primarily, the origin (i.e. site) for quick phases of nystagmus and saccades concerned most physiologists (LORENTE DE NÓ, 1933; SHIMAZU, this volume). It could be argued that until the work described in the next section was initiated, all prior data could be, and often were, reduced to the suggestion that both slow and rapid eye movements were generated by the pontine reticular formation and communicated directly via MLF pathways to the oculomotor and abducens nucleus (BAKER and BERTHOZ, 1977; RAPHAN and COHEN, 1978). That hypothesis is no longer acceptable.

In the last part of this paper we provide new evidence which requires re-evaluation of the abducens nucleus and its surround. Although we are not in favor of complicating oculomotor organization any more than it already is, to underemphasize the new data would be to repeat recent history in which some findings were slighted in favor of more attractive, but eventually less sound hypotheses. In the next section the individual neuronal elements observed, *to date*, within the confines of the abducens nucleus are described. The term parabducens nucleus and its future role in oculomotor literature is then discussed from that perspective.

THE ABDUCENS NUCLEUS

According to CAJAL (1909) the cat abducens nucleus consists of an ovoid group of cells in the dorsal pontine reticular formation bordered by the ascending tract of the facial nerve and contained within its hook.   He pointed out the difficulty of trying to limit rostrally or caudally the border of the abducens nucleus as it mixes with the longitudinal fasciculi and cells of the reticular substance.   CAJAL's Golgi studies show only motor cells (i.e. abducens motoneurons) in the abducens nucleus.   That such a situation might not be the case was first suggested by the absence of retrograde reaction product in some cells following HRP injection in the lateral rectus muscle (GACEK, 1974; confirmed by SPENCER and STERLING, 1977).   The first electrophysiological experiment which definitively differentiated abducens motoneurons from other neurons within the abducens nucleus was that of BAKER and HIGHSTEIN (1975; see BAKER, 1977 for more recent work).   Interestingly, the HRP studies suggested that abducens motoneurons were distributed more widely than anticipated on the basis of either Nissl or Golgi studies.   Our morphological and electrophysiological experiments have indicated that motoneurons may lie either lateral, medial or even superficial to the genu of the facial nerve (see Figures 5 and 6).   Thus, abducens motoneurons are scattered in a more or less centrifugal fashion encircling the arc of the seventh nerve as it courses in the dorsal pons.   Given such a dispersed population, the question arises as how to best define the boundaries of the abducens nucleus.   The problem is even of more concern when the extensive dendritic ramifications of individual motoneurons are taken into consideration (Figures 3, 4, 5, 11).   CAJAL's Golgi impregnations of cat abducens motoneurons showed extensive dendritic ramifications medial, lateral and especially posterior-lateral to the genu of the facial nerve.   He stated that "Many of the extensions of abducens motoneurons stay in the limitation of the nucleus, but many others go beyond it.   *It is a detail which has here, its importance*".   CAJAL, specifically pointed out dendrites which extended posterior and lateral and even crossed the facial nerve to terminate in or near what he called the dorsal vestibular nucleus.   In addition, he pointed out internal (i.e. medial) dendrites heading toward the MLF and articulating around the fascicles, as well as the anterior (i.e. ventral) dendrites which extended outside the nucleus to accompany the axons into the ventral reticular formation.

Similar extensive dendritic ramifications were observed by LORENTE DE NÓ (1933) in the mouse and these *characteristic features are evident* in all our reconstructed abducens motoneurons (Figure 5).   Both CAJAL and LORENTE DE NÓ suggested that the dendritic tree outside the defined boundaries of the abducens nucleus was equally as important to that inside the nucleus in respect to afferent input.   In this context we believe that many internuclear neurons clearly lie in the region containing the dendrites of the abducens motoneurons and they do so in order to receive the same afferent signal as the motoneurons.   Such an interdigitated arrangement is supported by our observation that reconstructed dendritic trees of putative internuclear neurons lying outside the defined boundaries of the abducens nucleus ramify throughout the nucleus (see Figure 11).   For our description of the different classes of neurons in the abducens nucleus we have drawn the boundaries of the abducens nucleus based upon cellular topography from Nissl stained sections.   Although determination of the border is rather arbitrary, it is not yet either crucial or limiting in respect to the parabducens concept, especially given our limited level of understanding the role(s) subserved by these various classes of neurons.

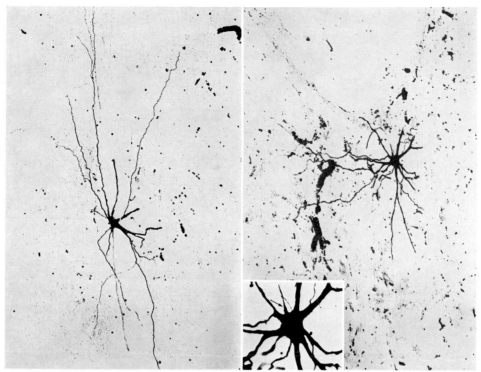

Fig. 3 Abducens motoneurons injected with HRP. Microphotograph of the axons and soma-dendritic trees of motoneurons located ventral (on the left) and dorsal (on the right) in the abducens nucleus. The inset on right shows the dorsal location of the axon hillock of the motoneuron at higher magnification. Note how the axon curves dorsally to bend under the genu before descending in the sixth nerve.

ABDUCENS MOTONEURONS

The foremost population of neurons in the abducens nucleus (and hopefully not the minority) are the abducens motoneurons themselves. Two antidromically identified cat abducens motoneurons injected with HRP are shown in Figure 3. Although the motoneuron on the left showed only 6 major dendrites, each ramified extensively and spread in the directions suggested by CAJAL and LORENTE DE NÓ. The dorsal-ventral extent of the dendritic tree was 2.7 mm. The abducens motoneuron shown on the right in Figure 3 was situated directly under the genu of the facial nerve. This motoneuron exhibited a more bushy dendritic tree and clearly had an axon directed dorsally towards the genu of the seventh nerve before it curved to descend ventrally to join the sixth nerve. The axon hillock of this motoneuron is shown in the inset at higher magnification. We have not yet observed axon collaterals from any antidromically identified abducens motoneuron (sample of about 30 HRP stained motoneurons). An interesting difference from the CAJAL Golgi material is that adult cat abducens motoneurons (Figure 3, 4 and 11) do not exhibit numerous dendritic spines. Considerable reabsorption of spine apparatus must take place between the young and adult material. Finally, motoneurons exhibit wide differences in size and shape (Van GEHUCHTEN, 1898; SPENCER and STERLING, 1977), and even fusiform motoneurons similar to the internuclear neurons shown in Figure 10 have been observed (McCREA and BAKER, 1978).

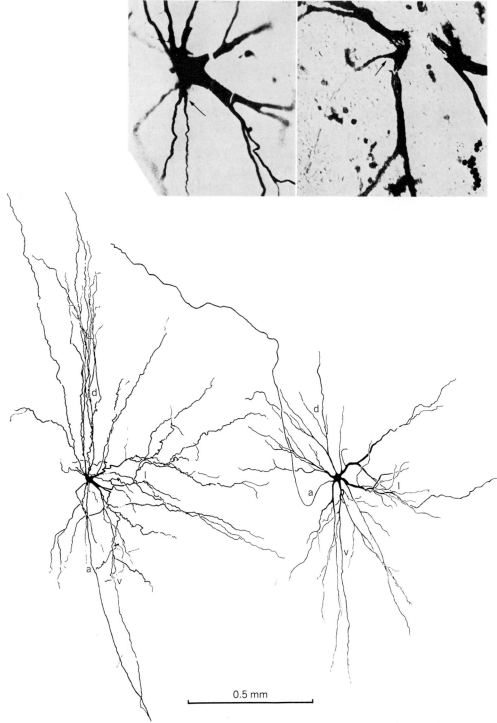

Fig. 4 Soma-dendritic profiles of a reconstructed abducens motoneuron and internuclear neuron. HRP was injected in an abducens motoneuron (on the left) and an internuclear neuron with an axon directed caudal in the medulla (on the right). a, axon of the two neurons, v, l and d indicate the ventral, lateral and dorsal directed dendritic trees, respectively. The upper two insets show the axon hillock of each cell at higher magnification.

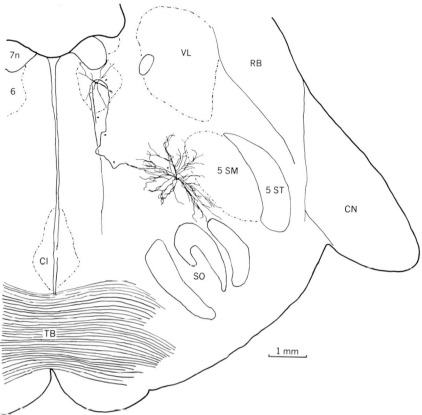

Fig. 5 A coronal brainstem section showing a reconstructed retractor bulbi motoneuron in the accessory abducens nucleus. The axonal trajectory of the retractor bulbi motoneuron has been marked with arrows. The axon of a partially reconstructed abducens motoneuron is also shown at the same coronal level.

RETRACTOR BULBI MOTONEURONS

Another class of motoneurons, referred to as retractor bulbi (or oculi) motoneurons, have been identified in the abducens nucleus.   According to recent work as many as 30 % of the motoneurons in the abducens nucleus innervate retractor bulbi muscle (SPENCER, 1978).   If such a high percentage is true then it suggests peripheral bifurcation of many abducens motoneurons.   The latter possibility is supported by our observation that axotomized abducens motoneurons prevented from reinnervating lateral rectus muscle may contact the retractor bulbi (DELGADO et al., 1978).   It is not yet clear whether a) retractor bulbi motoneurons from a separate and distinguishable class of cells within the abducens nucleus *and/or* b) whether some abducens motoneurons bifurcate peripherally in the orbit to innervate the retractor bulbi and lateral rectus muscle (CRANDALL et al., 1977; BAKER, 1977).   Recently, SPENCER (1978) has confirmed Van GEHUCHTEN's (1898) observation that "A specific nucleus for retractor bulbi motoneurons called *the accessory nucleus of the sixth nerve* is situated ventral and lateral to the abducens nucleus".   In addition, we also have documented TERNI's (1922) demonstration that motoneurons of the accessory abducens nucleus innervate retractor bulbi muscle by intracellular injection of HRP into antidromically identified motoneurons (Figure 5). Intriguingly, the axons of motoneurons in the accessory abducens nucleus ascend to traverse the abducens nucleus before descending ventrally in the sixth nerve. No axon collaterals were observed, thus suggesting that all motoneurons (at least those with axons in the sixth nerve) are without central collateralization. For the present, we must conclude that retractor bulbi muscle may be innervated by motoneurons located in both the accessory abducens as well as the abducens nucleus. Given the interest of this paper in citing the older literature, it is worth noting that LUGARO (1894), PACETTI (1896), SIEMERLING and BOEDEKER (1897) and GIANNULLI (1897) (from CAJAL, 1909 and Van GEHUCHTEN, 1898) had also observed the location of these multipolar cells in axotomized material and suggested their axons exited the brainstem with those of abducens motoneurons!

INTERNUCLEAR NEURONS IN THE ABDUCENS NUCLEUS

GRAYBIEL and HARTWIEG (1974) were the first to demonstrate in an unambiguous fashion the existence of neurons in the abducens nucleus sending axons toward the oculomotor complex. This fundamental finding has now been confirmed in many laboratories (for review, see BAKER, 1977) and one of the nicest studies to date has been the double labeling experiment of STEIGER and BÜTTNER-ENNEVER (1978). By the use of Evans blue in the lateral rectus muscle and HRP in the oculomotor complex, these authors were able to show the distribution of abducens (and/or retractor bulbi motoneurons) and ascending internuclear neurons in the abducens nucleus (Figure 6). Their results show a tendency for a rostral location of internuclear neurons, but for the most part clusters (i.e. groups) of internuclear neurons are *distributed* throughout the abducens nucleus. Especially noticeable is the distribution of internuclear neurons and abducens motoneurons as they curve laterally around the genu of the facial nerve.

The above morphological findings were confirmed by electrophysiological studies (BAKER and HIGHSTEIN, 1975) in which intracellular records were obtained from internuclear neurons antidromically identified from electrical stimulation of the oculomotor complex (as depicted in the diagram of Figure 7). The inset in the upper left shows an intracellular record from an antidromically identified internuclear neuron (Oc) and the absence of antidromic activation following supramaximal stimulation of the lateral rectus nerve (Abd). The widespread distribution of internuclear neurons has also received electrophysiological support. Finally, the intracellular injection of HRP (see Figures 4 and 11) has indicated the axonal trajectory of internuclear neurons to always be directed towards the MLF. In addition, internuclear neurons *do not have recurrent intrinsic axon collaterals* within the abducens nucleus. The latter finding, if it continues without exception in future work, may be an *essential* one for understanding the organization of horizontal eye movement.

Since their rediscovery, we have envisioned the ascending internuclear projection to be of significant importance for mediating *immediate* supranuclear conjugate eye movement signals to medial rectus motoneurons (i.e. to subserve the role assigned to the parabducens nucleus). Given the absence of axon collateralization in the abducens nucleus, these neurons could not provide the immediate supranuclear signal for horizontal eye movements to abducens motoneurons. HIGHSTEIN and BAKER (1978) demonstrated that stimulation at various sites along the ascending internuclear pathway (i.e. the abducens motor nucleus, MLF, etc) produced a powerful excitation in MR Mns (Figure 7, inset on the lower left). In addition, appropriate synaptic potentials, i.e. vestibular and reticular EPSPs and IPSPs

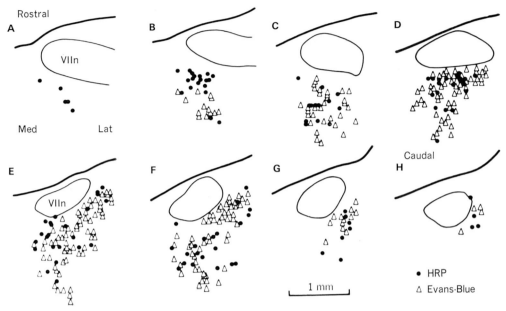

Fig. 6 Double labeling of internuclear and abducens motoneurons. HRP was injected in the oculomotor complex and Evans blue in the lateral rectus muscle. The distributions of motoneurons and internuclear neurons are shown at 240 micron intervals from the rostral to the caudal part of the abducens nucleus. (Summarized from Figure 3 in the paper of STEIGER and BÜTTNER-ENNEVER 1978 by permission of the authors).

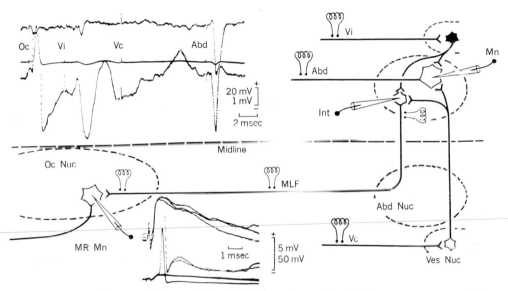

Fig. 7 Intracellular records from an identified internuclear and medial rectus motoneuron. The diagram schematically depicts the vestibular, internuclear and motoneuronal connections discussed in this paper. A specific internuclear pathway to medial rectus motoneuron in the oculomotor nucleus is shown. The inset on the upper left (from BAKER and HIGHSTEIN, 1975) shows antidromic activation (Oc), an EPSP-IPSP sequence following ipsilateral vestibular nerve stimulation (Vi), an EPSP following contralateral vestibular nerve stimulation (Vc) and the antidromic field potential following lateral rectus nerve stimulation (Abd). The inset in the lower lefthand part of the figure shows a monosynaptic EPSP in an antidromically identified medial rectus motoneuron following stimulation of the contralateral abducens nucleus.

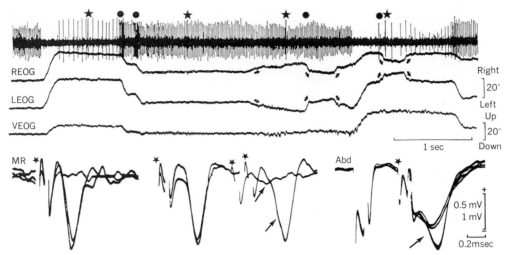

Fig. 8 Profile of activity in an identified internuclear neuron during conjugate and vergent eye
movements in the alert cat. The lower part of the figure shows antidromic activation of the internuclear neuron following stimulation of the oculomotor complex (on the left indicated by MR).
The next record shows a double shock to MR to point out the IS-SD invasion and then the
absence of a second spike at a critical condition-test interval of .75 msec. The last record shows
the ability of the unit potential to summate with the abducens (Abd) antidromic field potential.
The upper continuous record shows the activity of the internuclear neuron to be correlated with
only conjugate saccades or changes in eye position as opposed to those accompanying vergence
(latter part of the figure). The stars indicate points at which the neuron was antidromically
activated and the filled circles indicate conjugate saccades (on the left) to be compared with
similar amplitude and velocity eye movements during vergence (on the right).

were observed in the intracellular records from antidromically identified internuclear neurons (BAKER and HIGHSTEIN, 1975; HIGHSTEIN et al., 1976).   When coupled with the demonstration in the alert primate of unique horizontal burst-tonic signals recorded in the
MLF (KING et al., 1976; POLA and ROBINSON, 1978) it suggested that a specific class of
internuclear neurons could provide the MLF connection carrying the conjugate movement
signal.   The latter conjecture was confirmed in the alert cat paradigm (DELGADO-GARCIA
et al., 1977).   A representative record from an identified internuclear neuron responding
during horizontal conjugate eye movement is shown in Figure 8.   Antidromic identification was verified as shown by the lower set of records which, from left to right, point out a)
the all-or-none response, b) the critical double shock interval, c) the IS-SD inflection and
finally d) the summation of the unit potential with the abducens antidromic field potential.
The upper records clearly show the activity of the internuclear neuron (recorded in the
left abducens nucleus) to be correlated with the conjugate horizontal eye movement signal,
especially that shown in the right EOG.   Internuclear activity was not modulated during
vergence.   DELGADO-GARCIA et al. (1977) reached the conclusion that, qualitatively
speaking, there weren't any obvious differences between internuclear neurons and abducens motoneurons in respect to the information they provided during horizontal eye movement (i.e. they exhibit both eye velocity and position signals).   An important observation
in that study was that recording from numerous microelectrodes tracks throughout the
abducens nucleus and *its immediate surround* did not reveal, except for a few exceptions,
neuronal responses, other than described in Figure 8.

INTERNUCLEAR NEURONS WITH ROSTRAL
AND CAUDAL PROJECTIONS

In a recent oculomotor symposium (BAKER and BERTHOZ, 1977) the data from five separate studies estimated that about 30–40 % of the neurons in the abducens nucleus sent axons rostrally towards the oculomotor nucleus (similar percentages on MLF injections, MACIEWICZ et al., unpublished).   In addition, retrograde HRP studies have indicated that up to 5 % of the neurons in the abducens nucleus might also project to the cerebellum —most noticeably the flocculus (GRAYBIEL, 1977; KOTCHABHAKDI and WALBERG, 1977). We have confirmed the above finding, but more importantly, have recently found *substantial numbers of neurons, within and surrounding* the abducens nucleus which have axons directed caudally presumably terminating in the peri-hypoglossal nuclei and the dorso-medial medullary reticular formation.   The distribution of these neurons in representative rostral and caudal sections of the abducens nucleus is shown following a large (A) and small (B) injection of HRP in the prepositus nucleus (Figure 9).   Not only was there a bilateral distribution of cells throughout the abducens nucleus, but neurons were also scattered throughout the *peri-abducens area*.   A survey of all the published figures from the cat (see BAKER, 1977 for review) tends to suggest that there are not as many neurons surrounding the abducens nucleus following rostral (i.e. oculomotor) as compared to caudal HRP injections.   With respect to size and shape, internuclear neurons are a heterogenous population (Figure 10). It is worth noting that *all variations of cell form* i.e. fusiform, stellate, globiform, etc. are found following the caudal injections of HRP.   Fusiform and spindle shaped cell bodies are strikingly apparent.   In all cases, dendritic trees of retrogradely filled and intracellular injected abducens internuclear neurons ramify *in and around* the boundaries of the abducens nucleus (e.g. the internuclear neuron in Figure 4 was antidromically identified from ipsilateral

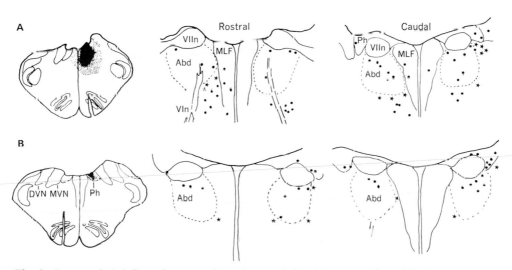

Fig. 9 Retrograde labeling of neurons in and around the abducens nucleus following HRP injection in the posterior medulla. A) a large injection of HRP in the prepositus and underlying dorsal medial reticular formation and B) a small injection confined to the prepositus nucleus. Rostral and caudal coronal sections through the abducens nucleus are shown. Cells were included from three consecutive sections (i.e. 150 microns). The dotted lines indicate our estimate of the boundary of the abducens nucleus and the neurons indicated by stars are those which lie in the peri-abducens region. (Further details in MCCREA and BAKER, 1978).

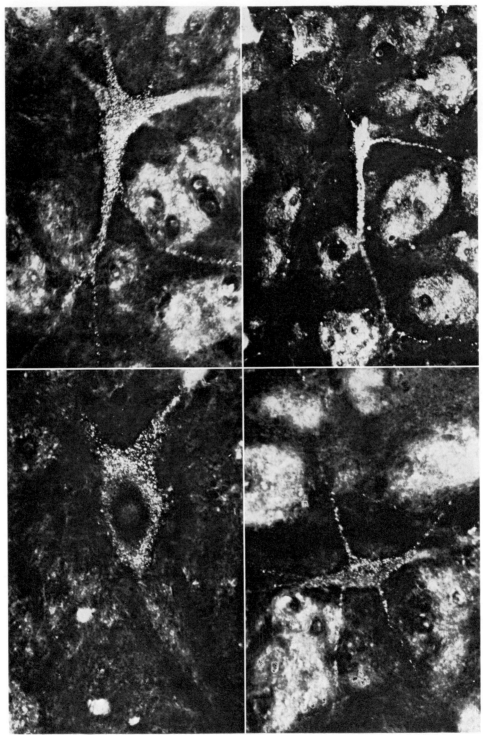

Fig. 10 Different size and shape of internuclear neurons as indicated by retrograde labeling following HRP injection in the descending MLF. All neurons at the same magnification and within the abducens nucleus.

caudal MLF stimulation).   Especially noticeable is how similar the internuclear neurons dendritic tree is organized when compared to that of the abducens motoneuron (Figure 4).   If one superimposes the two neurons (i.e. Mn and Int neuron), then the dendritic trees are coextensive *both inside and outside the boundaries* of the abducens nucleus (Figure 11). Recently, we have subdivided the internuclear neurons with caudally directed axons into four populations of cells based upon electrophysiological criteria (McCrea and Baker, 1978; see summary diagram in Figure 12).   First, there are neurons which descend to either the ipsilateral or contralateral prepositus nucleus, but not to both.   Second, there are cells which send axons both rostral and caudal in either the ipsi- or contralateral MLF,

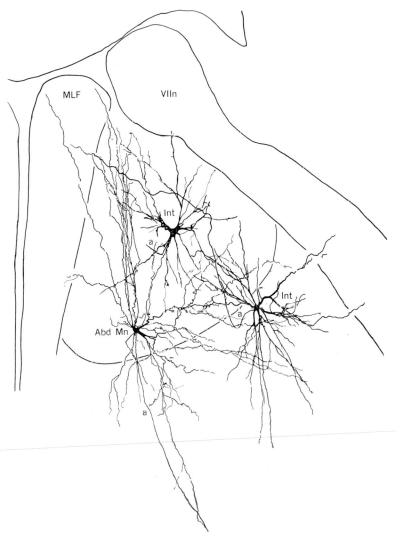

Fig. 11   Photographic superimposition of reconstructed internuclear neurons and an abducens motoneuron. The two internuclear neurons were antidromically identified from a rostral and caudal located stimulating electrode, respectively. The internuclear neuron with the caudally directed axon is situated outside the boundaries of the abducens nucleus whereas the one with the rostral axon was within its boundaries. Although the neurons were not located at the same coronal level, the superimposition shows an intimate overlapping of the dendritic trees, both within and outside the abducens nucleus.

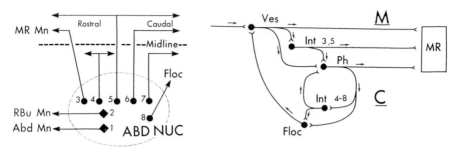

Fig. 12 Schematic diagrams representing the different classes of neurons within and around the abducens nucleus. The diagram on the left depicts each of the individual classes of neurons described within the abducens nucleus. Neurons labeled 3–7 are internuclear. Presumably, the axons of all neurons course in the MLF. The diagram on the right depicts multiple (M) and closed (C) loop pathways for internuclear neurons important for the medial rectus subdivisions. Only one internuclear neuron (i.e. 3) is shown to terminate directly on medial rectus motoneurons whereas all other internuclear neurons (4–8) are indicated to be involved in closed loop pathways with the prepositus, flocculus and vestibular nuclei. Use of multiple and closed loops is after that of LORENTE DE NÓ (1933 and 1938).

but not into both MLFs (there are a couple of exceptions). Finally following neuronal reconstruction after intracellular HRP injection, we have not, as yet, observed intrinsic axon collaterals from any antidromically identified internuclear neuron with either a rostral and/or caudal axonal trajectory. Thus far, 36 per cent of the caudally projecting neurons have bifurcating axons. By in large, the most frequently encountered internuclear neuron remains the one with its axon directed only rostrally in the contralateral MLF. Similarly those neurons with axons which bifurcate largely lie in the contralateral MLF. Although the prepositus nucleus is a very likely site we do not yet have definite data on axonal termination of caudally projecting neurons.

THE PARABDUCENS NUCLEUS

The coextensive dendritic trees of an abducens motoneuron and two internuclear neurons have been photographically superimposed in Figure 11. In this case, the Abd motoneuron and the internuclear neuron from Figures 3 and 4 have been placed in a coronal reconstruction of the Abd nucleus. In addition, an internuclear neuron with an axon directed rostrally towards the medial rectus subdivision has been included. This internuclear neuron and the abducens motoneuron are well within the cellular boundaries of the abducens nucleus. The internuclear neuron with the caudal axon was included because its soma would have to be described as being ventral and somewhat lateral to the boundaries of the Abd nucleus, but in any case, *the dendritic trees of all neurons overlap*, even though no two cells are within 500 microns of the other. In general, the latter dendritic overlap is true for *all sizes, shapes* and *locations of neurons* (McCREA and BAKER, unpublished). Given the working definition thus far of the parabducens nucleus (i.e. small associative cells which lie in the reticular gray adjacent to the abducens nucleus and intermingled with abducens motoneurons; CROSBY, see page 3) how could one attribute this term, to either one or the other of the two internuclear neurons shown in Figure 12? We believe that it would not be reasonable to use it to represent the class of internuclear neurons typified by the one shown near the center of the nucleus (i.e. those presumably carrying the specific horizontal eye movement signal to medial rectus motoneurons) because to do so would be both confusing and incorrect. These neurons are primarily (if not entirely) *within* the boundaries of the Abd nucleus. They are not located *parabducens*. On the other hand, if the term "parabducens" is saved for the internuclear neurons with their somata just outside the abducens nucleus, then it must be based on grounds other than morphological. Histological differentiation is out of the question because of the coextensive dendritic trees of all neurons and the similarity of axon projection (see Figure 12). The pertinent argument here though may eventually be the physiological observation which, to date, finds that nearly all neurons in the abducens nucleus carry some form of horizontal eye movement signal (see BAKER, 1977; DELGADO-GARCIA et al., 1977). *Even so, we clearly do not have any overwhelming morphological or physiological basis for reinstituting use of the term parabducens nucleus.* On the other hand, one can generate a stronger, but not yet compelling rationale for retaining the term on a conceptual basis. To illustrate this point, we have taken advantage of a simple, working viewpoint mentioned by LORENTE DE NÓ first in his classic vestibulo-ocular paper (1933) and later elaborated on in 1938. He divided all CNS circuitry into two types—namely, multiple M and closed C loops (Figure 12). The M loops ended directly on motoneuronal populations in parallel fashion. For example, there are direct vestibular, internuclear and prepositus pathways terminating on medial rectus motoneurons (see BAKER, 1977; BAKER and HIGHSTEIN, 1978; HIGHSTEIN and BAKER, 1978). In addition, the data presented here shows that internuclear pathways from the abducens nucleus terminate in the prepositus nucleus and that prepositus neurons likely reciprocate with axons back to the internuclear neurons as well as to the cerebellar cortex—especially the flocculus. The internuclear projection back to the prepositus nucleus closes the loop and another loop closure occurs back at the level of the vestibular nucleus. Except for the postulated specific monosynaptic internuclear pathway to the medial rectus motoneuron (and that does not exclude the internuclear neuron with a bifurcating axon), all other neurons described up till now both within and around, the Abd nucleus are elements of closed loops. Viewed by itself, the above connectivity exercise has little meaning; however, conceptually it presents the unifying concept that "the horizontal conjugate eye movement signal(s)" represented by internuclear neurons in and around the Abd nucleus are required by other brainstem and cerebellar structures for their own intrinsic operation. Fortunately it is not the purpose of this paper to elaborate on the various roles which these projections could subserve. In fact, they are potentially infinite being limited only by the number of roles which have been suggested for *each of the projection sites* itself. For the present, we are content with having provided morphological and physiological evidence that many brainstem areas receive horizontal eye movement signal(s) which originate directly from the abducens nucleus. Such signal(s) are easily generated by neurons within and extraneous to the abducens nucleus because of the overlapping dendritic trees both within and outside the boundaries of the Abd nucleus. *All neurons may be internuclear* (i.e. projection) as demonstrated by the absence of intrinsic axon collaterals as well as to date, of any neurons which may be classified as true interneurons (BAKER, 1977). Even in the absence of interneurons, it is no longer possible to visualize a simple role for the abducens nucleus (as we have up till now). Finally, if we assume the above suppositions about internuclear neurons to be true, then the "parabducens nucleus concept" could be restated as follows. The *parabducens nucleus consists of neurons, in and around* the Abd nucleus which distribute *unique* horizontal eye movement signal(s) to many nuclei. If that is the case then the parabducens nucleus function is to deliver a common signal(s) that may be used for quite different purposes depending on the projection site. Unfortunately, to do so would be to use "parabducens" quite differently then that originally envisioned by RILEY, CROSBY and others. For these authors, the parabducens nucleus was a *command center for the medial rectus motoneurons.* Given a paralysis of conjugate eye movement, such as that following a reticular lesion, they would certainly have placed the parabducens nucleus there (i.e. not in the abducens nucleus as all). Whereas, we would interpret the above problem as only a compromise of an *immediate supranuclear connection to the parabducens nucleus*. Also in contrast to prior usage, we do not envision the function of a internuclear cells in the "re-defined" parabducens nucleus to be command neurons. We find it more likely that they function as elements in circuits concerned with *something other than initiation of movement*. Compromise of their activity (whatever that might result in?) would not be the same as interfering with the postulated specific internuclear pathway to the medial rectus.

In conclusion, we believe that based on neuron location, size, distribution and termination, the parabducens nucleus concept cannot be justified on a morphological and physiological basis as originally defined by earlier authors. In spite of such reservation, we find the possibility of being able to refer to a 'parabducens role' and/or 'function' attractive especially if it turns out to be unique property of horizontal eye movement! However, to advocate now the use of 'parabducens nucleus' to refer collectively to neurons with a common eye movement signal would be premature. In fact, it would be based on as meager evidence as when the term was originally coined. The issue can only be resolved by understanding more completely the morpho-physiological profiles of the internuclear neurons *in and around* the abducens nucleus.

REFERENCES

BAKER, R.: Anatomical and physiological organization of brain stem pathways underlying the control of gaze. *In* BAKER, R. and BERTHOZ, A. (eds.): *Control of Gaze by Brain Stem Neurons*, pp. 207–233. Elsevier/North Holland Press, Amsterdam/New York (1977)

BAKER, R. and BERTHOZ, A. (eds.): *Control of Gaze by Brain Stem Neurons*. Elsevier/North Holland Press, Amsterdam/New York (1977)

BAKER, R. and HIGHSTEIN, S. M.: Physiological identification of interneurons and motoneurons in the abducens nucleus. *Brain Res., 83*: 292–298 (1975)

BAKER, R. and HIGHSTEIN, S. M.: The vestibular projections to medial rectus subdivision of the oculomotor complex. *J. Neurophysiol., 41*: 1629–1646 (1978)

BECHTEREW: Die Leitungsbahnen im Gehirn und Rückenmark (1899) (Cited from FRASER, 1901).

BENDER, M. B. (ed.): *The Oculomotor System*. Harper and Row, New York (1964)

BENDER, M. B. and SHANZER, S.: Oculomotor pathways defined by electrical stimulation and lesions in the brain stem of monkey. *In* BENDER, M. B.: *The Oculomotor System* p. 81–140, Harper and Row, New York (1964)

BENDER, M. B. and WEINSTEIN, E. A.: Effects of stimulation and lesion of the medial longitudinal fasciculus in the monkey. *Arch. Neurol. Psychiat., 52*: 106–113 (1964)

BENDER, M. B. and WEINSTEIN, E. A.: The syndrome of the medial longitudinal fasciculus. *Proc. Ass. Res. Nerv. Ment. Dis., 28*: 414–420 (1950)

BENNETT, A. H. and SAVILL, T.: A case of permanent conjugate deviation of the eyes and head, the result of a lesion limited to the sixth nucleus; with remarks on associated lateral movements of the eyeballs, and rotation of the head and neck. *Brain, 12*: 102–116 (1889)

BENVENUTI, E.: Sulla patologia del ponte di varolio: Contributo clinico e antomo-patologico, *Ann. Neurol., (Naples) 19*: 97–130 (1901)

BLOCQ, P. and GUINON, G.: Sur un cas de paralysie conjugée de la sixième paire. *Arch. Med. Exp. Anat. Path. (Par.), 3*: 74–89 (1891)

BRUCE, A.: A case of double paralysis of the lateral conjugate deviation of the eyes. *Rev. of Neurol. and Psych., 1*: 329–338 (1903)

BÜTTNER-ENNEVER, J. A. and HENN, V.: An autoradiographic study of the pathways from the pontine reticular formation involved in horizontal eye movements. *Brain Res., 108*: 155–164 (1976)

CARPENTER, M. B.: Central oculomotor pathways. *In* BACH-Y-RITA, P. COLLINS, C. C. and HYDE (eds.): *The Control of Eye Movements*, pp. 67–104. Academic Press, New York (1971)

CARPENTER, M. B. and HANNA, G. R.: Lesions of the medial longitudinal fasciculus in the cat. *Am. J. Anat.*, *110*: 307–331 (1962)

CARPENTER, M. B. and McMASTERS, R. E.: Disturbances of conjugate horizontal eye movements in the monkey. II. Physiological effects and anatomical degeneration resulting from lesions in the medial longitudinal fasciculus. *Arch. Neurol.*, *8*: 347–368 (1963)

CARPENTER, M. B., McMASTERS, R. E. and HANNA, G. R.: Disturbance of conjugate horizontal eye movements in the monkey. I. Physiological effects and anatomical degeneration resulting from lesions of the abducens nucleus and nerve. *Arch. Neurol.*, *8*: 231–247 (1963)

CARPENTER, M. B. and STROMINGER, N. L.: The medial longitudinal fasciculus and disturbances of conjugate horizontal eye movements in the monkey. *J. Comp. Neurol.*, *125*: 41–66 (1965)

COGAN, D. C., KUBIK, C. S. and SMITH, W. L.: Unilateral internuclear ophthalmoplegia. *Trans. Amer. Neuro. Assn.*, pp. 221–225 (1950)

COHEN, B.: Vestibulo-ocular relationships. In BACH-Y-RITA, P., COLLINS, C. C. and HYDE (eds.): *The Control of Eye Movements*, pp. 105–148. Academic Press, New York (1971)

COHEN, B. and HENN, U.: The origin of the quick phase of nystagmus in the horizontal plane. *Bibl. Ophthalmol.*, *82*: 36–55 (1972)

CRANDALL, W. F., WILSON, J. S. and GOLDBERG, S. J.: Branching axons to "Functionally independent" muscles in the cat oculomotor system. *Neuroscience Abst.*, *3*: 153 (1977)

CRAMNER, R.: Nystagmus related to lesions of the central vestibular apparatus and the cerebellum. *Ann. of Oto., Rhino & Laryng.*, *60*: 186–196 (1951)

CROSBY, E. C.: The application of neuroanatomical data to the diagnosis of selected neurosurgical and neurological cases. *J. Neurosurg.*, *7*: 566–583 (1950)

CROSBY, E. C.: Relations of brain centers to normal and abnormal eye movements in the horizontal plane. *J. Comp. Neurol.*, *99*: 437–479 (1953)

DELGADO-GRACIA, J., BAKER, R. and HIGHSTEIN, S. M.: The activity of internuclear neurons identified within the abducens nucleus of the alert cat. In BAKER, R. and BERTHOZ A. (eds.): *Control of Gaze by Brain Stem Neurons*, pp. 291–300, Elsevier/North Holland Press, Amsterdam/New York, (1977)

DELGADO-GARCIA, J. M., BAKER, R., ALLEY, K., and McCREA, R.: Anatomy and physiology of axotomized cat abducens motoneurons. Neuroscience Abst., 4, 603 (1978)

D'ESPINE, A. and DÉMOLE, V.: Tubercules de la protubérance. *Arch. Med. Enf. (Par.)*, *20*: 355–359 (1917)

DUVAL, M. and LABORDE, J. V.: De L'innervation des mouvements associés des globes oculaires. *J. Anat. Physiol. (Par.)*, *16*: 56–89 (1880)

FOVILLE,: Note sur une paralysie peu connue des certains muscles de l'oeil et sa liaison avec quelques points de l'anatomie et la physiologie de la protubérance annulaire. *Bulletin de la Société Anatomique. Paris (Second Series)*, *33*: 377–405 (1858)

FRASER, E. H.: An experimental research into relations of the posterior longitudinal bundle and Deiters' nucleus. *J. Physiol.*, *27*: 372–397 (1901)

FRASER, E. H.: Co-ordination paths in the posterior longitudinal bundle. *Rev. of Neurol. and Psychiatry*, *1*: 484–486 (1903)

FUCHS, A.: Role of vestibular and reticular nuclei in the control of gaze. In BAKER, R. and BERTHOZ, A. (eds): *Control of Gaze by Brain Stem Neurons*, pp. 341–348, Elsevier/North Holland, Amsterdam/New York (1977)

FUSE, G.: Über den abduzenskern der sauger. *Arbeiten aus dem hirnanatomischen Institut in Zürich*, *6*: 405–447 (1912)

GACEK, R. R.: Localization of neurons supplying the extraocular muscles in the kitten using horseradish peroxidase. *Exptl. Neurol.*, *44*: 381–403 (1974)

GAREL, J.: Nouveau fait de paralysie de la sixiéme paire avec deviation conjugée dans un cas d' hemiplegie alterne. *Rev. Med. (Par.)*, *2*: 593–599 (1882)

GRANTYN, A., GRANTYN, R. and ROBINÉ, K.-P.: Neuronal organization of the tecto-oculomotor pathways. In BAKER, R. and BERTHOZ, A. (eds.): *Control of Gaze by Brain Stem Neurons*, pp. 197–206, Elsevier/North Holland Press, Amsterdam/New York (1977)

GRAUX, G.: De la paralysie du moteur oculaire externe avec deviation conjugée. Thesis, 383, A. Parent, Paris, (1878)

GRAYBIEL, A. M.:   Organization of the oculomotor pathways in the cat and rhesus monkey. *In* BAKER, R. and BERTHOZ, A. (eds.):   *Control of Gaze by Brain Stem Neurons*, pp. 79–88, Elsevier/ North Holland Press, Amsterdam/New York (1977)

GRAYBIEL, A. M.:   Direct and indirect preoculomotor pathways of the brainstem: An autoradiographic study of the pontine reticular formation in the cat.   *J. Comp. Neurol.*, *175*: 37–78 (1977)

GRAYBIEL, A. M. and HARTWIEG, E. A.:   Some afferent connections of the oculomotor complex in the cat: An experimental study with tracer techniques.   *Brain Res.*, *81*: 543–551 (1974)

HIGHSTEIN, S. M. and BAKER, R.:   Excitatory synaptic termination of internuclear neurons of the abducens nucleus upon medial rectus motoneurons.   *J. Neurophysiol.*, *41*: 1647–1661 (1978)

HIGHSTEIN, S. M., MAEKAWA, K., STEINACKER, A. and COHEN, B.:   Synaptic input from the pontine reticular nuclei to abducens motoneurons and internuclear neurons in the cat.   *Brain Res.*, *12*: 162–167 (1976)

HOLMES, G.:   Palsies of the conjugate ocular movements.   *Brit. J. Ophthal.*, *5*: 241–250 (1921)

HUNNIUS: Zur Symptomaltologie der Bruckenerkrankurgen und uber die conjugirte Deviation der Augen bei Hirnkrankheiten Aus der medizinichen.   Abteilung des kolner Burgerhospital.   *Bonn. Cohen*, 1–91 (1881)

KING, W. M., LISBERGER, S. G. and FUCHS, A. F.:   Responses of fibers in medial longitudinal fasciculus (MLF) of alert monkeys during horizontal and vertical conjugate eye movements evoked by vestibular or visual stimuli.   *J. Neurophysiol.*, *39*: 1135–1149 (1976)

KOTCHABHAKDI, N. and WALBERG, F.:   Gerebellar afferents from neurons in motor nuclei of cranial nerves demonstrated by retrograde axonal transport of horseradish peroxidase.   *Brain Res.*, *137*: 158–163 (1977)

LANDOUZY, L.:   Étude des Convulsions.   These de Paris, p. 20 (1876)

LORENTE DE NÓ, R.:   Vestibulo-ocular reflex arc.   *Arch. Neurol and Psychiat.*, 30: 245–291 (1933)

LOKENTE DE NÓ, R.:   Analysis of the activity of the chains of internuncial neurons.   *J. Neurophysiol.*, *1*: 207–244 (1938)

LUTZ, A.:   Über die Bahnen der Blickwendung und deren Dissoziierung (nebst Mitteilung eines Falles von ophthalmoplegia internuclear ist anterior in Verbindung mit Dissoziierung der Bogengange), *Klin. Montsbl. Augenh.*, *70*: 213 (1923)

MACIEWICZ, R. J., EAGEN, K., KANEKO, C. R. S. and HIGHSTEIN, S. M.:   Vestibular and medullary brain stem afferents to the abducens nucleus in the cat.   *Brain Res.*, *123*: 229–240 (1977)

MCMASTERS, R. R., WEISS, A. H. and CARPENTER, M. B.:   Vestibular projections to the nuclei of the extraocular muscles.   *Am. J. Anat.*, *118*: 168–194 (1966)

MCCREA, R. and BAKER, R.:   Neurons in the oculomotor, trochlear and abducens nuclei project caudally in the MLF to the prepositus nucleus.   *Neuroscience Abstr.*, *4*: 602 (1978)

MUSKENS, L. J. J.:   An anatomico-physiological study of the posterior longitudinal bundle in its relation to forced movements.   *Brain, 36*: 352–426 (1913/1914)

NAUTA, W. J. H. and KUYPERS, H. G. J. M.:   Some ascending pathways in the brain stem reticular formation.   *In* JASPER, H. H. (eds.):   *The Reticular Formation*.   Chap. 1, pp. 3–30, Little, Brown and Company, Boston, 1958.

POLA, J. and ROBINSON, D. A.:   Oculomotor signals in medial longitudinal fasciculus of the monkey.   *J. Neurophysiol.*, *41*: 245–259 (1978)

RAMÓN Y CAJAL, S.:   Histologie du system nerveux de l'homme et des vertebres, (reprinted 1972) Tome 1 pp. 854–858, C. S. I. C., Madrid (1909)

RAPHAN, T. and COHEN, B.:   Brainstem mechanisms for rapid and slow eye movements.   *Ann. Rev. Physiol.*, *40*: 527–552 (1978)

RILEY, H. A.:   The central nervous system control of the ocular movements and the disturbances of this mechanism.   *Arch. Ophthal.*, *4*: 640–661 and 885–910 (1930)

RUSSELL, R. A.:   The origin and destination of certain afferent tracts in the medulla oblongata.   *Brain, 20*: 409 (1897)

SPENCER, R. F.:   Identification and localization of motoneurons innervating the cat retractor bulbi muscle.   *Neuroscience Abstr.*, *4*: 168 (1978)

SPENCER, R. F. and STERLING, P.:   An electron microscope study of motoneurons and interneurons in the cat abducens nucleus identified by retrograde intraaxonal transport of horseradish peroxidase.   *J. Comp. Neurol.*, 176: 65–86 (1977)

SPIEGEL, E. A. and SOMMER, I.: Neurology of the Eye, Ear, Nose and Throat. Grune and Stratton, New York (1944)

SPILLER, W. G.: Ophthalmoplegia internuclear anterior: A case with necrospy. *Brain, 47*: 345–357 (1924)

STEIGER, H. J. and BÜTTNER-ENNEVER, J.: Relationship between motoneurons and interneurons in the abducens nucleus: A double retrograde tracer study in the cat. *Brain Res., 148*: 181–188 (1978)

STRONG, O. S. and ELWYN, A.: *Human Neuroanatomy.* Chap. XIV, p. 212. The Williams & Wlkins Company (1943)

TERNI, T.: Ricerche sul nervo abducente e in special modo intorno al significato del suo nucleo accessorió d'origine. *Fol. neuro-biol., 12*: 227–327 (1922)

THOMAS: Dégénérscences secondaires à la section du faisceau longitudinal postérieur de la substance réticulée du bulbe. Compte rendus des séances de la Soc. de Biologie, 28 mai (1898)

THOMAS: Recherches sur le faisceau longitudinal posteriéur et la substance réticulée bulbo–protuberantielle. *Rev. Neurol.,* Vol. xi (1903)

TSUCHIDA: Über die Ursprangskerne der Augenbewegungsnerven. *Arbeiten aus dem hirnanatomischen. Institut in Zurich* (1906)

UEMURA, T. and COHEN, B.: Effects of vestibular nuclei lesions on vestibulo-ocular reflexes and posture in monkeys. *Acta Oto Laryngol., 315*: 1–71 (1973)

VAN GEHUCHTEN, A.: Recherches sur l'origine reele des nerfs moteurs craniens. I. Les nerfs moteurs oculaires. *J. de Neurologie et D'hypnologie, 3*: 114–129 (1898)

VAN GEHUCHTEN, A.: *Le systéme nerveux de l'homme.* lst Edition, J. van In ecio, Lierre (1893)

VAN GEHUCHTEN, A.: Les connexions centrales du noyau de Deiters et les masses grises voisines (Faisceau vestibulospinal, faisceau longitudinal posterieur, stries medullaries). *Nevraxe (Louvain), 6*: 19–73 (1904)

WARWICK, R.: Representation of extraocular muscles in the oculomotor nuclci of the monkey. *J. Comp. Neurol., 98*: 449–504 (1953)

DISCUSSION PERIOD

COHEN: I thought you made the point that none of the internuclear interneurons had collaterals, yet your types four and five appear to have them.   Is that correct?

BAKER: There are no recurrent collaterals terminating within the abducens nucleus.

COHEN: But some neurons do have collaterals?

BAKER: Yes.   One-third of the neurons have both a rostral and caudal projecting axon.   The collateralization likely takes place at the level of the medial longitudinal fasciculus and not within the abducens nucleus.   However, neurons do not have any recurrent intrinsic collaterals ending in the abducens nucleus.   All the information carried by these neurons leaves the abducens nucleus.

COHEN: When you put the horseradish peroxidase into the MLF, did you see any neurons in the region of the abducens nucleus which projected into the MLF and might then be considered to be parabducens neurons?

BAKER: No.   Most of the neurons, in fact, nearly all of the neurons, according to our definition of the boundaries of the abducens nucleus which, as I said, includes the expansive somadendritic tree of abducens and internuclear neurons were located within the abducens nucleus.

GRAYBIEL: How do you explain the classical result of cutting the VIth nerve and getting degeneration of everything in the nucleus?

BAKER: I don't know for certain.   Years ago morphologists were limited to the use of antiquated Marchi technique and that coupled with capricious fixation may have resulted in misinterpretation.   I don't think they misrepresented their data in any way which would be suggestive that they saw more than what was reported.   At that time, morphologists were being asked to generate anatomical support for a population of neurons to support a concept which physiologists and neurologists thought to be true; definitive evidence was beyond their technique's reach and that included the Nissl and axotomy studies which primarily were carried out in young material.   If a chromolytic response is desired, then it may be easy to find if you're looking for it, especially in young animals.

EXCITATORY AND INHIBITORY PREMOTOR NEURONS RELATED TO HORIZONTAL VESTIBULAR NYSTAGMUS*

Hiroshi SHIMAZU

*Department of Neurophysiology, Institute of Brain Research
School of Medicine, University of Tokyo
Tokyo, Japan*

The vestibuloocular reflex system reacts by producing rhythmic ocular movements—nystagmus—on stimulation of the peripheral labyrinth. The rhythm is formed centrally, but the origin of the rhythm, especially the role of the vestibular nuclei and the reticular formation in generation of nystagmus, has long been a subject of controversy. The function of these two structures related to nystagmus was first explicitly described by LORENTE DE NÓ (1933), who stated that the vestibular nuclei set up a continuous series of excitatory impulses (the slow phase) and that the production of the rhythm of nystagmus, i.e., of the quick component, needs more neurons than those used in the production of the slow component. On the basis of anatomical studies and lesion experiments, he concluded that these additional neurons lie in the reticular formation and proposed two neuron systems, V.N. (vestibular neuron) and Q (reticular neuron), explaining the production of the rhythm of nystagmus (Fig. 1):

"The group V. N. sets up a continuous series of impulses that produce the discharge of the motor cells M and at the same time excite the neuron system Q. After a certain time Q discharges and inhibits the effect of the V. N. impulses; therefore, muscle M relaxes. After the discharge, Q enters into a refractory state, the inhibition ceases, and, therefore, the impulse V. N. again set up a contraction M which increases until Q discharges. The cyclic process continues as long as V. N. impulses are produced (LORENTE DE NÓ, 1933)."

SPIEGEL and PRICE (1939) confirmed LORENTE DE NÓ's observation that a certain lesion in the reticular formation impaired vestibular nystagmus, inducing tonic eye deviation instead of the rhythmic reaction on labyrinthine stimulation. But this effect was found only in the initial postoperative stage, and vestibular nystagmus reappeared especially if concomitant lesions of the medial longitudinal fasciculus were avoided. It was thereby suggested that the nystagmic rhythm is produced in the vestibular nuclei. Since then, however, BENDER and his colleagues (BENDER and SHANZER, 1964; GOEBEL et al., 1971; COHEN and HENN, 1972) found that distinct oculomotor dysfunctions caused by a small lesion in the paramedian zone of the monkey pontine reticular formation persisted even long after the postoperative stage. On the basis of stimulation and lesion experiments using acute and chronic preparations, they proposed that the paramedian pontine reticular formation plays an important role in generation of nystagmus as well as the control of horizontal conjugate gaze.

Recently abundant knowledge has accumulated, suggesting that both the reticular formation and the vestibular nuclei (and also other structures) participate in generation of nystagmic rhythm of ocular motor activity. A variety of neurons whose activity is closely related to eye movements have been found in the reticular formation (DUENSING and

---

* This study was supported by a grant from Japan Ministry of Education.

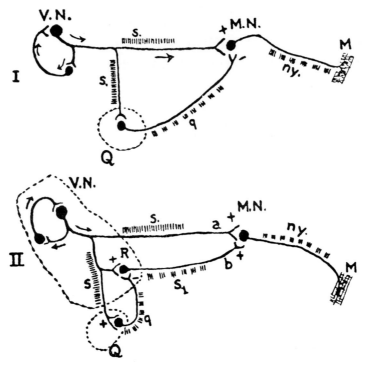

Fig. 1 Diagrams proposed to explain the production of the rhythm of nystagmus. I. Vestibular nuclei (V.N.) (including reticular relays) set up a continuous stream of impulses s, which on the one hand excite the motoneuron (M.N.) and on the other hand excite the system of neurons Q. which set up a discontinuous series of inhibitory impulses (q). II. V.N. includes internuncial neurons R and explains the production of the rhythm without inhibition of motoneurons. (from LORENTE DE NÓ R.: *Arch. Neurol. Psychiat. (Chic.)*, *30*: 245–291, Copyright 1933, American Medical Association)

SCHAEFER, 1957; SPARKS and TRAVIS, 1971; COHEN and HENN, 1972; LUSCHEI and FUCHS, 1972; KELLER, 1974; HIKOSAKA and KAWAKAMI, 1977), the vestibular nuclei (DUENSING and SCHAEFER, 1958; HORCHOLLE and TYČ-DUMONT, 1968; LUSCHEI and FUCHS, 1972; MILES, 1974; KELLER and DANIELS, 1975; KELLER and KAMATH, 1975; FUCHS and KIMM, 1975) and the prepositus hypoglossi nucleus (BAKER et al., 1976).   Even in the same structure, however, there are various types of neuron exhibiting different patterns of impulse activity in relation to eye movements.   So far little evidence has been provided what types of neuron in what structures are immediately premotor and terminate directly on ocular motoneurons to cause nystagmus.   This is crucial to understand the functional role of each structure in the generation of nystagmus and to advance future analyses of the interaction between different structures forming complex neuronal chains such as in Figure 1.   This review will deal with spike activity of premotor axons in the abducens nucleus which correlates with postsynaptic events in abducens motoneurons underlying their nystagmic modulation.   The location of the immediate premotor neurons will also be discussed on the basis of physiological evidence for their direct connection with motoneurons and their characteristic impulse activity causing postsynaptic potential changes.

SYNAPTIC EVENTS IN ABDUCENS MOTONEURONS
DURING VESTIBULAR NYSTAGMUS

Nystagmus was induced by high frequency (400/sec) electric stimulation of the vestibular nerve in the encéphalé isole cat under local anesthesia. Intracellular recording from abducens motoneurons during nystagmus revealed a rhythmic change of the membrane potential, i.e. a slow progression in the depolarizing direction followed by a quick hyperpolarization, while the abducens nerve activity on the same side showed an alternation of a slow excitation and a quick suppression (Fig. 2B) (Maeda et al., 1972). When the direction of nystagmus was reversed, the rhythmic change in the intracellular potential consisted of a quick depolarization followed by a slow progression in the hyperpolarizing direction (Fig. 2D). For convenience, a progression of the membrane potential in the depolarizing or hyperpolarizing direction will be simply called "depolarization" or "hyperpolarization", respectively. In Figure 2, the membrane was hyperpolarized during the silent phase of abducens nerve discharge with reference to the prestimulatory potential level (Fig. 2A and C). However, this does not directly indicate the existence of inhibitory postsynaptic potentials (IPSPs) in the hyperpolarizing phase, since the hyperpolarization may be produced by reduction of the excitation which tonically maintains the prestimulatory membrane potential at a certain depolarized level.

The synaptic mechanism of the depolarization and hyperpolarization was examined by passing currents through the recording microelectrode (Maeda et al., 1971) or electrophoretic injection of Cl^- ions into the motoneuron (Maeda et al., 1972). Figure 3 shows an example of the latter effect. The effectiveness of Cl^- injection was judged in each neuron by reversal of the IPSP induced by a single-shock stimulation of the ipsilateral vestibular nerve into a depolarizing potential (Fig. 3C and D) (Baker et al., 1969). Under this

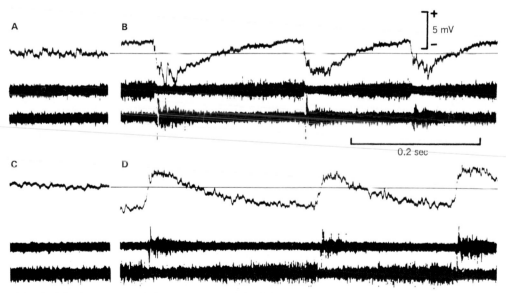

Fig. 2 Membrane potential changes in a left abducens motoneuron associated with rhythmic motor nerve discharges during nystagmus (B and D). Horizontal lines indicate the membrane potential levels recorded before stimulation as shown in A and C, respectively. Each of A–D represents intracellular record (top), left (middle) and right (bottom) abducens nerve discharges. Stimulation was applied to right (B) and left (D) vestibular nerve (Maeda et al., 1972).

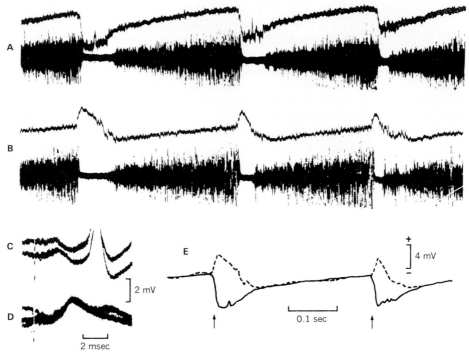

Fig. 3 Effects of electrophoretic injection of Cl⁻ ions into the motoneuron on the nystagmic modulation of the membrane potential. *A* and *B*: changes in the membrane potential of an abducens motoneuron (top) and abducens nerve discharges (bottom) on the same side. *A*: control record. *B*: record obtained during reversal of the IPSP to a depolarizing potential due to Cl⁻ injection. *C*: IPSP (and rebound excitation) induced in the motoneuron by single shocks to the ipsilateral vestibular nerve. *D*: the same as in *C* but after Cl⁻ injection. *E*: superimposed traces of intracellular potential curves in A (solid line) and those in B (broken line). Moment of quick cessation of nerve discharges (left arrow) in each trial is taken as the standard of time and the potential at the end of slow depolarization phase is taken as the reference level for superposition. In this particular case the period of the beat in each trial was by chance the same. Calibration and time scale for *E* apply to *A* and *B* (MAEDA et al., 1972).

condition the rhythm of the membrane potential associated with periodic nerve activities exhibited a characteristic pattern (Fig. 3B); the slow depolarization was followed by an additional, steep depolarization at the time of abrupt cessation of nerve impulses, instead of the hyperpolarization consistently found in the control record (Fig. 3A). Figure 3E depicts two potential traces obtained before (solid line) and after (broken line) Cl⁻ injection. These two traces were superimposed by taking the moment of abrupt cessation of nerve discharges as the standard of time in two trials (arrow in Fig. 3E). It is clear from these superimposed traces that the onset of steep depolarization after Cl⁻ injection was coincident with the onset of steep hyperpolarization in the control trace. The diverging point of the two potential curves was approximately synchronous with abrupt cessation of nerve discharges. These results indicate that there is an abrupt production of the IPSP at the quick hyperpolarization phase. The steep depolarization recorded after Cl⁻ injection turned relatively slowly in the hyperpolarizing direction and then met the slowly depolarizing curve of the control trace at about 100 msec or more after the diverging point (Fig. 3E). This period indicated the duration of active inhibition due to production of the IPSP relating to the potential rhythm. In Figure 3B the membrane potential level at the peak of each repolarization after Cl⁻ injection was distinctly deeper than the peak of the preceding slow depolarization. Therefore, the progression of the membrane potential to a hyperpolarizing direction in the control trace was attributed not only to production of the IPSP but also to reduction of the EPSP (disfacilitation). Since the IPSP did not contribute to the later phase of slow depolarization, the depolarization was mainly caused by an increase in excitatory postsynaptic potentials (EPSPs) (see Fig. 5B).

Similar analyses were performed for the potential sequence consisting of a quick depolarization followed by a slow hyperpolarization shown in Fig. 2D. The quick depolarization was not reversed to a hyperpolarization when the IPSP was inverted by electrophoretic injection of Cl^- ions, indicating that an increase in the EPSP underlies it. However, a reduction of the amplitude of the quick depolarization occurred during reversal of the IPSP, which indicated a contribution of disinhibition to the quick depolarization. The later phase of slow hyperpolarization was caused not only by a decrease in the EPSP but also by a slow increase in the IPSP (MAEDA et al., 1972) (see Fig. 5B′).

A previous study of HORCHOLLE-BOSSAVIT and TYČ-DUMONT (1969) failed to reveal postsynaptic inhibition of abducens motoneurons during nystagmus, but suggested a presynaptic inhibition at the silent period of the motoneurons. However, BAKER and BERTHOZ (1974) found EPSP-IPSP sequences related to nystagmus in the trochlear motoneurons in good agreement with the present data.

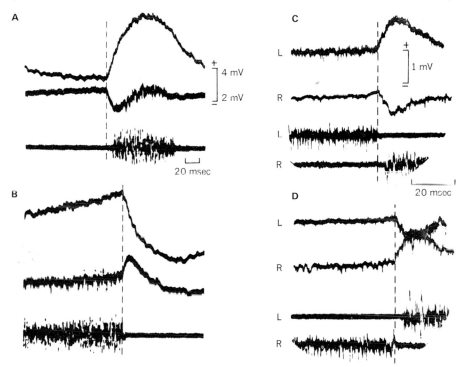

Fig. 4 Temporal relation between intracellular potentials of an abducens motoneuron and extracellular field potentials in the abducens nucleus at the quick phase of nystagmus. A: simultaneous recording of intracellular (top) and extracellular potentials (middle) and abducens nerve discharges (bottom) on the same side at the quick excitatory phase. B: same arrangement as in A, but for the quick inhibitory phase of the motoneuron (HIKOSAKA, MAEDA, NAKAO, SHIMAZU and SHINODA, 1977). C and D: simultaneous recording of field potentials in the bilateral abducens nuclei (top and second traces) and of discharges in the bilateral abducens nerves (third and bottom traces). L and R represent recording side, left and right respectively. Repetitive stimulation was applied to right (C) and left (D) vestibular nerve. Vertical broken bars indicate the reference line for timing (MAEDA et al., 1972).

To investigate how the postsynaptic activities of the population of abducens motoneurons are reflected in the extracellular field potentials, the temporal relationship between
intra- and extracellular potential at the quick phase was examined for a large number of
nystagmic beats (HIKOSAKA et al., 1977 b).   Figure 4A exemplifies, from top to bottom,
simultaneous recording of a steep depolarization in the abducens motoneuron, the negative
field potential recorded close to the penetrated motoneuron and abducens nerve discharges
on the same side at the quick excitatory phase of the motoneuron.   Figure 4B shows similar
recordings at the quick inhibitory phase of the motoneuron.   The results showed that the
onset of the negative or positive field potential at the quick phase was synchronous with the
steep depolarization or hyperpolarization of motoneurons, and could therefore be utilized
as an indicator to determine the onset of the steep change in the membrane potential of the
population of motoneurons at the quick phase.   With the microelectrodes inserted into the
left and right abducens nuclei, the field potentials associated with alternating, rhythmic
activities in the abducens nerves were simultaneously recorded and their time relation was
directly compared.   As shown in Figure 4C and D, the onsets of both deflections were
found to be highly synchronous (MAEDA et al., 1972).

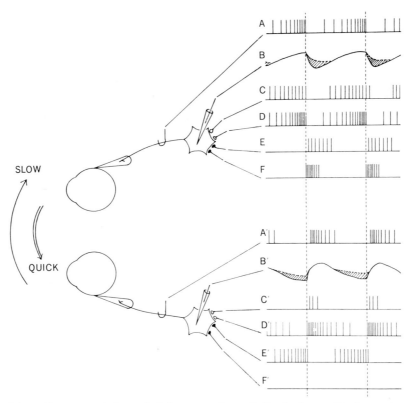

Fig. 5 Schematic representation of abducens motor activity during vestibular nystagmus and
related presynaptic impulses. *A, A'*: abducens nerve impuses. *B, B'*: membrane potential of
abducens motoneuron. Solid line indicates the actual membrane potential change and hatched
area represents component IPSPs. *C, C'*: impulses of monosynaptic V_c axon. *D, D'*: those of
axons disynaptically activated from the contralateral vestibular nerve. *E, E'*: those of monosynaptic V_i axon. *F, F'*: those of inhibitory burst axon. Four groups of axons were presumed
to make excitatory (open symbols) and inhibitory (filled symbols) synapses with the motoneuron.
Right abducens motoneuron (top) shows slow excitation followed by quick inhibition and left
motoneuron (bottom) slow inhibition followed by quick excitation.

It was therefore concluded that at the quick phase the onset of depolarization in moto-neurons on one side and that of hyperpolarization in contralateral motoneurons were synchronous. The component synaptic potentials causing membrane potential changes related to nystagmus and the time relation between motoneuron activities on both sides are schematically shown in Figure 5A, B and A′, B′. The suppression of slow phase nerve discharges at the quick phase was synchronous with the onset of quick hyperpolarization of the motoneuron, but the onset of quick phase nerve discharges on the contralateral side was always later than the onset of quick depolarization of the motoneuron by 5–10 msec. This striking delay time was first demonstrated by LORENTE DE NÓ (1934). This delay was attributed to the time required for the quick depolarization to reach the firing threshold of the motoneuron (MAEDA et al., 1972).

NYSTAGMUS-RELATED IMPULSES OF PRESYNAPTIC AXONS IN THE ABDUCENS NUCLEUS

Unit spikes of axons projecting to the abducens nucleus and responding to horizontal rotation of the head were recorded within the nucleus. Their discharge pattern related to vestibular nystagmus was investigated with reference to PSP changes of abducens moto-neurons as monitored by the field potentials in the same nucleus (HIKOSAKA et al., 1977 b). There were four groups of presynaptic axons whose activity was tightly related to moto-neuronal PSPs (Fig. 5).

Axons monosynaptically activated from the contralateral vestibular nerve (monosynaptic V_c axons)

The axons in this group, like abducens motoneurons, increased their firing frequency with contralateral horizontal angular acceleration and decreased it with ipsilateral accele-ration, suggesting that the axons originated from contralateral secondary vestibular type I neurons in the horizontal canal system. During nystagmus they fired periodically in phase with slow depolarization in abducens motoneurons (Fig. 5C), suggesting their excitatory action on motoneurons. Averaged time course of successive discharge frequency in the slow excitatory phase of motoneurons (Fig. 6A, filled circles) showed little tendency to increase in frequency towards the end of the slow phase. It is therefore unlikely that gradually increasing EPSPs in abducens motoneurons are attributed merely to simple synaptic transmission from this group of axons to motoneurons. The discharge pattern of these axons was similar to that of type I vestibular plus saccade (pause) units in the vestibular nuclei (FUCHS and KIMM, 1975; KELLER and DANIELS, 1975). A decrease or cessation of tonic discharges at the onset of steep hyperpolarization of abducens motoneurons obviously contributes to the disfacilitation observed in the motoneurons during intracellular recording (see above) and plays an important role in production of the quick inhibitory phase.

At the quick depolarization phase of motoneurons, this group of axons was less active (Fig. 5C′, filled circles in Fig. 6B). The synaptic action of these axons may contribute to a small fraction of the postsynaptic activity, though their total synaptic action depends on their relative proportion in the population which is so far unknown.

Similarly, excitatory axons of secondary vestibular neurons projecting to the contralat-eral trochlear nucleus were reported to reveal discharge patterns closely correlated to both the slow and quick phases of nystagmus (BAKER and BERTHOZ, 1974). It was suggested that excitatory vestibular neurons activated monosynaptically from the labyrinth could generate, or—minimally—assist in the production of, the slow and quick phases in oblique motoneurons.

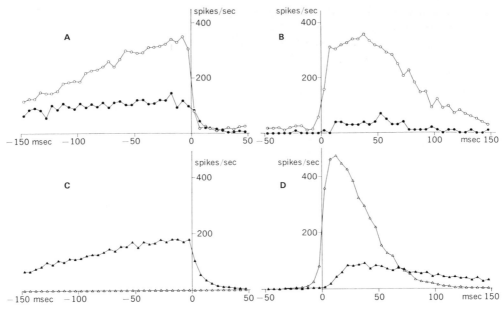

Fig. 6 Averaged time course of successive discharge frequency in four groups of presynaptic axons during vestibular nystagmus. *A*: slow excitatory phase of motoneuron. *B*: quick excitatory phase. *C*: slow inhibitory phase. *D*: quick inhibitory phase. Filled circles: monosynaptic V_c axons. Open circles: axons disynaptically activated from the contralateral vestibular nerve. Filled triangles: monosynaptic V_i axons. Open triangles: inhibitory burst axons (HIKOSAKA et al., 1977b).

Axons disynaptically activated from the contralateral vestibular nerve

The response to horizontal rotation of this group of axons was qualitatively similar to the above group: these axons were also activated from the contralateral horizontal canal, but the activation was disynaptic. During the slow depolarization phase of motoneurons, the discharge frequency increased approximately linearly and the maximum frequency at the end of the slow phase attained 200–650/sec (mean: about 350/sec) (Fig. 6A, open circles). These response characteristics were in the mathematical sense an integrated form of steady input to the vestibular nuclei. In all axons in this group, tonic discharges were silenced or abruptly decreased in frequency at the onset of the steep hyperpolarization in motoneurons (Fig. 5D).

At the onset of the quick depolarization phase, a burst of spikes was observed in these axons (Fig. 5D'). The onset of the burst was synchronous with that of the motoneuronal depolarization (Fig. 6B, open circles) and the discharge frequency in each burst attained its peak (200–450/sec) at 5–10 msec after the onset. The discharges were maintained at maximum frequency for 50–60 msec and continued for more than 150 msec with gradually decreasing frequency. The discharge pattern was quite similar in every respect to that of abducens motoneurons (burst-tonic type, LUSCHEI and FUCHS, 1972), except that the onset of burst activity in this group of axons clearly preceded motor nerve discharges.

Assuming that impulses of these axons impinge upon abducens motoneurons, the EPSP produced in motoneurons at both the slow and quick phases could mainly be caused by excitatory synaptic action of this group of axons. Likewise, disfacilitation observed in the quick hyperpolarization phase of motoneurons may be attributed to reduction of synaptic action of these axons as well as the monosynaptic V_c axons described above.

Axons monosynaptically activated from the ipsilateral vestibular nerve (monosynaptic V_i axons)

The axons in this group increased their firing frequency with ipsilateral horizontal angular acceleration and decreased it with contralateral acceleration, indicating that the axons originated from ipsilateral secondary vestibular type I neurons in the horizontal canal system. During nystagmus they fired periodically in phase with slow hyperpolarization in abducens motoneurons (Fig. 5E′). The spike frequency increased quasi-linearly during the slow phase (filled triangles in Fig. 6C). The maximum frequency reached close to 200/sec on the average at the end of the slow phase, and abruptly decreased at the onset of the quick depolarization of motoneurons. These axons were presumed to be inhibitory in nature, and gradually increasing IPSPs in motoneurons (Fig. 5B′) were attributed to synaptic action of these axons. Abrupt suppression of tonic discharges of these axons at the onset of steep depolarization of the motoneurons should cause disinhibition observed in motoneurons with intracellular study (MAEDA et al., 1972), and assist the production of burst activity in motoneurons.

Nearly half of the axons in this group exhibited a train of spikes (50–150/sec) at the quick hyperpolarization phase of motoneurons (Fig. 5E). Although its onset was usually slightly later than the onset of the quick hyperpolarization phase, the discharges lasted for 150 msec or more which approximated the duration of IPSPs in motoneurons at the quick inhibitory phase (Fig. 6D, filled triangles). This suggests an important contribution of these axons in production of quick inhibition of motoneurons. A similar suggestion was made for the role of inhibitory axons of secondary vestibular neurons projecting to the ipsilateral trochlear nucleus in the production of nystagmus in the oblique system (BAKER and BERTHOZ, 1974).

Axons related only to the quick inhibitory phase of motoneurons (inhibitory burst axons)

The axons in this group responded to horizontal rotation, indicating their receiving input from the horizontal canal. However, the response of these axons to horizontal rotation was quite different from that of V_e or V_i axons. The spikes never showed such a gradual increase or decrease in frequency during angular acceleration as the type I or II response, but were induced consistently in a high frequency burst fashion during contralateral horizontal angular acceleration. The spike burst occurred periodically and was tightly related to the quick inhibitory phase of motoneurons in per-rotatory nystagmus. During ipsilateral angular acceleration the spikes were completely suppressed. Another contrast between this group of axons and V_e or V_i axons was less relation of the former with primary vestibular afferents. Single shock stimulation of the vestibular nerve was less effective in evoking spikes from this group of axons. Double or triple shocks to the contralateral vestibular nerve induced spikes with long, variable latencies. The threshold of vestibular nerve stimulation for evoking spikes was much higher in this group than that for activation of V_e or V_i axons. These characteristics suggest their origin outside the vestibular nuclei and polysynaptic connections with primary afferents (PRECHT and SHIMAZU, 1965).

During nystagmus the firing frequency in a burst increased abruptly at the onset of the quick hyperpolarization of motoneurons (Fig. 5F) and the maximum frequency of intraburst spikes attained 700–800/sec (approximately 500/sec on the average) (Fig. 6D, open triangles). The discharge frequency decreased fairly abruptly with little tonic component and the burst activity rarely lasted more than 80 msec, much shorter than the duration of spike train of monosynaptic V_i axons. The results suggest that this group of axons were inhibitory in nature and that the early part of the IPSP at the quick inhibitory phase of motoneurons is mainly attributed to the synaptic action of this group of axons, though monosynaptic V_i axons also contribute to production of the IPSP, especially in the later phase of inhibition.

It was a remarkable contrast with other axons projecting to the abducens nucleus that this group of axons was silent during the slow phase (Fig. 5F′, open triangles in Fig. 6C).

LOCATION OF IMMEDIATE PREMOTOR NEURONS RELATED TO VESTIBULAR NYSTAGMUS

In the preceding section the characteristic time course of PSPs in abducens motoneurons during vestibular nystagmus was explained by presumed synaptic action of four groups of axons on motoneurons. This section will deal with an origin of each group of axons and evidence for their direct connection with motoneurons.

Origin of nystagmus-related monosynaptic V_c and V_i axons

Monosynaptic V_c axons are likely to originate from excitatory type I neurons in the contralateral vestibular nuclei, since stimulation of the contralateral vestibular nerve induces disynaptic EPSPs in abducens motoneurons and the interneurons in this pathway are located in the rostral part of the medial vestibular nucleus on the contralateral side (BAKER et al., 1969; HIGHSTEIN, 1973). However, in the study described above no evidence has been provided for the *termination* of nystagmus-related monosynaptic V_c axons in the motor nucleus. Moreover, GRANT et al. (1976) reported that no neurons in the medial vestibular nucleus, activated antidromically from the contralateral abducens nucleus and monosynaptically from the ipsilateral horizontal canal, revealed a nystagmus-related pattern of spike activity. The apparent discrepancy may be resolved by observing spike activity of vestibular neurons whose axons are proved to terminate in the contralateral abducens nucleus.

In a recent study of SCHOR, NAKAO and SHIMAZU (1977), extracellular unit spikes recorded in the rostral part of the medial vestibular nucleus were identified as type I neurons in the horizontal canal system on the basis of their response to rotation and their monosynaptic response to stimulation of the ipsilateral vestibular nerve. Neurons sending their axons to the contralateral abducens nucleus were selected by their antidromic response to microstimulation (less than 15 μA) in the nucleus. The use of such low intensity microstimulation demonstrated that applied currents did not spread to adjacent structures such as the medial longitudinal fasciculus. This technique, however, could not distinguish between an axon which terminated within the abducens nucleus and a passing fiber which merely traversed the nucleus. During successive tracks through the contralateral abducens nucleus, the vestibular type I neuron could typically be activated from a variety of scattered sites within the nucleus, with intervening ineffective sites. This suggested that the axon branched extensively and terminated within the nucleus. More direct evidence for the excitatory connection of a projecting vestibular neuron with abducens motoneurons was obtained by the use of post-spike averaging of abducens nerve discharges triggered from spikes of a single vestibular neuron. The validity of this technique was fully described elsewhere (HIKOSAKA et al., 1978b). These identified vestibular type I neurons projecting to the contralateral abducens nucleus were found almost invariably to exhibit a rhythmic modulation of their spike activity during vestibular nystagmus (Fig. 7A). The discharge pattern was similar to that of monosynaptic V_c axons recorded in the contralateral abducens nucleus (see above).

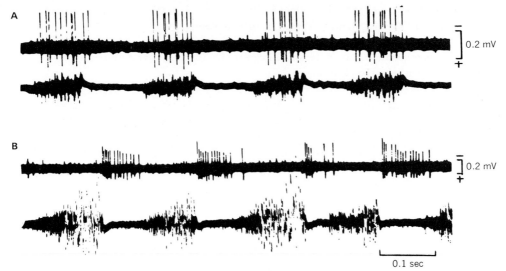

Fig. 7 Nystagmic modulation of spike activity of horizontal type I and type II neurons recorded in the medial vestibular nucleus. *A*: spikes of a type I neuron projecting to the contralateral abducens nucleus. *B*: spikes of a type II neuron. Bottom record in A and B represents abducens nerve discharges on the contralateral side (unpublished observations of NAKAO, SCHOR and SHIMAZU).

A similar study was performed on secondary type I neurons in the medial vestibular nucleus which projected to the ipsilateral abducens nucleus. By the aid of antidromic microstimulation technique for tracing the course of the axon and post-spike averaging of abducens nerve discharges, the direct inhibitory action of these vestibular neurons on ipsilateral abducens motoneurons was confirmed. Most of the neurons thus identified showed a nystagmic modulation of firing. The discharges were in phase with the slow inhibitory period of ipsilateral abducens motoneurons and exhibited a similar pattern to that of monosynaptic V_i axons recorded in the ipsilateral abducens nucleus.

The nystagmic modulation of activity in the secondary vestibular neurons was caused by a periodic production of IPSPs at the onset of the quick phase (HIKOSAKA, NAKAO and SHIMAZU, unpublished observation). As a candidate for inhibitory interneurons responsible for this periodic inhibition, vestibular type II neurons were selected for study (SCHOR et al., 1977), since they have been suggested as inhibitory neurons acting on type I neurons in the same nucleus (SHIMAZU and PRECHT, 1966). Type II neurons in the medial vestibular nucleus, characterized by their response to horizontal rotation (increased firing with contralateral angular acceleration and decreased firing with ipsilateral acceleration), were further selected by their activation at short latencies from the contralateral labyrinth. Most of these neurons had a nystagmic rhythm, showing an abrupt increase in discharge frequency at the onset of the quick inhibitory phase of contralateral abducens motoneurons, when type I neurons were showing a quick suppression of activity (Fig. 7B).

The firing pattern of vestibular type II neurons during nystagmus was consistent with the hypothesis that they are contributing to inhibition of type I activity at the quick phase. This was more directly confirmed by post-spike averaging of the membrane potential of a type I neuron triggered from spikes of a single type II neuron, revealing an IPSP with a monosynaptic latency. It is thus reasonable to conclude that the vestibular type II neurons mediating commissural inhibition play a role in the origin of the nystagmic modulation of activity observed in type I neurons which project to the abducens nuclei and contribute to the nystagmic rhythm of motoneurons.

Origin of nystagmus-related axons disynaptically activated from the contralateral vestibular nerve

The following structures will be considered as candidates for the origin of this group of axons, because a population of neurons in these structures are known to receive disynaptic excitatory input from the labyrinth; the vestibular nuclei (PRECHT and SHIMAZU, 1965; KELLER and KAMATH, 1975), the prepositus hypoglossi nucleus (BAKER and BERTHOZ, 1975), the reticular formation (PETERSON et al., 1975) and the abducens nucleus (BAKER and HIGHSTEIN, 1975).

a) The vestibular nuclei. KELLER and KAMATH (1975) differentiated between head rotation-related neurons and eye movement-related neurons in the monkey vestibular nuclei. During sinusoidal angular head rotation, the firing frequency of the former was approximately proportional to head rotational velocity and that of the latter was closer to being in phase with eye position than with head velocity. The head rotation-related neurons received monosynaptic input and most eye movement-related neurons disynaptic input from the ipsilateral vestibular nerve. Thus, the latter neurons could be an origin of burst-tonic excitatory input to abducens motoneurons, yet their real motor destination has not been elucidated. In studies in our laboratory, we have been so far unable to find neurons in the medial vestibular nucleus having discharge characteristics shown in Fig. 5D and D′ and Fig. 6A and B (open circles) which project to the contralateral abducens nucleus and receive disynaptic activation from the ipsilateral horizontal canal.

b) The prepositus hypoglossi nucleus and the reticular formation. When the recording microelectrode was shifted slightly medially so as to record from the prepositus hypoglossi nucleus and the underlying reticular formation (Fig. 8), many neurons were found to respond to sinusoidal horizontal head rotation with characteristics similar to those of abducens motoneurons (FUKUSHIMA et al., 1977). Figure 9A exemplifies an averaged response of a prepositus type II neuron to head rotation (bottom) together with averaged activity in the ipsilateral abducens nerve (middle) under decerebrate condition. The phase lag relative to angular acceleration obtained with different neurons varied considerably (Fig. 9B), and covered the whole range between the phase of vestibular nucleus neurons and that of abducens motoneurons described by SHINODA and YOSHIDA (1974). Similar results were reported by BLANKS et al. (1977). However, when the phase lag of individual neurons obtained at a certain stimulus frequency was plotted against that of *simultaneously* recorded abducens nerve discharges (Fig. 9C), a great majority of the points (filled circles) fell along the line with the slope of unity. It was thereby suggested that most prepositus type II neurons have proper phase characteristics for eye movements and may correspond to the burst-tonic type of neurons found in this structure of naturally behaving animal (BAKER et al., 1976), which resemble ocular motoneurons in their discharge pattern.

Since previous works showed that prepositus neurons projected to the oculomotor complex (GRAYBIEL and HARTWIEG, 1974; BAKER and BERTHOZ, 1975) and the abducens nucleus (MACIEWICZ et al., 1977), it seemed worth investigating whether the premotor axons recorded in the abducens nucleus, which received disynaptic input from the contralateral horizontal canal and showed nystagmic modulation of firing frequency (Fig. 5D and D′), originated from the prepositus hypoglossi nucleus. This possibility was examined by HIKOSAKA, IGUSA and IMAI (1978), who reported that most prepositus neurons identified as type II by horizontal rotation exhibited nystagmus-modulated discharge pattern in

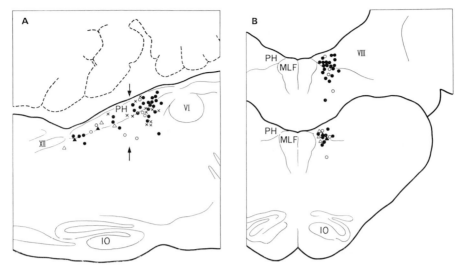

Fig. 8 Anatomical location of prepositus and reticular neurons which responded to horizontal head angular acceleration. *A*: schematic drawing of a sagittal section of the brain stem at 1.5 mm lateral to the midline. Circles and triangles represent type II and type I neurons respectively. Filled symbols represent neurons with phase lag similar to the abducens nerve. Open symbols represent neurons having phase lag smaller than that of the abducens nerve discharge. Crosses represent type II neurons whose phase relationship to the abducens nerve was not examined and are plotted only in A. *B*: transverse sections at the levels of about 1.5 mm (upper section) and 3.5 mm (lower section) caudal to the abducens nucleus. Neurons which lay rostral to the level indicated by arrows in A are replotted on upper section and those located caudal to the arrows are on lower section. VI, abducens nucleus; VIII, vestibular nuclei; XII; hypoglossal nucleus; PH, prepositus hypoglossi nucleus; MLF, medial longitudinal fasciculus; IO, inferior olive (FUKUSHIMA et al., 1977).

phase with the ipsilateral abducens nerve activity.   However, at the quick excitatory phase of motoneurons, the prepositus neuron began to fire approximately at the onset of abducens nerve discharge and distinctly later than the onset of motoneuronal depolarization which was reflected in the negative field potential (Fig. 4A).   This explains well the precedence of firing of prepositus neurons to eye movement (BAKER et al., 1976), but may not support a causal role in production, of at least the initial part, of the quick depolarization in motoneurons.   Moreover, prepositus type II neurons related to horizontal vestibular nystagmus could not be antidromically activated following microstimulation in any part of the ipsilateral abducens nucleus.   It was therefore suggested that prepositus neurons anatomically found to project to the ipsilateral abducens nucleus would not correspond to nystagmus-related type II neurons in the horizontal canal system.   Some neurons located in the reticular formation ventral to the prepositus hypoglossi nucleus also exhibited nystagmus-related firing, but their timing of activity relative to the quick phase and the absence of antidromic response to microstimulation in the abducens nucleus were similar to the behavior of prepositus neurons.   In spite of such negative evidence, however, further study with different techniques is needed to reveal the role of these structures in eye movements.

   c) **Interneurons in the abducens nucleus**. The axons of interneurons in the abducens nucleus are known to project to the contralateral oculomotor complex by anatomical (GRAYBIEL and HARTWIEG, 1974) and electrophysiological studies (BAKER and HIGHSTEIN, 1975).   These neurons receive disynaptic excitatory input from the contralateral vestibular nerve (BAKER and HIGHSTEIN, 1975) and have a monosynaptic excitatory effect on the contralateral medial rectus motoneurons (HIGHSTEIN, 1977).   Such neuronal

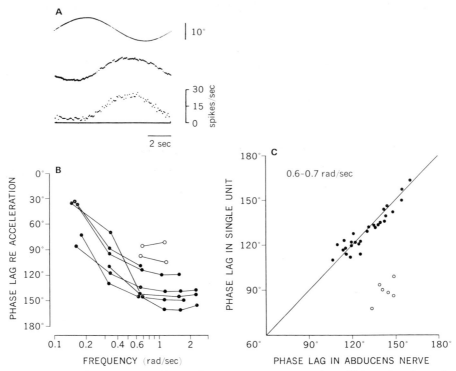

Fig. 9 Response of prepositus and reticular type II neurons to sinusoidal acceleration. *A*: an example of averaged response of a single neuron to 10 successive cycles at 0.62 rads/sec. Traces from the top give head position, averaged activity in ipsilateral abducens nerve and averaged firing rate of the unit. Ipsilateral head position is indicated as upward displacement. *B*: phase lag relative to angular acceleration plotted against stimulus frequency for 8 neurons. Symbols are the same as in C. *C*: comparison between phase lag of single unit response and that of simultaneously recorded abducens nerve response for 34 neurons at stimulus frequency of 0.6– 0.7 rads/sec. Although individual units show variations in their phase lags, most neurons (filled circles) have phase lag similar to that of the abducens nerve. Open circles represent neurons with phase lag distinctly smaller than that of abducens nerve discharge (FUKUSHIMA et al., 1977).

organization and the intimate relationship of their activity with eye movement (DELGADO-GARCIA et al., 1977) suggested the possibility that at least a part of the axons recorded within the abducens nucleus, which received disynaptic input from the contralateral horizontal canal and exhibited nystagmus-related discharges (Fig. 5D and D′), might originate from the abducens interneurons. This possibility was investigated in the study of NAKAO and SASAKI (1978), leading to positive evidence that the firing pattern of identified abducens interneurons were in every respect similar to that of such axons as shown in Fig. 5D and D′. Especially noted was that the onset of burst discharges of abducens interneurons observed at the quick excitatory phase of motoneurons in the same nucleus was approximately synchronous with the onset of the motoneuronal depolarization, and distinctly preceded abducens nerve discharges (Fig. 10).

A crucial problem is, however, to find the termination of axon collaterals of the abducens interneurons on abducens motoneurons. So far no physiological evidence for it has been provided. Morphologically, the absence of axon collaterals of interneurons within the abducens nucleus was strongly suggested (see BAKER, 1977). If this is true, the immediate premotor neurons forming a major excitatory input for nystagmic modulation of abducens

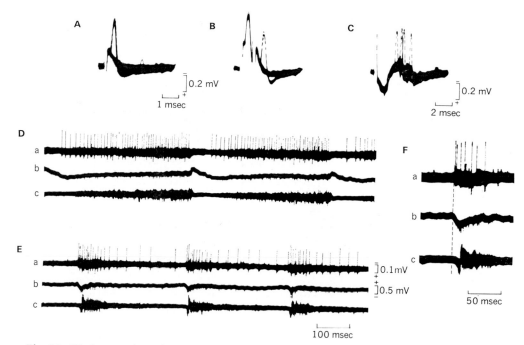

Fig. 10 Discharges of an interneuron in the abducens nucleus during nystagmus. *A–C*: identification of the neuron. *A and B*: responses to single shock stimulation at threshold-straddling intensity (A) and double shocks at suprathreshold (B) of the contralateral MLF. *C*: responses to stimulation of the contralateral vestibular nerve. *D*: stimultaneous recording of spike potentials of the interneuron (a), the field potential in the abducens nucleus (b) and abducens nerve discharges (c) on the same side during nystagmus. *E*: same as in D, but the direction of nystagmus was reversed. *F*: same as in E, but with expanded time scale. The vertical broken line indicates the onset of negative field potential (NAKAO and SASAKI, 1978).

motoneuron activity are to be looked for in other structures, especially in the paramedian pontine reticular formation (see Comments).

Origin of inhibitory burst axons

HIKOSAKA and KAWAKAMI (1977) explored the pontine and medullary reticular formation to find the somatic origin of inhibitory burst axons projecting to the abducens nucleus. Identification of each neuron was accomplished by observing the burst activity at the quick phase of nystagmus and the antidromic response to microstimulation in the abducens nucleus.   Effective stimulus sites to induce antidromic responses were fairly well confined to the abducens nucleus (Fig. 11B).   Patch-like distribution of effective stimulus sites in the abducens nucleus, with intervening ineffective sites (Fig. 11A), suggested that the axon gave off many branches and terminated within the nucleus.   Thus identified inhibitory burst neurons were located in the dorsomedial part of the pontomedullary reticular formation mainly caudal to the level of the abducens nucleus and exclusively contralateral to the abducens nucleus to which their axons projected (Fig. 12).

To confirm that these neurons are *inhibitory premotor* neurons and form synaptic contact with abducens motoneurons, the spike potentials of an antidromically identified burst neuron were employed to trigger a post-spike average of the membrane potential of contralateral abducens motoneurons (HIKOSAKA et al., 1978 b), revealing unitary IPSPs with monosynaptic latencies (Fig. 11C and D).   Each inhibitory burst neuron was estimated

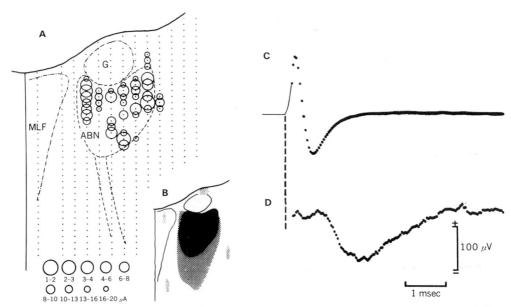

Fig. 11 Axonal branching in the abducens nucleus of a single inhibitory burst neuron and its synaptic effect on the abducens motoneuron. *A*: distribution of effective sites for antidromic activation of a contralateral burst neuron in the frontal plane through the abducens nucleus. Threshold currents for antidromic activation were determined at every 100 μm in each electrode track (dots). The diameter of each circle indicates the threshold current as shown below the drawing. Dots without circles indicate ineffective sites with stimulus currents of 20 μA. *B*: approximate extent of most frequently effective sites for antidromic activation (solid area) and relatively frequently effective sites (hatched area) obtained from 25 inhibitory burst neurons (HIKOSAKA and KAWAKAMI, 1977). *C*: averaged extracellular spikes of a single burst neuron used for post-spike average of the membrane potential recorded intracellularly from a contralateral abducens motoneuron. Initial parts of the spike drawn by a solid line was reconstructed from spontaneous spikes recorded with another oscilloscope. *D*: averaged unitary IPSP triggered by spikes shown in C (360 sweeps). Vertical broken line indicates the onset of triggering spike (unpublished observations of HIKOSAKA, NAKAO and SHIMIZU).

to make monosynaptic connections with approximately 60 per cent of the motoneuron pool. This was in good agreement with the extensive distribution of axonal branches of a single inhibitory burst neuron in the abducens nucleus (HIKOSAKA and KAWAKAMI, 1977).

The location of inhibitory burst neurons found in these studies was consistent with the anatomical findings with horseradish peroxidase (MACIEWICZ et al., 1977) and radioactive tracer technique (GRAYBIEL, 1977) that cells in the dorsomedial reticular formation caudal to the abducens nucleus project fibers to the contralateral abducens nucleus.   Electrophysiologically, a group of neurons in the paramedian pontine reticular formation has been reported to exhibit a high frequency burst of spikes prior to fast eye movements (DUENSING and SCHAEFER, 1957; SPARKS and TRAVIS, 1971; LUSCHEI and FUCHS, 1972; COHEN and HENN, 1972; KELLER, 1974).   On the basis of close functional correlation of their activity with eye movement, these neurons were presumed to provide an excitatory motor command signal for fast eye movements.   However, until the destination of the axon of each burst neuron is studied at the single neuron level, few conclusions can be drawn on the functional relationship between these burst neurons and inhibitory burst neurons described here.

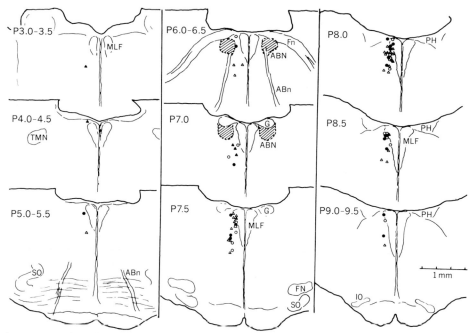

Fig. 12 Location of inhibitory burst neurons. Numbers following P indicate stereotaxic frontal planes. *Circles*: neurons identified by antidromic activation from the contralateral abducens nucleus. *Triangles*: neurons not identified by antidromic stimulation. *Filled symbols*: recording sites marked by the dye. *Open symbols*: recording sites estimated by measuring distances from the marked spot with the aid of the scale of the micromanipulator. ABN (hatched area), abducens nucleus; ABn, abducens nerve; FN, facial nucleus; Fn, facial nerve; G, genu of the facial nerve; IO, inferior olive; MLF, medial longitudinal fasciculus; PH, prepositus hypoglossi nucleus; SO, superior olive; TMN, trigeminal motor nucleus (HIKOSAKA and KAWAKAMI, 1977).

COMMENTS

We have shown evidence that the immediate premotor neurons participating in nystagmic modulation of abducens motoneuron activity are located in both the reticular formation and the vestibular nuclei. The finding that a group of burst neurons in the reticular formation are inhibitory in nature and immediately premotor (HIKOSAKA et al., 1977b; HIKOSAKA and KAWAKAMI, 1977; HIKOSAKA et al., 1978b) is surprisingly consistent with the original idea of LORENTE DE NÓ (1933) (Fig. 11). Moreover, he suggested that the neuron system Q in Fig. 1 is located in the neighborhood of the abducens nucleus. The location also agrees well with that of the identified inhibitory burst neurons.

The inhibition at the quick phase of vestibular type I neurons projecting to the contralateral abducens nucleus obviously causes disfacilitation in the motoneurons, thus contributing to suppression of motoneuron activity in addition to active inhibition due to reticular inhibitory burst neurons. The inhibition and disfacilitation of motoneurons occur approximately synchronously (MAEDA et al., 1972). The well coordinated timing of impulse frequency change observed in reticular and vestibular neurons at the quick phase of nystagmus suggests the existence of significant reticulo-vestibular interaction. The quick phase inhibition of vestibular type I neurons is unlikely to originate from the ipsilateral reticular inhibitory burst neurons via axon collaterals of the contralaterally projecting fibers, because no antidromic response was observed in the identified inhibitory burst neurons following stimulation of the ipsilateral vestibular nuclei (IMAI et al., 1977).   Instead, vestibular type II neurons mediating commissural inhibition were demonstrated to be an origin of nystagmic modulation of type I neuron activity.   Simultaneous excitation at the quick phase of vestibular inhibitory type II neurons and reticular inhibitory burst neurons on the same side seems to be of functional importance, yet common excitatory input to these two kinds of neurons has not been identified.

With respect to the reticulo-vestibular interaction, anatomical studies have shown that the nucleus reticularis pontis oralis and caudalis project to the vestibular nuclei with an ipsilateral preponderance (HODDEVIK et al., 1975; see also GRAYBIEL, 1977).   In addition, GRAYBIEL (1977) has found that the corresponding reticular area projects to the ipsilateral abducens nucleus (see also BÜTTNER-ENNEVER and HENN, 1976) and peri-abducens reticular area, the latter in turn projecting to the contralateral vestibular nuclei as well as the abducens nucleus.   The nucleus pontis oralis and caudalis area appears to correspond to the paramedian pontine reticular formation controlling the horizontal eye movements (BENDER and SHANZER, 1964) and the peri-abducens reticular area to the location of inhibitory burst neurons (Fig. 12).   These anatomical data attract us to exploring these regions to find specific connections between individual reticular neurons identified functionally by their discharge pattern related to nystagmus and vestibular type I or II neurons.

The neuronal organization of the vestibulooccular reflex system is still far from elucidation.   We know very little about how functionally different neurons are coupled with each other to provide proper function.   The following remarks may be most befitting to the conclusion: "The whole vestibular system has revealed itself as constituted by numerous chains of neurons, reciprocally connected in many ways and having their links in various anatomic nuclei.   All the chains work in intimate collaboration and all are necessary for the production of the normal reflex reaction" (LORENTE DE NÓ, 1933).

ACKNOWLEDGEMENTS

The author is indebted to Drs. HIKOSAKA, NAKAO and SCHOR for permission to refer to unpublished results.

REFERENCES

BAKER, R.:   Anatomical and physiological organization of brain stem pathways underlying the control of gaze.   In BAKER, R. and BERTHOZ, A. (eds.):   Control of Gaze by Brain Stem Neurons.   pp. 207–222.   Elsevier, Amsterdam-New York (1977)

BAKER, R. and BERTHOZ, A.:   Organization of vestibular nystagmus in oblique oculomotor system.   J. Neurophysiol., 37: 195–217 (1974)

BAKER, R. and BERTHOZ, A.:   Is the prepositus hypoglossi nucleus the source of another vestibuloocular pathway?   Brain Res., 86: 121–127 (1975)

BAKER, R., GRESTY, M. and BERTHOZ, A.:   Neuronal activity in the prepositus hypoglossi nucleus correlated with vertical and horizontal eye movement in the cat.   Brain Res., 101: 366–371 (1976)

BAKER, R. and HIGHSTEIN, S. M.:   Physiological identification of interneurons and motoneurons in the abducens nucleus.   Brain Res., 91: 292–298 (1975)

BAKER, R. G., MANO, N. and SHIMAZU, H.:   Postsynaptic potentials in abducens motoneurons induced by vestibular stimulation.   Brain Res., 15: 577–580 (1969)

BENDER, M. B. and SHANZER, S.:   Oculomotor pathways defined by electrical stimulation and lesions in the brainstem of monkey.   In BENDER, M. B. (ed.):   The Oculomotor System.   pp. 81–140.   Harper and Row, New York (1964)

BLANKS, R. H. I., VOLKIND, R., PRECHT, W. and BAKER, R.:   Responses of cat prepositus hypoglossi neurons to horizontal angular acceleration.   Neuroscience, 2: 391–403 (1977)

BÜTTNER-ENNEVER, J. A. and HENN, V.: An autoradiographic study of the pathways from the pontine reticular formation involved in horizontal eye movements. *Brain Res.*, *108*: 155–164 (1976)

COHEN, B. and HENN, V.: The origin of quick phases of nystagmus in the horizontal plane. *Bibl. ophthal.*, *(Basel) 82*: 36–55 (1972)

DELGADO-GARCIA, J., BAKER, R. and HIGHSTEIN, S. M.: The activity of internuclear neurons identified within the abducens nucleus of the alert cat. *In* BAKER, R. and BERTHOZ, A. (eds.): *Control of Gaze by Brain Stem Neurons.* pp. 291–300. Elsevier, Amsterdam-New York (1977)

DUENSING, F. and SCHAEFER, K. P.: Die Neuronenaktivität in der Formatio reticularis des Rhombencephalons beim vestibulären Nystagmus. *Arch. Psychiat. Nervenkr.*, *196*: 265–290 (1957)

DUENSING, F. and SCHAEFER, K. P.: Die Aktivität einzelner Neurone im Bereich der Vestibulariskerne bei Horizontalbeschleunigungen unter besonderer Berücksichtigung des vestibulären Nystagmus. *Arch. Psychiat. Nervenkr.*, *198*: 225–252 (1958)

FUCHS, A. F. and KIMM, J.: Unit activity in vestibular nucleus of the alert monkey during horizontal angular acceleration and eye movement. *J. Neurophysiol.*, *38*: 1140–1161 (1975)

FUKUSHIMA, Y., IGUSA, Y. and YOSHIDA, K.: Characteristics of responses of medial brain stem neurons to horizontal head angular acceleration and electrical stimulation of the labyrinth in the cat. *Brain Res.*, *120*: 564–570 (1977)

GOEBEL, H. H., KOMATSUZAKI, A., BENDER, M. B. and COHEN, B.: Lesions of the pontine tegmentum and conjugate gaze paralysis. *Arch. Neurol.*, *24*: 431–440 (1971)

GRANT, K., GUERITAUD, J. P., HORCHOLLE-BOSSAVIT, G. and TYČ-DUMONT, S.: Horizontal vestibular nystagmus. II. Activity patterns of medial vestibular neurones during nystagmus. *Exp. Brain Res.*, *26*: 387–405 (1976)

GRAYBIEL, A. M.: Direct and indirect preoculomotor pathways of the brainstem: An autoradiographic study of the pontine reticular formation in the cat. *J. Comp. Neurol.*, *175*: 37–78 (1977)

GRAYBIEL, A. M. and HARTWIEG, E. A.: Some afferent connections of the oculomotor complex in the cat: an experimental study with tracer technique. *Brain Res.*, *81*: 543–551 (1974)

HIGHSTEIN, S. M.: Abducens and oculomotor internuclear neurons: relation to gaze. *In* BAKER, R. and BERTHOZ, A. (eds.): *Control of Gaze by Brain Stem Neurons.* pp. 153–162. Elsevier, Amsterdam-New York (1977)

HIGHSTEIN, S. M.: Synaptic linkage in the vestibulo-ocular and cerebellovestibular pathways to the VIth nucleus in the rabbit. *Exp. Brain Res.*, *17*: 301–314 (1973)

HIKOSAKA, O., IGUSA, Y. and IMAI, H.: Firing pattern of prepositus hypoglossi and adjacent reticular neurons related to vestibular nystagmus in the cat. *Brain Res.*, *144*: 395–403 (1978a)

HIKOSAKA, O., IGUSA, Y., NAKAO, S. and SHIMAZU, H.: Direct inhibitory synaptic linkage of pontomedullary reticular burst neurons with abducens motoneurons in the cat. *Exp. Brain Res.*, *33*: 337–352 (1978b)

HIKOSAKA, O. and KAWAKAMI, T.: Inhibitory reticular neurons related to the quick phase of vestibular nystagmus—their location and projection. *Exp. Brain Res.*, *27*: 377–396 (1977a)

HIKOSAKA, O., MAEDA, M., NAKAO, S., SHIMAZU, H. and SHINODA, Y.: Presynaptic impulses in the abducens nucleus and their relation to postsynaptic potentials in motoneurons during vestibular nystagmus. *Exp. Brain Res.*, *27*: 355–376 (1977b)

HODDEVIK, G. H., BRODAL, A. and WALBERG, F.: The reticulovestibular projection in the cat. An experimental study with silver impregnation methods. *Brain Res.*, *94*: 383–399 (1975)

HORCHOLLE, G. and TYČ-DUMONT, S.: Activités unitaires des neurones vestibulaires et oculomoteurs an cours du nystagmus. *Exp. Brain Res.*, *5*, 16–31 (1968)

HORCHOLLE-BOSSAVIT, G. and TYČ-DUMONT, S.: Phénoménes synaptiques du nystagmus. *Exp. Brain Res.*, *8*: 201–218 (1969)

IMAI, H., HIKOSAKA, O. and IGUSA, Y.: Axonal projection of reticular inhibitory burst neurons and their target cells in the cat (in Japanese). *J. Physiol. Soc. Japan*, *39*: 321 (1977)

KELLER, E. L.: Participation of medial pontine reticular formation in eye movement generation in monkey. *J. Neurophysiol.*, *37*: 316–332 (1974)

KELLER, E. L. and DANIELS, P. D.: Oculomotor related interaction of vestibular and visual stimulation in vestibular nucleus cells in alert monkey. *Exp. Neurol. 46*: 187–198 (1975)

KELLER, E. L. and KAMATH, B. Y.: Characteristics of head rotation and eye movement-related neurons in alert monkey vestibular nucleus. *Brain Res.*, *100*: 182–187 (1975)

LORENTE DE NÓ, R.: Vestibulo-ocular reflex arc. *Arch. Neurol. Psychiat. (Chic.), 30*: 245–291 (1933)

LORENTE DE NÓ, R.: Observation on nystagmus. *Acta oto-laryng. (Stockh.)*, *21*: 416–437 (1934)

LUSCHEI, E. S. and FUCHS, A. F.: Activity of brain stem neurons during eye movements of alert monkeys. *J. Neurophysiol.*, *35*: 445–461 (1972)

MACIEWICZ, R. J., EAGEN, K., KANEKO, C. R. S. and HIGHSTEIN, S. M.: Vestibular and medullary brain stem afferents to the abducens nucleus in the cat. *Brain Res.*, *123*: 229–240 (1977)

MAEDA, M., SHIMAZU, H. and SHINODA, Y.: Inhibitory postsynaptic potentials in the abducens motoneurons associated with the quick relaxation phase of vestibular nystagmus. *Brain Res.*, *26*: 420–424 (1971)

MAEDA, M., SHIMAZU, H. and SHINODA, Y.: Nature of synaptic events in cat abducens motoneurons at slow and quick phase of vestibular nystagmus. *J. Neurophysiol.*, *35*: 279–296 (1972)

MILES, F. A.: Single unit firing patterns in the vestibular nuclei related to voluntary eye movements and passive body rotation in conscious monkeys. *Brain Res.*, *71*: 215–224 (1974)

NAKAO, S. and SASAKI, S.: Firing pattern of interneurons in the abducens nucleus related to vestibular nystagmus in the cat. *Brain Res.*, *144*: 389–394 (1978)

PETERSON, B. W., FILION, M., FELPEL, L. P. and ABZUG, C.: Responses of medial reticular neurons to stimulation of the vestibular nerve. *Exp. Brain Res.*, *22*: 335–350 (1975)

PRECHT, W. and SHIMAZU, H.: Functional connections of tonic and kinetic vestibular neurons with primary vestibular afferents. *J. Neurophysiol.*, *28*: 1014–1028 (1965)

SCHOR, R. H., NAKAO, S. and SHIMAZU, H.: Responses of medial vestibular nucleus neurons during vestibular nystagmus. *Neurosci. Abstr.*, *3*: 545 (1977)

SHIMAZU, H. and PRECHT, W.: Inhibition of central vestibular neurons from the contralateral labyrinth and its mediating pathway. *J. Neurophysiol.*, *29*: 467–492 (1966)

SHINODA, Y. and YOSHIDA, K.: Dynamic characteristics of responses to horizontal head angular acceleration in vestibuloocular pathway in the cat. *J. Neurophysiol.*, *37*: 653–673 (1974)

SPARKS, D. L. and TRAVIS, R. P.: Firing patterns of reticular formation neurons during horizontal eye movements. *Brain Res.*, *33*: 477–481 (1971)

SPIEGEL, E. A. and PRICE, J. B.: Origin of the quick component of labyrinthine nystagmus. *Arch. Oto-Laryngol.*, *30*: 576–588 (1939)

DISCUSSION PERIOD

WILSON: This is a brief comment rather than a question. The location of your inhibitory and excitatory neurons is very much the same as the area where there also is a concentration of neurons inhibiting neck motoneurons. It makes you wonder to what extent some of these neurons might be involved in both vestibulo-ocular and vestibulo-spinal pathways.

SHIMAZU: Well, the location of the inhibitory and excitatory vestibular and reticular neurons projecting to the abducens nucleus seem to intermingle with the location of neurons controlling neck motoneurons. But I do not know whether there are neurons projecting to both the neck and eye motor nucleus and whether the neurons controlling the neck have the same functional characteristics as the neurons controlling the eye have.

WILSON: It's a general area which I think may be involved in both neck and eye control.

SHIMAZU: Yes, I agree.

BAKER: Where do you believe the excitatory burst neurons are located?

SHIMAZU: We have tried to find burst or burst-tonic type of excitatory premotor neurons around the abducens nucleus and rostral or caudal to it, but so far we were unable to find their origin. We found burst-tonic neurons in various areas near the abducens nucleus, but could not demonstrate their projection to the abducens nucleus or termination on motoneurons. Your question is still our current research project and I do not think I have a proper answer at the present moment.

COHEN: In the area that Ann GRAYBIEL showed, the projections to the abducens nucleus appear to be somewhat more rostral in the pontine reticular formation than the region in which you found the inhibitory burst neurons. Have you looked in that rostral area for possible projections to the abducens nucleus? Or to abducens motoneurons?

SHIMAZU: Yes. We looked for neurons in the pontine reticular formation rostral to the abducens nucleus, because that area seemed to us to be one of the most probable regions in view of anatomy. As I told you, we have not yet found burst or burst-tonic neurons which make direct excitatory connection with abducens motoneurons. But I expect some neurons located in this region should project directly to the abducens nucleus and it is interesting to see the behavior of possible premotor neurons in this area during nystagmus.

VESTIBULAR COMPENSATION: A DISTRIBUTED PROPERTY OF THE CENTRAL NERVOUS SYSTEM*

Rodolfo LLINÁS and Kerry WALTON

*Department of Physiology and Biophysics, New York University Medical Center
New York, NY*

INTRODUCTION

While many topics in neurophysiology could in fact be regarded as representative of the important influence of Rafael LORENTE DE NÓ and David LLOYD, the study of vestibular compensation is one which touches on the work of both these distinguished scientists. Few phenomena in the central nervous system are as remarkable and as deep rooted in both motor performance and sensory reorganization as vestibular compensation. For among the special senses, vestibular input is the only one where the bilateral complementarity of function is essential for survival. Thus, while the unilateral loss of olfaction, vision or audition leaves the animal relatively unimpaired, a unilateral lesion of the vestibular nerve renders the animal completely defenseless and incapable of survival.

It is, therefore, not surprising that the nervous system responds to this lesion in such a manner as to generate the efficient postural and dynamic compensation which is commonly observed (cf. SCHAEFFER and MEYER, 1974). In addition, because vestibular damage can be inflicted in a very precise manner and because the deficiencies that follow and the steps in their compensation are uniform from one animal to the next, it is one of the paradigms of choice in the study of response of the central nervous system to lesions (cf. EIDELBERG and STEIN, 1974). In our particular experimental animal, the rat, vestibular compensation following lesion under ether occurs in a matter of hours (LLINÁS et al., 1975) at least as far as correction of the abnormal posture of head and limbs is concerned; compensation of abnormal eye movements takes somewhat longer (Fig. 1). Furthermore, this paradigm is of general interest since considerable data are available regarding the morphology and neurophysiology of the brain areas which are *prima facie* implicated in this compensation. Thus, electrophysiology of the brain stem, including the oculomotor, vestibular, and associated cerebellar and precerebellar nuclei, is the best understood area in our field today.

In the present paper, in addition to a brief description of our main findings regarding the implication of the inferior olive and cerebellar nuclei in vestibular compensation, we will present some new findings relating to the redistribution of activity at these levels, both immediately following vestibular lesion and after its compensation. From this set of experiments we conclude that vestibular compensation is not the product of an altered activity in a particular pathway, but rather the product of a concerted reorganization of activity involving a much broader region of the nervous system than would be expected from present knowledge of the brain stem. Because our results imply a broad distribution of the functional modifications producing and maintaining this compensation, we wish to refer to this phenomenon as a distributed process. We will further give reasons for how this may be more in agreement with our present understanding of nervous system function.

---

* Research was supported by USPHS grant NS-13742 from the National Institute of Neurological and Communicative Disorders and Stroke.

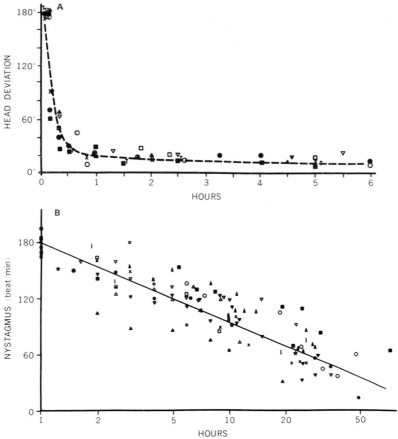

Fig. 1 Time course of vestibular compensation in the rat. *A*: Compensation of head tilt follow-ing hemilabyrinthectomy in 8 animals. *B*: Decrease in rate of spontaneous nystagmus following hemilabyrinthectomy in 14 animals. Note semilogarithmic scale in B. (from LLINÁS and WALTON, 1977)

General description of vestibular compensation

As stated above, recovery of function following unilateral injury to the peripheral vestib-ular apparatus occurs rapidly and is remarkably complete.   Compensation has been stud-ied in man (FLUUR, 1960; PFALTZ and KAMATH, 1970; PFALTZ et al., 1973) and has been a subject of experimental investigation since the last century (cf. BECHTEREW, 1883).   In these studies the investigators have found that this process can be divided into three distinct stages as defined by the presence of characteristic behavior patterns (McCABE and RYU, 1969).   In the first or "critical" stage, beginning immediately after hemilabyrinthectomy or neurotomy, the animals exhibit severe symptoms of imbalance including rapid sponta-neous nystagmus, severe head deviation and forced circling or rolling toward the deaffer-ented side (see Fig. 2A).   The second or "acute" stage is marked by a rapid partial recov-ery of asymmetry (Fig. 2B), while during the last or "compensatory" stage the animal's recovery is maximum (Fig. 2C).   The duration of each period is species-dependent (cf. SCHAEFER and MEYER, 1974) as is the level of recovery achieved.

Recent electrophysiological investigations of the vestibular nucleus (VN) of cat have found that characteristic changes in the activity in this nucleus are associated with each of these stages.   The most salient findings are that there is a decrease in spontaneous activity

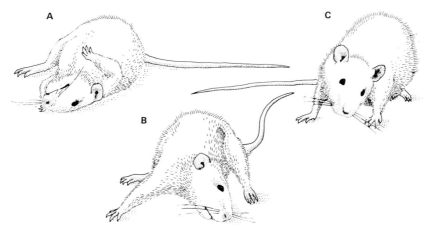

Fig. 2 Postural characteristics of rat following left hemilabyrinthectomy. *A*: Critical stage immediately following lesion. Animal is very unstable and tends to roll toward the lesioned side. *B*: Acute stage in the same animal 20 min following the lesion. Animal assumes a more stable posture characterized by tilting, twisting of head to lesioned side, extension of contralateral forelimb and a wide stance. *C*: Compensatory stage in same animal two weeks following lesion. This particular animal is as stable as a normal animal but has a larger head-tilt than the majority of compensated rats. Basic posture in drawings was traced from photographs.

in the deafferented vestibular nuclei which begins immediately after hemilabyrinthectomy and lasts, in the cat, for several days (GERNANDT and THULIN, 1952; SHIMAZU and PRECHT, 1966; PRECHT et al., 1966; McCABE and RYU, 1969; McCABE et al., 1972; PRECHT, 1974) and that normal activity is restored in the compensatory stage (PRECHT et al., 1966; McCABE and RYU, 1969; McCABE et al., 1972). GERNANDT and THULIN (1952), recording immediately following neurotomy in decerebrate or lightly anesthetized cats, found that this reduction or elimination of spontaneous activity in the deafferented VN was not affected even by great horizontal angular acceleration. However, activity could be recorded from the intact nucleus. Here the response of type I neurons to natural vestibular stimulation was not significantly altered.

Similar results for the deafferented side in the critical stage (3 hrs) have been reported by SHIMAZU and PRECHT (1966); however, they did not observe a cessation of activity. A slight increase in spontaneous discharge frequency was found in the intact side where the threshold of type I neurons to horizontal angular acceleration was elevated while the maximum firing frequency did not change. This increase in spontaneous activity was attributed to decreased inhibitory input from the lesioned side. The change in the deafferented nucleus was investigated further (PRECHT et al., 1966) where recordings were made from decerebrate and decerebellate cats in the acute (3–4 days) and the compensatory (30–45 days) stages.

During the acute stage, as in the critical stage, the number of spontaneously active cells, their rate of activity, and the frequency response of type I cells to acceleration were all below normal. These increased still more in the compensatory stage, although type I spontaneous activity was still lower on the deafferented side than on the intact side, and the maximum discharge frequency of type I cells during ipsilateral natural stimulation was about one-third normal. These authors interpreted their findings in terms of changes in the VN themselves. The reappearance of spontaneous activity, for example, was attributed to inherent mechanisms at the level of the vestibular nuclei; increased biochemical sensitivity of the type I neurons and sprouting of afferent fibers were mentioned as possible mechanisms.   Functional changes in the type I neurons were also proposed as the basis for an observed lowered threshold for commissural inhibition, while the decreased maximum firing rate is explained in terms of inhibitory influences from the contralateral canal. It is important to note that, although the animals in this study did recover normal vestibulo-ocular function, postural abnormalities remained.   PRECHT et al. suggested that the remaining asymmetry could reflect the low level of spontaneous activity on the deafferented as compared to the intact side. These results underline the importance of restored vestibular symmetry in achieving full compensation and suggest that these animals were not, in fact, in the compensatory stage.

McCABE and RYU (1969) recorded unit activity from the medial VN (MVN) during all three stages of compensation.   In contrast to the findings of PRECHT et al. (1966) and GERNANDT and THULIN (1952), no active cells could be found in the MVN on either side during the critical stage (1 and 2 days).   In the acute stage (7 days) low to moderate activity was recorded on the intact side and "scant" or no activity on the deafferented side. Normal activity returned to both sides by the compensatory stage (30 days).   Unfortunately, the findings reported in this paper are difficult to evaluate as no quantitative treatment of the data was given nor were records of neuronal activity shown.   Furthermore, the postural and oculomotor characteristics of each particular animal were not provided.

The results briefly reviewed above cannot be directly compared since the recordings were made from different areas with the VN and at different times after peripheral lesion. Nevertheless, a correlation can be made between the presence or absence of symmetrical VN activity and the behavioral characteristics of the critical, acute and compensated stages. Interpretation of the data concerned with the activity in the intact VN in the critical and acute stages is difficult at this time as no change (GERNANDT and THULIN, 1952), a small increase (SHIMAZU and PRECHT, 1966), lower than normal activity (PRECHT et al., 1966) and no activity (McCABE and RYU, 1966, 1972) have all been reported.   The main question does not lie here, however, but concerns defining the systems and mechanisms by which vestibular balance is restored.

To pursue the importance of changes in the functional properties of the vestibular neurons themselves, DIERINGER and PRECHT (1977) have studied the characteristics of synaptic function in the vestibular nuclei of hemilabyrinthectomized frogs.   They report that neurons in the partially deafferented nucleus in chronic preparations (≤ 60 days) have increased excitability and increased synaptic efficacy of the commissural system when compared to acute preparations (≤ 12 hrs).   The improved synaptic transmission was characterized by a lower threshold, shorter rise time, and increased amplitude of EPSPs elicited by stimulation of the contralateral eighth nerve.

Although changes in the properties of neurons within the deafferented vestibular nucleus itself may play a role in compensation, other systems are equally if not more important. Thus, in an effort to define the neurological basis for compensation, early studies involved for the most part the ablation or lesioning of various central nervous system structures known to be associated with vestibular function.   Although these results were not in complete agreement, those structures other than the vestibular nuclei most often found to play a role in the rapid and complete acquisition of compensation were the spinal cord (FISCHER, 1930; KOLB, 1955), the cerebellum (LANGE, 1891; DEMETRIADES and SPIEGEL, 1927), the cerebellar nuclei (CARPENTER et al., 1959; DOW, 1938a), and the visual system (DOW, 1938b Van HOLST, 1955).   Recent experiments have sought to extend and clarify the contribution of each of these structures.

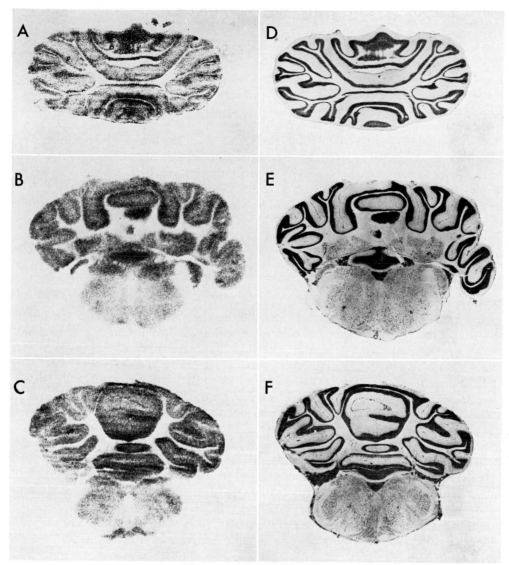

Fig. 4   Normal animal. Autoradiographs (A–C) and histological sections (D–F). *A and D*: Horizontal section through the cerebellar cortex (rostral is up). Note difference in grain density between the vermis and hemispheres. *B and E*: Transverse section at the level of the cerebellar nuclei (CB) and the vestibular nuclei (VN). Note that the grain density in the CB is close to that in the molecular level of the cortex. *C and F*: Transverse section at the level of the inferior olive. Note that the density in the inferior olive is close to that in the molecular layer. *D–F*: Nissl stained tissue.

4B, 8A, and 9A) nuclei.   The inferior olive is also demarcated; in Figs. 4C and 8C its several subnuclei are clearly indicated.   Also visible in these few examples are the nucleus of the spinal trigeminal tract (Fig. 4C) and the cochlear nucleus (Figs. 4B and 9A).   Neither axons nor dendrites take up appreciable amounts of glucose.   For this reason, fiber tracts and the molecular layer of the cerebellar cortex are very light.   In fact, in some brain stem sections the edge is not well defined; see Fig. 4C for example.   This is especially so for those sections in which the spinal tract of the trigeminal nerve runs on the lateral surface of the brain stem.

The distribution of radioactivity in sections made from the brains of experimental animals will not be described in detail in this paper.   Rather, we will consider only those areas in which a significant change in activity is seen following vestibular lesion.   Although a quantitative study of these results is in progress, a qualitative analysis will be given here. Accordingly, differences in activity levels of particular structures (e.g. VN) between different animals (e.g normal and compensated) will be noted only when the ratios between these structures and the background density of the sections are markedly different in the two animals.

Uncompensated animals

Immediately after hemilabyrinthectomy, during the critical stage when the animals are uncompensated, the distribution of activity within the brain stem and cerebellum is significantly different from that seen in normal animals.   In the cerebellar cortex the posterior vermis is slightly darker than other areas.   This increased radioactivity can be seen in both horizontal (Fig. 5A) and transverse (Fig. 5C and D) sections.   Activity in the cerebellar nuclei (CB) is also above normal levels (Fig. 5B) (this is especially apparent if one compares the CB/cortex ratio in normal and uncompensated animals), with the largest increase seen bilaterally in the dentate nuclei.   Increased activity is also seen in the interpositus and fastigial nuclei, however.   Further, nuclei ipsilateral to the lesion seem more active than those on the contralateral side.

The most outstanding change from the control is seen in the vestibular nuclei themselves (Figs. 5C and 8B), where activity in the deafferented nucleus is well below that on the intact side.   This is consistent with electrophysiological findings of decreased spontaneous activity in the first stages following peripheral vestibular lesion (GERNANDT and THULIN, 1952; SHIMAZU and PRECHT, 1966), but activity is, however, present in the intact VN.   In the ventral brain stem (Fig. 5D), activity levels in the inferior olive are increased slightly above normal.   Note that the medial and dorsal accessory and principal subnuclei can be distinguished.   These autoradiographs show that immediately following peripheral nerve lesion, a considerable change in the distribution of activity can be seen.   Even greater changes are seen in compensated animals.

Compensated animals

Autoradiographs taken of tissue from animals in the compensatory stage give a clear indication of which brain stem and cerebellar structures have activity above normal levels and may be considered to contribute to the active maintenance of compensation.   The most important feature is that the activity in the deafferented vestibular nucleus has increased so as to equal that on the intact side (Fig. 6B, C).   Moreover, the amount of radioactivity is higher on both sides than is seen in normal or uncompensated animals.

In the cerebellum, the posterior vermis is very active, as can be seen both in horizontal

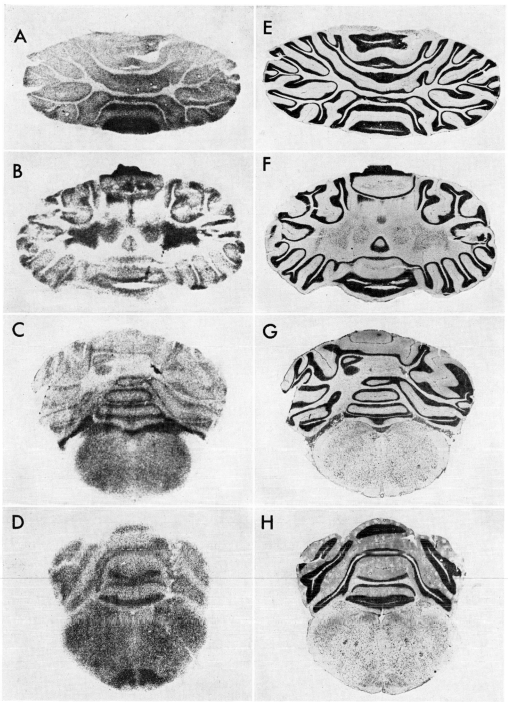

Fig. 5 Animal in the critical stage immediately following left hemilabyrinthectomy. Autoradiographs (A–D) and histological sections (F–H). *A and E*: Horizontal section through the cerebellar cortex (rostral is up). Note density of radioactivity in posterior vermis. *B and F*: Horizontal section at the level of the cerebellar nuclei (rostral is up). Note density in the dentate and interpositus nuclei. *C and G*: Transverse section at the level of the vestibular and prepositus nuclei. Note high density of grains on the right side. *D and H*: Transverse section at the level of the inferior olive. Note density in this nucleus is higher than normal. *E–H*: Nissl stained tissue.

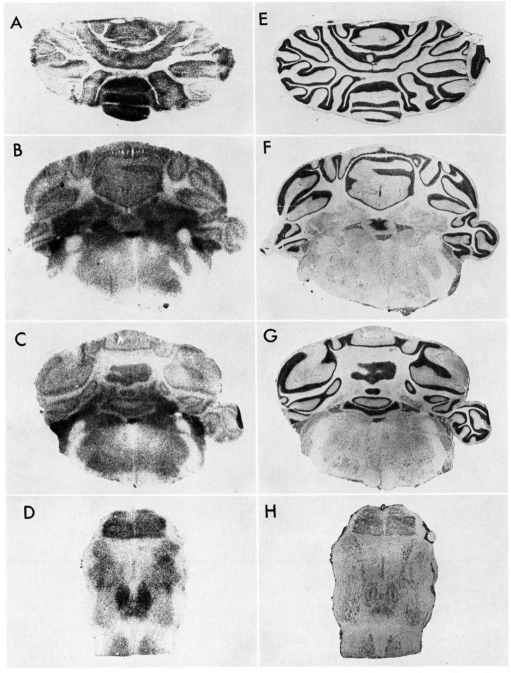

Fig. 6 Animals in the compensatory stage following left hemilabyrinthectomy. Autoradiographs (A–D) and histological sections (E–H). *A and E*: Horizontal section through the cerebellar cortex (rostral is up). Note high grain density in the posterior vermis. *B and F*: Transverse section at the level of the cerebellar nuclei and the medial and lateral vestibular nuclei. Note that the grain density in the vestibular nuclei on both sides is very similar and the cerebellar nuclei are dark (black areas are choroid plexus). *C and G*: Transverse section at the level of the vestibular nuclei. Note the grain density is close to equal on the two sides. *D and H*: Horizontal section (rostral is up) at the level of the inferior olive and lateral reticular nucleus. Note high density of inferior olive and activity in the reticular nuclei. *E–H*: Nissl stained tissue.

(Fig. 6A) and in transverse (Fig. 8C) sections. There is also increased activity in the lobus simplex (Fig. 6A).

As in the uncompensated animal, radioactivity levels in the cerebellar nuclei are above normal (Figs. 6B and 9C); this is especially marked in both dentate nuclei. The fastigial nuclei, although not as active as the lateral nuclei, are still above normal levels. There are two findings of particular interest in these autoradiographs. First, the radioactivity in the dentate nuclei is much higher than that found in normal animals. The increase may be due, in part, to cerebellar disinhibition, but this is difficult to determine for, although there is no increased activity in those lobules projecting to this nucleus, a decrease in activity is not easily discernible. Second, the vermal cortex is very dark, while the fastigial nuclei are the least active of the CB. It is possible that the relatively low level of activity here may be due to Purkinje cell inhibition.

Activity in the inferior olive is also above normal levels (Figs. 6D and 8C). In the Fig. 8C the subnuclei can be clearly distinguished, and the medial accessory and principal subnuclei are especially dark.

A group of cells in the region of the lateral reticular nucleus (LRN) and the Nucleus ambiguus can be distinguished in compensated animals. This reticular area is not usually noticeable in autoradiographs of normal animals.

The compensatory stage is marked by increased activity in the posterior vermis, cerebellar nuclei (especially the dentate), and reticular nuclei. These results suggest that increased activity very likely contributes to maintaining the compensatory state, in part by supporting the activity in the deafferented VN. This can be tested by determining whether the radioactivity in these structures returns to normal levels when compensation is lost.

Decompensated animals

The distribution of activity in animals decompensated following chemical lesion of the inferior olive (Fig. 7) looks very similar to that seen in uncompensated animals. Once again the activity in the vestibular nuclei is asymmetrical (Fig. 7C). The activity on the deafferented side is below normal, and that of the intact nucleus is very close to normal. The distribution of activity in the cerebellar cortex has also decreased, as has that in the reticular nuclei (Fig. 7A). A close look at the histological sections at the level of the inferior olive (Fig. 7D) reveals that only glial cells remain while no radioactivity is visible in this region of the corresponding autoradiograph (Fig. 7A). This verifies that significant glucose uptake is limited to neuronal elements.

The results in Figure 7 shows that the increase in activity seen during the critical and compensatory stages is indeed part of the compensatory process and, for this reason, is lost along with compensation.

Summary of results

These findings support and extend investigations at the behavioral and electrophysiological levels. In fact, they serve to bridge the gap between these two approaches in that spontaneous activity levels can be measured in several brain regions during a particular behavioral state. The progressively changing behavioral manifestations of the compensation process are a result not of activity in a small area of a single nucleus which can be monitored by electrodes, but of the concerted activity of the brain stem and cerebellum.

A primary finding of this study is that decompensation causes asymmetry in the vestibular nuclei. This can be seen at the level of the medial nuclei (Fig. 8). By comparing Figures 8A, B and C, a progressive change in activity is seen. Not only has the ipsilateral

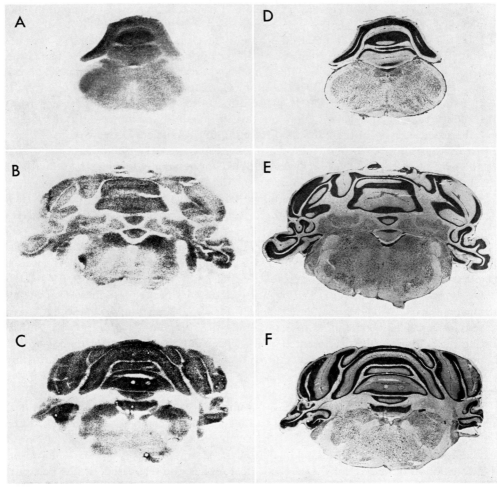

Fig. 7 3-Acetylpyridine decompensated animal. Vestibular compensation (from left labyrinthectomy) was lost in this animal following injection of 3-acetylpyridine and harmaline. Autoradiographs (A–C) and histological sections (D–F). *A and D*: Transverse section at the level of the inferior olive and posterior vermis. Note the light grain density and absence of cells (D) in the inferior olive. *B and E*: Transverse section at the level of the cerebellar nuclei and medial and lateral vestibular nuclei (VN). Note that grain density in the cerebellar nuclei is relatively low and that the right VN is darker than the left. *C and F*: Transverse section at the level of the medial and superior VN. Note that right VN has a higher grain density than the left. *D–F*: Nissl stained tissue.

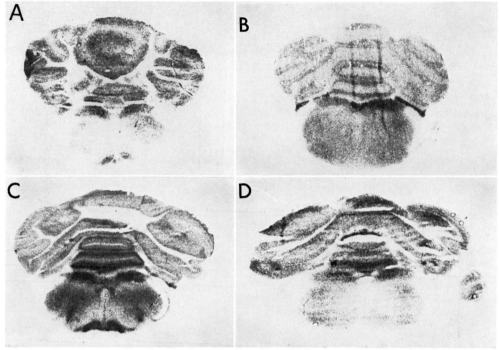

Fig. 8 Changes in the vestibular nuclei with vestibular compensation and decompensation following left hemilabyrinthectomy. Autoradiographs of transverse sections at the level of the medial vestibular nuclei. *A*: Normal animal. *B*: Critical stage. Note density of grains in nuclei contralateral to the lesioned side. *C*: Compensatory stage. Note that the high grain density is present in the vestibular nuclei on both sides. Also activity can be seen in reticular nuclei on both sides. *D*: Decompensated animal. Note the higher grain density on the side contralateral to the lesion.

activity decreased, but contralateral activity has increased (compare 8A and B) in the critical stage. It has been suggested that this is due to a loss of inhibition of the commissural system (PRECHT, 1974). However, additional work is needed before we can determine if a change of such magnitude can be produced in this way. During the compensatory stage, bilateral symmetry returns to the vestibular nuclei (Fig. 8C); in addition, their level of activity appears above normal. Finally, in decompensated animals vestibular symmetry is lost and the increased activity in the brain stem and cerebellum returns to normal (Fig. 8D).

The changes in the activity of the cerebellar nuclei during the compensation process can be seen in Figure 9. The most striking finding is that the activity of all three nuclei is above normal in the compensating animals (Fig. 9B and C) and that, among these nuclei, the dentate is the darkest and the fastigial the lightest. These results suggest that the inferior olive, lateral reticular nucleus and other reticular nuclei, as well as the vestibular nuclei themselves, may contribute to this increased activity.

A view of vestibular compensation

These findings support the view that vestibular compensation results from the combined activity of many brain stem and cerebellar structures. Accordingly, following the loss of primary input to one vestibular nucleus, the level of spontaneous and evoked activity is severely decreased, if not eliminated entirely. Symmetry of function is lost and the animal

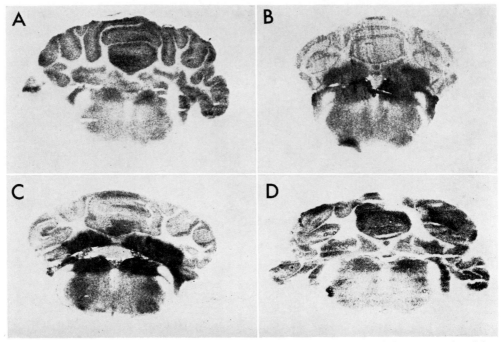

Fig. 9 Changes in the cerebellar nuclei with vestibular compensation and decompensation following left hemilabyrinthectomy. Autoradiographs of transverse sections. *A*: Normal animal. *B*: Critical stage. Note that the cerebellar nuclei have a high grain density. *C*: compensatory stage. Note high density in cerebellar nuclei, especially the dentate. *D*: Decompensated animal. Note that cerebellar nucleus activity is relatively low and comparable to normal animal (A).

is virtually helpless. Correlated with the return of function is an increased activity in the deafferented nucleus and in other structures. This reappearance of activity must have a structure, and it must contain information concerning the position of the head in space and vestibulo-ocular function. This is necessary since maintaining the compensatory state is an active, continuous, process in which the nervous system must create, from moment to moment, a mime of the normal vestibular input. Although input from the intact vestibular apparatus may contribute to this reconstruction, information provided by other sensory systems may be more important (see PFALTZ and KAMATH, 1970; PUTKONEN et al., 1977).

We picture then that in vestibular compensation, input from muscle, joint and cutaneous receptors would first be integrated in the brain stem precerebellar and prevestibular nuclei. This information would then proceed to the cerebellar and vestibular nuclei and from the cerebellum to the vestibular nuclei. Descending inputs from, for example, the cerebral cortex and visual centers would influence the output of vestibular neurons as well. Thus, there would be no "new" inputs to the deafferented nucleus, but those systems normally influencing the functioning of this nucleus would modulate their input by the synaptic sprouting or increased activity in such a way so as to correct for the postural and oculomotor abnormalities which would otherwise result from the peripheral lesion. Accordingly, those motor systems most involved in the compensatory process would be the vestibulo-spinal and reticulo-spinal tracts. (A more detailed discussion may be found in LLINÁS and WALTON, 1979.)

In order to provide a summary of this scheme, some of the pathways are represented in Figure 10. It should be understood, however, that we do not view this scheme as a set of loops but rather as a means to demonstrate a distributed property arising from integrated

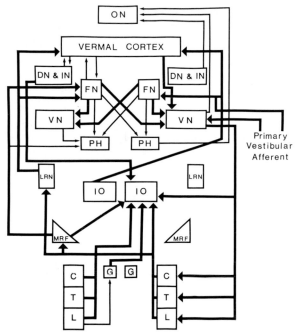

Fig. 10 A schematic representation of some of the major structures involved in the compensation of postural and oculomotor asymmetry following left hemilabyrinthectomy in rats. Some bilateral pathways are shown on only one side for the sake of clarity. ON, oculomotor nuclei; DN, dentate nucleus; IN, interpositus nucleus; FN, fastigial nucleus; VN, vestibular nuclei; PH, prepositus nucleus; IO, inferior olive; MRF, medial reticular formation; LRN, lateral reticular nucleus; G, nucleus gracilis; C, T, L, cervical, thoracic and lumbar spinal cord.

activity at many levels. In short, as stated in the title, we maintain the conviction that vestibular compensation is one of the best examples of what is known as a distributed property (PELLIONISZ and LLINÁS, 1979) as opposed to the product of serial acts of particular neuronal loops. This topic will be treated in more detail in the Discussion.

DISCUSSION

There is no doubt, we are sure, that the present general conceptions regarding the function of the nervous system still lack much crucial data relating form and function in the brain. Thus, although present neurobiological research still continues to be dominated by classical reflexological concepts, some general reevaluation of its tenets does seem to be called for.

Basically, one of our main conceptual stands regarding the general character of brain organization is the parallel nature of its neuronal circuits. Nevertheless, we continue to treat such circuits as simple loops reducible in principle to a small category of "representative elements". There are, however, two main reasons why this approach, although extremely productive in the past, may become sterile. One of them relates to the fact that a description of a sequential loop (where many cells are collapsed into a typical "neuronal net") destroys, by definition, the parallel nature of nerve net function. In other words, while it is correct that a particular input may have a specific and quite determined internal projection, the purely sequential description of the events which follow its activation does not give any true insight into the nature or significance of the "message" carried by that particular fiber.

Essentially, the study of such reflexology may be described as an extension of electro-anatomy, the basic assumption being that in describing the sequence of events triggered, at single cell level, by a given input, one defines the network function.   Such an approach has not been as fruitful (in retrospect) as was originally expected.   This outcome is not altogether surprising if we consider that the parallel distribution of activity in the brain is probably the most salient of its morphological characteristics.   There is no question that while morphologically the above statement is easy to accept, it is very difficult to formulate into clear functional research design.   It is also true, however, that until we agree that messages in the brain are not serially organized, but rather, are organized in a parallel fashion, we will not develop the necessary tools and conceptology for confronting such problems.   It is very likely, on the other hand, that rather than finding a totally new technological approach capable of reorganizing our experimental approach, we may have to develop hybrid techniques and new conceptual tools, such as tensor network theory (PELLIONISZ and LLINÁS, 1979), which, in a piecemeal fashion, take account of different aspects of the spatial distribution of activity.   With these thoughts in mind, we have attempted to study what we consider to be a classical paradigm: compensation from the abnormal posture which follows unilateral vestibular lesion.

Factors influencing vestibular compensation

Even the crudest compilation of the various lesions which may delay or reverse vestibular compensation indicates that this compensation is the product of activities in which many levels of integration coalesce.   It involves the participation of afferents from the hindlimbs to the all pervasive neck input, but is not restricted to proprioception since it also may require some of the special senses.   Furthermore, in comparing how the different verte-brates must compensate vestibular lesions (cf. SCHAEFER and MEYER, 1974), one finds that while the final compensatory state is basically comparable the detailed mechanisms by which this final compensation is attained may differ from one species to another.   In fact, the mechanisms may be as different as is the mode of locomotion or the general organi-zation of movement in the various species.

The general aim here, however, is to attempt a broad summary of those regions of the nervous system that are necessary and sufficient for vestibular compensation since, although the system is obviously "distributed", it is finite.   Experiments suggest that, at least at first approximation, vestibular compensation requires primarily, as has been indicated electro-physiologically, an increase in the background activity of the deafferented vestibular nucleus.

The problem is to define how, in the absence of vestibular nerve input, the deafferented nucleus can reconstruct activity dynamically equivalent to its contralateral counterpart. Evidently the vestibular nucleus itself may do so while its remaining inputs are largely un-altered.   A better statement may be, however, that in order to generate vestibular compen-sation the rest of the nervous system must modify its emphasis onto the deafferented vestib-ular nucleus in such a manner as to equalize the difference between the two vestibular nuclei. The difference between these two statements is important.   One may assume, for instance, that vestibular compensation can be produced by the modified effectiveness of, let us say, the synaptic efficiency of a given input.   There is, however, no input which can alone produce vestibular compensation.   In addition, a synaptic overemphasis by any particular input would probably require a complete reorganization of such input with respect to the other, equally important, vestibular inputs and, thus, a general change in motor response.   Such is apparently not the case; for the most part vestibular com-pensated animals behave, following normal vestibular stimulation, in a manner quite similar to non-lesioned individuals.

More to the point, the experiments described above indicate that such compensation is produced by an increased activity not simply in the vestibular nucleus, but rather in a large number of nuclei across the brain stem. This is also the case in animals which compensate in the absence of the cerebellar cortex. However, beyond the inferior olivary nucleus, an equally large increase of activity was found in the cerebellar nuclei, concomitantly with the acquisition of this compensation, suggesting a wide reorganization of CNS activity. In addition, the nervous system elevates the activity of the deafferented nucleus in a continuous manner. This is clearly demonstrated following injection of radioactive sugars. Thus, in the various animals studied, the background radioactivity in brain stem seems always to be higher in the compensated animals than in their uncompensated or normal counter parts. Equally interesting, the inferior olive showed a bilateral increase in activity in the compensated animal.

Approach to study of distributed systems in the central nervous system

If indeed single cell activity in the nervous system does not truly reflect the overall properties of the ensemble, how do we go about studying such properties in a more precise manner than may be determined by radioactive sugar and in a manner more global than may be achieved by the study of many single individual cells with microelectrodes?

In a recent theoretical paper (PELLIONISZ and LLINÁS, 1979), we have discussed the possibility of studying distributed properties in the brain by means of tensor theory. Basically, the approach may be described as follows. We consider that peripheral messages coming into the nervous system via a pathway actually represent frequency vectors which are meant to "specify", in concert with other inputs, an internal functional status. This internal status is the result of input connectivity with the postsynaptic elements (the connectivity matrix). The connectivity matrix determines vector-to-vector transformation, which represents central status and which converts a set of input spikes into output firing. Our theory indicates that the vector-vector transformation is performed by the *network tensor*. Since tensors are reference-frame invariant mathematical relations among vectors, with this approach cerebellar function is interpretable in the multidimensional vector-space of the cerebellar tensor. In fact, the trajectories in this cerebellar vector space set the "natural rails" for motor coordination. In short then, the cerebellar anatomy implements the tensorial property through neuronal connectivity, cerebellar tuning then being generated by the interplay at cerebellar nuclear level between the status vector (mossy fiber input to cerebellar nuclei and cortex) and the coordination vector (generated by the Purkinje cell output).

However, the important point here in relation to the role of the cerebellum in the acquisition of motor skills, as exemplified by vestibular compensation, is that according to the present results we must consider the cerebellar nuclei as serving to correct for gross modifications of posture while the cerebellar cortex probably relates more specifically to a fine tuning of given corrections. This is in accordance with our new views regarding cerebellar function, since in our scheme we simply assume that, as stated above, the inputs to the cerebellar nuclei represent status vectors which relate to the gross distribution of overall activity. These status vectors must activate the cerebellar nuclei in order to generate an overall balance between the two vestibular nuclei. The status vectors would continue on to the cortex to specify the Purkinje cell system and thus refine, via the Purkinje cell (to the coordination vector), the coordination characteristic of a normal rat. It is quite clear that while animals devoid of cerebellar cortex can compensate the gross motor abnormalities which follow vestibular lesion, they are ataxic not only in regard to their normal gait but also in the way they respond to vestibular stimuli. We would then say that the difference between compensation of a normal and a cerebellar-decorticate animal is that the former is capable of rather sophisticated dynamic vestibular response while the latter, although compensated for the major posture abnormalities, is not capable of such fine tuning.

This set of experiments in which we attempted to define the change in the spatial distribution of neuronal activity concomitant with the changing behavioral state of the animal bore out previous conclusions: in particular, that vestibular compensation requires a complex modification of many aspects of brain stem and spinal function (LLINÁS and WALTON, 1979). They also support the view that vestibular compensation is a distributed property of the nervous system.

REFERENCES

ALBUS, J. S.: A theory of cerebellar function. *Math. Biosci., 10*: 25–61 (1971)

AZZENA, G. B.: Role of the spinal cord in compensating the effects of hemilabyrinthectomy. *Arch. Ital. Biol., 107*: 43–53 (1969)

AZZENA, G. B., MAMELI, O., and TOLU, E.: Vestibular nuclei of hemilabyrinthectomized guinea pigs during decompensation. *Acta Ital. Biol., 114*: 389–398 (1976)

BECHTEREW, W.: Ergebnisse der Durchaschneidung des N. acusticus, nebst Erörterung der Bedeutung der semicirculären Canäle für das Korpergleichgewicht. *Pflüg. Arch. ges. Physiol., 30*: 312–347 (1883)

CARPENTER, M. B., FABREGA, H. and GLINSMANN, W.: Physiological deficits occurring with lesions of labyrinth and fastigial nuclei. *J. Neurophysiol., 22*: 222–234 (1959)

COURJON, J. H., JEANNEROD, M., Ossuzio, I. and SCHMID, R.: The role of vision in compensation of vestibulo-ocular reflex after hemilabyrinthectomy in the cat. *Exp. Brain Res., 28*: 235–248 (1977)

DÉMÉTRIADES, T. D. and SPIEGEL, E. A.: Zur Frage der Bedeutung des Kleinhirns für die Entwicklung von Spontannystagmus. *Zeitschr f. z. Hals-, Nas.-u. Ohrenheilk., 19*: 250–257 (1927)

DIERINGER, N. and PRECHT, W.: Modification of synaptic input follwing unilateral labyrinthectomy. *Nature, 269*: 431–433 (1977)

Dow, R. S.: Effect of lesions in the vestibular part of the cerebellum in primates. *Arch. Neurol. & Psychiat., 40*: 500–520 (1938a)

Dow, R. S.: The effects of unilateral and bilateral labyrinthectomy in monkey, baboon and chimpanzee. *Am. J. Physiol., 121*: 392–399 (1938b)

ECCLES, J. C.: An instructive-selection theory of learning in the cerebellar cortex. *Brain Res., 127*: 327–352 (1977)

EIDELBERG, E. and STEIN, D. G.: Functional recovery after lesions of the nervous system. *Neurosci. Res. Prog. Bull., 12*: 191–303 (1974)

FISCHER, M. H.: Körperstellung und Körperhaltung bei Fischen, Amphibien, Reptilien und Vogeln. In *Hb. Norm. Pathol. and Physiol., Vol. 15 (1)*, pp. 97–159, Springer, Berlin (1930)

FLUUR, E.: Vestibular compensation after labyrinthine destruction. *Acta Oto laryng., 52*: 367–375 (1960)

GERNANDT, B. E. and THULIN, C.-A.: Vestibular connections of the brain stem. *Am. J. Physiol., 171*: 121–127 (1952)

GILBERT, P. F. C.: Theory of memory that explains function and structure of cerebellum. *Brain Res., 70*: (1) 1–18 (1974)

GILBERT, P.: How cerebellum could memorize movements. *Nature, 254* (5502): 688–689 (1975)

GILBERT, P. F. C. and THACH, W. T.: Purkinje cell activity during motor learning. *Brain Res., 128*: 309–328 (1977)

HADDAD, G. M., HADDAD, M., FRIENDLICH, A. R. and ROBINSON, D. A.: Compensation of nystagmus after VIIIth nerve lesion in vestibulo-cerebellectomized cats. *Brain Res., 135*: 192–196 (1977)

HOSHINO, K. and POMPEIANO, O.: Crossed responses of lateral vestibular neurons to macular labyrinthine stimulation. *Brain Res., 131*: 152–157 (1977)

ITO, M.: Cerebellar control of the vestibular neurons: Physiology and pharmacology. *Prog. in Brain Res.*, *37*: 377–390 (1972)

KENNEDY, C., DES ROSIERS, M. H., JEHLE, J. W., REIVICH, M., SHARP, F. and SOKOLOFF, L.: Mapping of functional neural pathways by autoradiographic survey of local metabolic rates with (^{14}C) dexyglucose. *Science*, *187*: 850–853 (1975)

KOLB, G.: Untersuchungen ueber zentrale Kempensation und Kempensationsbewegungen einseitig entstateter Froesche. *Z. vergl. Physiol.*, *37*: 136–160 (1955)

LACOUR, M., ROLL, J. J. P. and APPAIX, M.: Modifications and development of spinal reflexes in the alert baboon (*Papio papio*) following a unilateral vestibular neurotomy. *Brain Res.*, *113*: 255–269 (1976)

LANGE, B.: Inwieweit sind die Symptone, welche nach Zerstörung des Kleinhirns beobachtet werden, auf Verletzungen des Acusticus zurückzuführen? *Pflüg. Arch. ges. Physiol.*, *50*: 612–625 (1891)

LLINÁS, R. (ed.): *Neurobiology of Cerebellar Evolution and Development.* American Medical Association, Chicago (1969)

LLINÁS, R. and WALTON, K.: Significance of the olivo-cerebellar system in compensation of ocular position following unilateral labyrinthectomy. *In* BERTHOZ, A. and BAKER, R. (eds.): *Control of Gaze*, pp. 399–408, Elsevier, Amsterdam (1977)

LLINÁS, R. and WALTON, K.: The place of the cerebellum in motor learning. *In* BRAZIER, M. A. B. (ed.): *Brain Mechanisms in Memory and Learning*, pp. 17–36, Raven Press, New York (1979)

LLINÁS, R., WALTON, K., HILLMAN, D. E. and SOTELO, C.: Inferior olive: Its role in motor learning. *Science*, *190*: 1230–1231 (1975)

McCABE, B. F. and RYU, J. H.: Experiments on vestibular compensation. *Laryngoscope (St. Louis)*, *79*: 1728–1736 (1969)

McCABE, B. F., RYU, J. H. and SEKITANI, T.: Further experiments on vestibular compensation. *Laryngoscope (St. Louis)*, *82*: 381–396 (1972)

MARR, D.: A theory of cerebellar cortex. *J. Physiol.*, *202*: 437–470 (1969)

PELLIONISZ, A. and LLINÁS, R.: Brain modeling by tensor network theory and computer simulation. The cerebellum: distributed processor for predictive coordination. *Neuroscience*, *4*: 323–348 (1979)

PFALTZ, C. R. and KAMATH, R.: Central compensation of vestibular dysfunction. I. Peripheral lesions. *Pract. Oto-rhino-laryng.*, *32*: 335–349 (1970)

PFALTZ, C. R., PIFFKO, P. and MISHRA, S.: Central compensation of vestibular dysfunction. II. Neuronal and central lesions. *Otorhino-laring. int.*, *35*: 71–82 (1973)

PLUM, F., GJEDDE, A. and SAMSON, F. E.: Neuroanatomical functional mapping by the radioactive 2-deoxy-D-glucose method. *Neueosci. Res. Prog. Bull.*, *14*: 457–518 (1976)

PRECHT, W.: Characteristics of vestibular neurons after acute and chronic labyrinthine destruction. *In* KORNHUBER, H. H. (ed.): *Handbook of Sensory Physiology*, Vol. 6, part 2, *Vestibular System*, pp. 451–462, Springer, Berlin (1974)

PRECHT, W., SHIMAZU, H. and MARKHAM, C. H.: A mechanism of central compensation of vestibular function following hemilabyrinthectomy. *J. Neurophysiol.*, *29*: 996–1010 (1966)

PUTKONEN, P. T. S., COURJON, J. H. and JEANNEROD, M.: Compensation of postural effects of hemilabyrinthectomy in the cat. A sensory substitution process? *Exp. Brain Res.*, *28*: 249–257 (1977)

ROBINSON, D. A.: Adaptive gain control of vestibulo-ocular reflex by the cerebellum. *J. Neurophysiol.*, *39*: 954–969 (1976)

SANCHEZ ROBLES, S. and ANDERSON, J. H.: Compensation of vestibular deficits in the cat. *Brain Res.*, *147*: 183–187 (1978)

SCHAEFER, K. P. and MEYER, D. L.: Compensatory mechanisms following labyrinthine lesions in the guinea pig. A simple model of learning. *In* ZIPPEL, H. P. (ed.): *Memory and Transfer of Information*, pp. 203–232, Plenum, New York (1973)

SCHAEFER, K. P. and MEYER, D. L.: Compensation of vestibular lesions. *In* KORNHUBER, H. H. (ed.): *Handbook of Sensory Physiology*, Vol. 1/2, part 2, *Vestibular System*, pp. 463–490, Springer, Berlin-Heidelberg-New York (1974)

SHARP, F. R.: Relative cerebral glucose uptake of neuronal perikarya and neuropile determined with 2-deoxyglucose in resting and swimming rat. *Brain Res.*, *110*: 127–139 (1976a)

SHARP, F. R.: Rotation induces increases of glucose uptake in rat vestibular nuclei and vestibulo-cerebellum. *Brain Res.*, *110*: 141–151 (1976b)

SHARP, F. R., KAUER, J. S. and SHEPHERD, G. M.: Local sites of activity-related glucose metabolism in rat olfactory bulb during olfactory stimulation. *Brain Res.*, *98*: 596–600 (1975)

SHIMAZU, H. and PRECHT, W.: Inhibition of central vestibular neurons from the contralateral labyrinth and its mediating pathway. *J. Neurophysiol.*, *29*: 467–492 (1966)

SOKOLOFF, L.: Relation between physiological function and energy metabolism in the central nervous system. *J. Neurochem.*, *29*: 13–26 (1977)

WILSON, V. J. and PETERSON, B. W.: Peripheral and central substrates of vestibulospinal reflexes. *Physiolog. Rev.*, *58*: 80–105 (1978)

ELECTROPHYSIOLOGICAL AND DYNAMICS STUDIES OF VESTIBULOSPINAL REFLEXES*

Victor J. WILSON

The Rockefeller University
New York, NY

INTRODUCTION

Stimulation of the labyrinth by movement of the head results in reflexes that, briefly put, maintain the visual image by stabilizing the eyes in space during the head movement and also act to stabilize the position of the head in space. The mechanisms by means of which the vestibular system executes these reflexes have been the subject of numerous investigations for many years. Over this period we have accumulated extensive anatomical and physiological information about most stages of the system at which information is processed, starting with the canal ampullae and the maculae in the labyrinth and ending with the various efferent pathways by which vestibular activity is transmitted to the extraocular, body and limb muscles. As we will see later, however, critical information about the processing that leads to compensatory vestibular reflexes is still lacking.

This paper deals only with the pathways by which activity originating in the labyrinth exerts its influence on limb and axial muscles, with emphasis on its action on the neck muscles that move the head (more comprehensive reviews of vestibular physiology can be found in Kornhuber, 1974, Wilson and Peterson, 1978, and Wilson and Melvill Jones, 1979). I will first review some of the pertinent data obtained by anatomica land single-unit electro physiological studies. As recent work has shown, these methods alone will not enable us to understand even relatively simple vestibulospinal reflexes. The latter part of the paper will deal with some other approaches which may advance our knowledge further.

CONNECTIONS BETWEEN LABYRINTH AND SPINAL CORD

The vestibular nuclei

As described by Brodal and Pompeiano (1957) the vestibular nuclear complex in the pontomedullary region of the brain stem consists of our principal nuclei—the superior, lateral (Deiters'), medial and descending—and of some minor cell groups. Vestibular afferent fibers terminate widely in this complex, from which, after processing and integration with a variety of other inputs, vestibular activity is activity is distributed to other regions of the central nervous system.

The nuclei projecting to the spinal cord are the lateral, medial and descending (see next section), shown by degeneration methods to receive both canal and macular input (Brodal, 1974). Canal afferents terminate in the rostral and perhaps caudal parts of the descending and medial nuclei, and to some extent in the medial part of the lateral nucleus (Stein and Carpenter, 1967; Gacek, 1969). Utricular afferents terminate in the lateral nucleus

* Work in the author's laboratory supported by N.I.H. grant NS 02619, and NSF grant BMS 75–00487 to Dr. B.W. Peterson.

and the rostral part of the descending, and perhaps in the medial nucleus; saccular afferents in the lateral and descending nuclei (STEIN and CARPENTER, 1967; GACEK, 1969). As first pointed out by LORENTE DE NÓ on the basis of Golgi methods (1933a), and confirmed by subsequent authors, there may be overlap in the vestibular nuclei between the area of termination of afferents from different canals, or of afferents from canals and maculae. The question arises, what kind of signal is transmitted by second—or higher order vestibular neurons? This can be answered partially by stimulating branches of the vestibular nerve and recording from neurons in the nuclei. In view of the overlap revealed by anatomical techniques, it is remarkable that when different ampullary nerves are stimulated selectively (SUZUKI et al., 1969a), second-order neurons in a variety of preparations typically respond monosynaptically to stimulation of only one ipsilateral canal nerve (see WILSON and PETERSON, 1978). There may be convergence on some higher-order neurons, and natural stimulation reveals that many neurons respond to angular acceleration in the plane of more than one canal, or to angular acceleration and tilt (e.g. CURTHOYS and MARKHAM, 1971). Such convergence is presumably mediated by complex connections. The fact remains that many second-order neurons receive a direct input from only one ampulla (there has been little testing for monosynaptic convergence of ampullary and macular afferents). In other words, there may be fairly selective, direct pathways linking particular receptors in the labyrinth with specific targets in the brain stem or spinal cord.

The reticular formation

There is no evidence, anatomical or physiological, that primary vestibular afferents terminate in the reticular formation, but there is considerable evidence that pontine and medullary reticular neurons respond to natural vestibular stimulation, as first shown by DUENSING and SCHAEFFER (1960), and respond to stimulation of the vestibular nerve with a latency that is at least disynaptic (PETERSON et al., 1975). The importance of vestibular input to the reticular formation for vestibulospinal reflexes will become clear later. For the moment it is important to note that activity reaching the reticular formation must do so *via* the vestibular nuclei.

The vestibulospinal and reticulospinal tracts

The most direct connections between vestibular nuclei and spinal cord are provided by the lateral and medial vestibulospinal tracts (LVST and MVST). The LVST arises in the lateral nucleus and extends, ipsilaterally, as far as the sacral spinal cord (BRODAL, 1974). Many of its axons branch to widely separated segmental levels, e.g. cervical and lumbar (ABZUG et al., 1974), while others are more narrowly distributed (RAPOPORT et al., 1977a). The different roles of these two types of axons are not understood.

One function of the LVST is to transmit labyrinthine activity to the spinal cord. Degeneration experiments and study of the properties of identified LVST neurons show that within the lateral nucleus the imput from the labyrinth is found mainly ventrally (WALBERG et al., 1958; WILSON et al., 1967; ITO et al., 1969). There is also a tendency for LVST neurons with long axons to be located dorsally in the lateral nucleus, and for neurons with shorter axons to be located ventrally (see WILSON, 1972). The result of this distribution of afferent fibers and efferent neurons is that the LVST is more likely to relay activity from the labyrinth directly to the cervical than to the lumbar cord.

The MVST arises in the medial, descending and lateral nuclei, courses bilaterally, and terminates predominantly in the upper cervical segments (BRODAL, 1974; AKAIKE et al., 1973a; RAPOPORT et al., 1977a). A very large proportion of neurons with their axons in the MVST are activated monosynaptically by stimulation of vestibular afferent fibers

(WILSON et al., 1968; AKAIKE et al., 1973a; RAPOPORT et al., 1977a) and this tract therefore serves as a direct relay between the labyrinth and the rostral cervical spinal segments.

While the VSTs are the most direct link between labyrinth and spinal cord, they are by no means the only one. As pointed out by LLOYD (1941; see particularly his Fig. 15) vestibular activity which enters the pontomedullary reticular formation eventually reaches the spinal cord both by long reticulospinal fibers and by the bulbospinal correlation system, i.e. by propriospinal fibers that receive their input from fibers originating in the brain stem. The labyrinthine input to the reticulospinal tracts (RST), and the organization of the tracts themselves, is discussed in some detail in the chapter by PETERSON. At this time, we need only to know that antidromically identified RST neurons do receive input from the labyrinth, with a latency that is *at least* disynaptic. They can relay this input to all spinal levels, because RST axons can extend as far as the sacral region.

Labyrinthine actions on motoneurons

Before considering the effects that are produced in motoneurons by stimulation of the labyrinth it is useful to review briefly the spinal connections of VSTs and RSTs. Most of this information has been obtained by localized stimulation within the vestibular nuclei and reticular formation.

a) Spinal connections of descending tracts. The LVST, which is well known to have excitatory actions on the extensor musculature (BRODAL et al., 1962), has been studied by stimulation of the lateral vestibular nucleus (e.g. LUND and POMPEIANO, 1968; WILSON and YOSHIDA, 1969a; GRILLNER et al., 1970). This tract makes monosynaptic excitatory connection with many ipsilateral dorsal neck motoneurons and with some types of hindlimb extensor motoneurons (particularly quadriceps and gastrocnemius). Excitatory actions on other hindlimb and on most forelimb extensor motoneurons, as well as inhibitory actions on flexor motoneurons, are carried out via interneurons. Contralateral actions on limb motoneurons, which are similar to ipsilateral effects, are also produced via segmental interneurons (HONGO et al., 1975).

The connections and functions of the MVST remained unknown until stimulation of the medial vestibular nucleus revealed that this tract contained inhibitory fibers that acted monosynaptically on dorsal neck motoneurons (WILSON and YOSHIDA, 1969b; see also AKAIKE et al., 1973b). These observations have now been extended by a technique not subject to the difficulties of localizing the action of stimulating currents applied within the brain (RAPOPORT et al., 1977b). In these experiments, which utilized a method first used in the central nervous system by JANKOWSKA and ROBERTS (1972), the spontaneous or glutamate-driven firing of single neurons in the vestibular nuclei was recorded extracellularly and the spikes were used to trigger an averaging program while recording intracellularly from neck motoneurons: only polysynaptic events time-locked to the triggering spike show up in the average. An example of the results is shown in Figure 1. The axon of this neuron was fired by microstimulation near C3 motoneurons (Fig. 1 A1) and the neuron was monosynaptically excited by stimulation of the ipsilateral vestibular nerve (Fig. 1A 2). The neuron was inhibited by stimulation of the contralateral vestibular nerve (Fig. 1B), illustrating the well-known phenomenon of commissural inhibition (SHIMAZU and PRECHT, 1966). Fig. 1C and D show the IPSP evoked by the activity of this vestibular neuron in two neck motoneurons. With this technique we could show that inhibitory neurons acting on neck motoneurons were present in the medial and descending vestibular nuclei.

The MVST contains not only inhibitory but also excitatory fibers (AKAIKE et al., 1973b), and its fibers make monosynaptic connections not only with neck but also with other axial

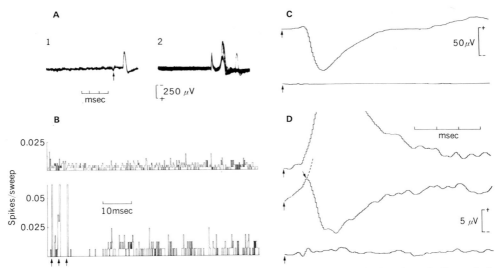

Fig. 1 Properties of an inhibitory neuron in the vestibular nuclei and of unitary IPSPs evoked by activity of this neuron in two motoneurons. *A1*: antidromic spike of neuron evoked by a 8 μA stimulus (at upward arrow) to the electrode in C_3 neck extensor motoneuron pool. *A2*: monosynaptic response of the neuron to stimulation of the ipsilateral vestibular nerve at 1.4 times N_1 threshold. *B*: upper trace shows spontaneous activity of the neuron as a PST histogram (440 sweeps). Lower trace shows effect of a 150 μA triple shock to the contralateral vestibular nerve (150 sweeps). *C*: unitary IPSP evoked in one motoneuron by activity of the inhibitory neuron; lower trace, extracellular record. *D*: unitary IPSP (middle trace) evoked in another motoneuron. IPSP was reversed by injection of 10 nA hyperpolarizing current and part of this reversed IPSP is shown in the upper trace. Downward arrow in middle trace shows divergence between IPSPs recorded with and without current injection. Lower trace, extracellular record. All records in C and D are average of 600–1000 sweeps; upward arrows indicate time of discriminator output pulses (from RAPOPORT et al., 1977b).

motoneurons.   The tract seems not to have direct excitatory or inhibitory connections with limb motoneurons.

The RSTs also exert direct actions on spinal motoneurons.   Stimulation experiments show there is monosynaptic excitation of axial motoneurons and of some limb flexor and extensor motoneurons, as well as disynaptic inhibition of other limb motoneurons (GRILLNER and LUND, 1968; GRILLNER et al., 1971; WILSON and YOSHIDA, 1969a; WILSON et al., 1970).   More recent work has also revealed that there are inhibitory reticulospinal fibers that make synapses with neck motoneurons (PETERSON et al., 1976).   In addition to such short-latency actions, there are also less direct effects on motoneurons and on spinal reflex pathways (ENGBERG et al., 1968; JANKOWSKA et al., 1968).

b) Labyrinth-spinal connections. Two questions that arise are first, how closely is the labyrinth coupled to different types of motoneurons, and second, which tracts are utilized to relay vestibular afferent information to the musculature.   The answers can be partly predicted from the connections of the tracts described in part 'a'.   They have been clarified further by experiments in which stimulation of the vestibular nerve or of its branches was combined with intracellular recording from motoneurons and with lesions that selectively damage the LVST or MVST.

In sufficiently excitable preparations, e.g. in decerebrate cats, stimulation of the vestibular nerve evokes synaptic potentials in limb motoneurons.   In forelimb motoneurons these potentials are polysynaptic (MAEDA et al., 1975), as is very likely the case for hindlimb motoneurons.   This is due to a combination of two factors: connections between VST

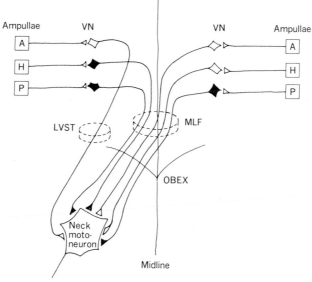

Fig. 2 Connections between ipsilateral and contralateral ampullae and neck motoneurons. A, H, P, are anterior, horizontal and posterior ampullae; VN, vestibular nuclei. Inhibitory neurons and their terminals shown in black, excitatory in white (from WILSON and MAEDA, 1974).

fibers and limb motoneurons are mainly longer than monosynaptic, and relatively few VST neurons projecting to hindlimb segments receive monosynaptic input from the laby-rinth (see above). Tract lesions show that these polysynaptic, i.e. longer than disynaptic, connections are due to the LVST (MAEDA et al., 1975). From our knowledge of the ex-tent and organization of the two vestibulospinal tracts, we can be sure that the same is true for connections between labyrinth and hindlimb motoneurons.

Considering the close relation between labyrinth and head movement, it is not surpris-ing that connections between labyrinth and neck, and some other axial, motoneurons are very direct, i.e. disynaptic. The pathways that are known best are those that link the semi-circular canal ampullae with neck motoneurons; they have been studied by selective stimu-lation of individual ampullary nerves and by tract interruption (WILSON and MAEDA, 1974). Figure 2 summarizes the results of these experiments. Recording from motoneu-rons innervating biventer cervicis or complexus, dorsal neck muscles that extend the head (REIGHARD and JENNINGS, 1935; RICHMOND and ABRAHAMS, 1975) shows that the typical motoneuron receives disynaptic input from most or all of the six bilateral semicircular canals. The central pathways, consisting of the specifically-innervated second order neurons described earlier, are excitatory from both anterior canals and from the contralateral hori-zontal canal; they are inhibitory from the ipsilateral horizontal canal and from both poste-rior canals. This pattern of connections is fully consistent with the movements evoked by stimulation of the same canals (SUZUKI and COHEN, 1964), or produced when the canals are activated by natural stimuli. Almost all of this direct input to neck motoneurons is relayed by the MVST: this is true both for the inhibitory connections and for the contra-lateral excitatory ones. Only the excitation from the ipsilateral anterior canal is due to the LVST.

The disynaptic connections between canals and neck motoneurons are precisely organiz-ed and consistent with reflexes expected during movement, but they are weak: the EPSPs are typically not larger than 500μV. Nevertheless, they build up when short trains of stimuli are used instead of single shocks and are strong enough to cause short-latency motor nerve discharge or EMGs (EZURE et al., 1978; WILSON, PETERSON, FUKUSHIMA, HIRAI and UCHINO, see below).

Macular inputs to neck motoneurons have been less thoroughly studied than canal input, perhaps because it is more difficult to achieve selective stimulation of a macula or of its nerve than of an ampullary nerve (see however SUZUKI et al., 1969b, and HWANG and POON, 1975). We have approached this problem by surgically destroying, to the extent possible, most of vestibular ganglion, leaving intact only the cell bodies of saccular or utricular afferents (WILSON et al., 1977); selective preservation was easier to achieve for the saccular than for the utricular nerve. After the damaged afferents had degenerated, the remaining nerve was stimulated in acute experiments. In this way we showed that stimulation of both the utricular and the saccular nerve evoked short-latency potentials, some of them disynaptic, in neck motoneurons. Again, this result is consistent with the equilibrium function of the maculae, well known for the utricle and recently established for the mammalian sacculus by FERNANDEZ et al. (1972). The tracts involved in the pathways from maculae to cord have not been completely worked out. Potentials of contralateral origin are due to the MVST, because AKAIKE, FANARDIJIAN, ITO and OHNO (1973) showed that *all* disynaptic potentials evoked by stimulation of the contralateral vestibular nerve are abolished by section of this tract. Very likely ipsilateral excitatory potentials are at least in part due to the LVST because utricular and saccular afferents both have terminations in the lateral nucleus (STEIN and CARPENTER, 1967; GACEK, 1969).

Experiments such as the ones that produce the diagram of Figure 2 concentrate on very direct connections, which may be disynaptic or short polysynaptic pathways. These are not the only connections present, however. For example, small EPSPs or IPSPs are still seen in neck motoneurons after the VSTs are cut (WILSON and MAEDA, 1974). These synaptic potentials have latencies of 3.5–5 msec, in comparison to disynaptic latencies which are shorter than 2.5 msec. The tracts producing late activity, which may be the reticulospinal tracts, seem to play an important role in vestibulospinal reflexes.

Summary

Electrophysiological and neuroanatomical studies tell us that receptors in the labyrinth are linked to spinal motoneurons by short reflex arcs. The afferent input first relays in the vestibular nuclei, where a certain amount of information processing takes places. From the brain stem the most direct output to motoneurons is *via* two vestibulospinal tracts, both of which make monosynaptic connections with motoneurons, particularly with neck motoneurons. The MVST is mainly a pathway to neck and other axial motoneurons, the LVST to limb motoneurons. The disynaptic connections between semicircular canals and neck motoneurons, while not powerful, are precisely organized and their pattern is consistent with that of vestibulocollic (vestibulo-neck) reflexes. Vestibular activity can also be relayed by other tracts, particularly the reticulospinal tracts. While the labyrinth-reticular formation-motoneuron pathway does not have a disynaptic component, it can produce rather short latency activity.

DYNAMICS OF VESTIBULOSPINAL REFLEXES

We now ask the question, to what extent do the various vestibulospinal pathways that have been identified, as described in the first half of this paper, explain the dynamics of vestibulospinal reflexes? Our recent experiments have been addressed to this point. Before reviewing the pertinent literature and describing these experiments, it is necessary to briefly describe some studies on vestibulo-ocular reflexes. Although the first systematic dynamic analysis of a vestibular reflex was on the vestibulospinal system (PARTRIDGE and KIM, 1969, described further below) most of the advances in the field first came from work on the vestibulo-ocular system.

The pathways of the vestibulo-ocular reflex consist of direct excitatory and inhibitory fibers and parallel, more complex circuits. The direct fibers are both in and outside the MLF, the complex circuits have long been believed to be in the reticular formation (LORENTE DE NÓ, 1933b; COHEN, 1974). What is the relative importance of these two components of the reflex arc? As pointed out by SKAVENSKI and ROBINSON (1973), because the semicircular canals are stimulated by acceleration and over a wide range give a response related to velocity, another integration must be performed if the motor system is to generate an output related to the change in head position, something it must do for the proper reflex to be executed. The dynamic properties of the vestibulo-ocular reflex, and of the components that may be performing this integration, have been widely studied by the powerful method of linear systems analysis. In this way, by applying horizontal sinusoidal oscillation to alert monkeys, SKAVENSKI and ROBINSON (1973) showed that above 1 Hz much of the integration was performed by the orbital mechanics. Below this frequency the integration must take place in the brain stem. SKAVENSKI and ROBINSON (1973) postulated that the vestibulo-ocular reflex pathway as a whole consists of a "neural integrator" in parallel with the direct pathways, the integrator making a smaller and smaller contribution to the response with increasing frequency. The neural integration appears to take place downstream from second order vestibular neurons, at least in decerebrate cats. Under many conditions these neurons respond to angular acceleration with a phase very similar to that of vestibular afferent fibers (e.g. Melvill JONES and MILSUM, 1970, 1971; SHINODA and YOSHIDA, 1974). SHINODA and YOSHIDA (1974), working in decerebrate cats, studied the dynamic responses of various elements of the horizontal canal-abducens pathway starting with second-order neurons. Their results (see their Figure 14) show that starting with frequencies of 0.16 Hz there is an increasing phase lag between second-order vestibular neuron firing and abducens nerve discharge. Thus phase lag reaches 40–60° between 0.05 and 0.35 Hz, approaching one step of integration.

The frequency response of a vestibulospinal reflex was first studied in decerebrate cats by PARTRIDGE and KIM (1969) who stimulated the whole vestibular nerve with pulse trains whose frequency was modulated sinusoidally, and recorded the tension of triceps surae. There was no phase lag between input and output below 0.1 Hz, and an increasing lag as the frequency of modulation was increased: about 45° at 1.0 Hz, about 90° at 4.0 Hz. When the lag due to the muscle, obtained by stimulating the muscle nerve, was subtracted, there remained little or no central phase lag at any of these frequencies. Perhaps this result was due to the method of stimulation chosen. Rather different results have been obtained by subsequent investigators who also used decerebrate cats, but used natural stimulation while recording from neck or forelimb muscles.

An early description of BERTHOZ and ANDERSON (1971a, b) showed that both in the forelimb and neck musculature there was a considerable phase lag with reference to acceleration when the decerebrate cat was stimulated sinusoidally by lateral tilt (linear acceleration) and horizontal oscillation (angular acceleration). Central phase lag in the horizontal vestibulocollic reflex, with reference to primary afferents, ranged from 50° to about 30° between 0.1 and 1.0 Hz. More recently there have been two rather complete analyses of the reflex responses of decerebrate cats to horizontal angular acceleration, that of EZURE and SASAKI (1978; see also EZURE et al., 1976) on vestibulocollic reflexes and that of ANDERSON et al. (1977) on forelimb reflexes.

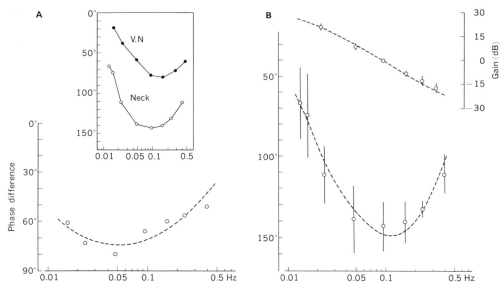

Fig. 3 Dynamic properties of the vestibulocollic reflex. *A*: averaged phase differences between vestibular nucleus neurons and neck motor units. The best fit curve is drawn with the method of least squares (dashed line). Inset, upper curve from data of SHINODA and YOSHIDA, 1974; lower curve, present data of neck motor unit responses. *B*: dashed lines indicate reconstruction of the gain and phase lag of the vestibulocollic reflex system on the basis of the calculated transfer function. Gain normalized at 0.1 Hz (from EZURE and SASAKI, 1978).

EZURE and SASAKI oscillated cats at 0.015–0.4 Hz while recording either EMGs of single motor units or compound EMGs of dorsal neck muscles. They observed a phase lag between angular acceleration and response even larger than that previously observed in the vestibulo-ocular reflex (inset of Figure 3A, Figure 3B). When the phase of the response of second-order neurons (as measured by SHINODA and YOSHIDA, 1974) is subtracted from the phase of the reflex response, a big central phase lag remains (Figure 3A). This central lag is as large as 70–80° between 0.02 and 0.1 Hz, and decreases to about 50° at 0.04 Hz. ANDERSON et al. (1977), who did similar experiments but recorded from triceps brachii, calculated the central phase lag by subtracting the response of vestibular afferents from their results (their Figure 7): the lag rose from 40° at 0.15Hz to 85° at 1 Hz. By using vertical angular acceleration and subtracting the contribution of macular afferents SOECHTING et al. (1977) deduced that reflex pathways originating in the vertical canals have similar dynamic characteristics.

There are differences between the results of EZURE and SASAKI and ANDERSON et al. that could be due to the fact that they recorded in neck and forelimb muscles respectively. Both groups agree, however, that there is a pronounced central phase lag which cannot be produced by direct relays between vestibular nuclei and motoneurons. They suggest that an integrator is present in the vestibulospinal reflex, probably in the reticular formation. The system may resemble that suggested by SKAVENSKI and ROBINSON (1973) for the vestibuloocular reflex: the output of a complex circuit, including the integrator, may reach motoneurons via the reticulospinal tracts, in parallel with the direct VSTs.

In the horizontal vestibulocollic reflex, where in response to acceleration in one direction the contralateral neck muscles contract, the direct tract involved is the MVST, the excitatory link between the vestibular nuclei and contralateral neck motoneurons. EZURE et al. (1978) studied the role of this tract by cutting the MLF caudally in the brain stem.

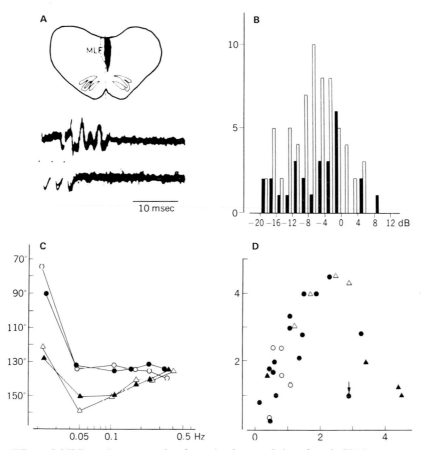

Fig. 4 Effect of MLF section upon the dynamic characteristics of neck EMG response. *A*: a typical lesion. Two recordings in the lower part of A are compound EMG potentials from the right neck extensor muscles evoked by stimulation of the contralateral horizontal canal nerve (trains of three pulses are indicated by dots). The EMG activity which is seen in the control record (above) is not present after the MLF cut (below). *B*: Distribution of the gain of motor unit response at 0.17 Hz. White columns: before the cut (mean±S.D.: −6.75±6.14 dB; n—65). Filled columns: after the cut (mean±S.D.: −6.26±7.47 dB; n=27). *C*: phase characteristics of compound EMG response from 2 cats. Phase lags (ordinate in degrees) are plotted with open symbols (before the cut) and filled symbols (after the cut) against angular frequency (abscissa). *D*: relation between the spontaneous activity (abscissa) and gain (ordinate) of compound EMG response. The data are from two cats, open and filled symbols represent the data before and after the cut respectively. The point indicated with an arrow shows data obtained immediately after the cut (from EZURE et al., 1978)

This procedure abolishes disynaptic EPSPs in motoneurons contralateral to the stimulated horizontal ampullary nerve (WILSON and MAEDA, 1974). The results are illustrated in Figure 4. As Figure 4A shows, the cut abolishes the short latency compound EMG in the contralateral dorsal neck muscles. Phase data from two cats after such a cut are shown in Figure 4C (circles and triangles). Within the frequency range studied (0.017 to 0.4 Hz) cutting the MLF had no effect on phase. Measurement of the gain of the response of individual motor units showed no difference in the distribution of gains before and after the cut.

It must be appreciated that these experiments on the vestibulocollic reflex were performed with the head immobilized, i.e. in the open loop mode. This is a very different condition from the normal closed loop mode where the movement of the head that follows activation of the labyrinth is, in turn, detected by the labyrinth. Nevertheless, two conclusions emerge. First, in the open loop mode the dynamics of the vestibulocollic reflex (and of vestibulospinal reflexes in general) are quite similar to the dynamics of vestibulo-ocular reflexes. Second, for the vestibulocollic reflex of the highly excitabled decerebrate cat loss of the MVST has no appreciable influence in the low to mid frequency range (up to 0.4 Hz). One hypothesis is that, as suggested by SKAVENSKI and ROBINSON (1973) for the vestibulo-ocular reflex, the MVST becomes more important at higher frequencies. We have tested this hypothesis as part of our recent work on the vestibulocollic reflex, which is described next.

Studies on the vestibulocollic reflex of the decerebrate cat

This presents some results of recent experiments by our group (V. J. WILSON, B. W. PETERSON, K. FUKUSHIMA, N. HIRAI, Y. UCHINO), which will be described in more detail in the near future. For these experiments we chose to use not natural stimulation but activation of ampullary nerves, very likely of nerve terminals, with modulated continuous current. Among the reasons we adopted this approach, which bypasses the receptor, are the ease with which an extended frequency range of sinusoidal or square wave stimuli can be used, and the lessened difficulty for extracellular, and eventually intracellular, single neuron recording. So far we have stimulated only one of a pair of coplanar canals. We assumed, however, that electrical modulation of one labyrinth would activate the integrator that is activated by natural stimulation. Our results have proved this assumption correct.

Bipolar electrodes were implanted near the horizontal or anterior ampullary nerve (SUZUKI et al., 1969a) in locations where eye movements were evoked by trains of pulses. The animal was subsequently decerebrated and the caudal part of the cerebellum was aspirated to expose the floor of the fourth ventricle. One wire of the implanted electrode pair was used for monopolar polarization, with a distant electrode connected to the base plate or to nearby muscle. We recorded compound EMGs of dorsal neck muscles on the side contralateral to the stimulated canal. In many experiments second-order vestibular neurons were studied. They were identified by their response to single shocks to the appropriate ampullary nerve. Sometimes the activity of muscle and neurons was recorded simultaneously; in other instances neuron activity was studied in decerebrate animals immobilized with Flaxedil.

The modulating stimulus wave forms were generated by a PDP 11–45 computer which drove a constant current stimulator (designed by Mr. M. ROSETTO). The output of this stimulator ranged over positive and negative values about any selected midpoint. That is, the nerve, or nerve terminals, were successively depolarized and hyperpolarized. It will be appreciated that a sine wave delivered in this fashion mimics the effect of sinusoidal horizontal angular oscillation.

We used two different stimulating methods. In both cases we were able to record simultaneously the activity of a single neuron and the rectified EMGs from two different muscles. With the first stimulating program we were able to select a sine or square wave at one of several available frequencies. The stimulus was divided into 512 segments and the number of spikes or the rectified EMG was averaged for each bin over a selected number of cycles. For sinusoidal stimuli the binned data were then fitted with a DC term and a sinusoid at the fundamental frequency of the response by the method of least squares. When responses were truncated, because elements in the circuit fell below threshold, fitting was done only over the non-truncated portion. Phase difference was measured from the peak negativity of the stimulus to the peak of the fitted sine wave.   Responses to square waves were analyzed by eye.

The second stimulating procedure was derived from the method of VICTOR et al. (1977). The stimulus consisted of nine superimposed sinusoids of equal amplitude representing the harmonics of a common fundamental.   The frequencies were chosen to minimize interference between them, and distortion.   For each cycle of the fundamental an integral number of cycles of each of the other frequencies was delivered.   With this program the data were binned over 64 points per cycle for each frequency.   Phase and gain of the fundamental component of the response to each frequency were determined by Fourier analysis.   This stimulating procedure has several advantages, two of which are relevant to our present experiments.   First, it has the effect of linearizing the system (see VICTOR et al., 1977).   Responses evoked by superimposed sine waves were usually more sinusoidal than responses evoked by a single frequency of stimulation.   This was especially true at higher frequencies (1 Hz and above) where responses to single frequencies sometimes had prominent early phasic components.   Second, determining the responses to all the frequencies simultaneously minimizes the difficulties caused by shifts in the excitability of the preparation.   Most of the present results were obtained with superimposed sine wave stimulation.

It was shown previously that the vestibulo-ocular (e.g. SHINODA and YOSHIDA, 1974) and vestibulocollic (EZURE and SASAKI, 1978) reflexes are sufficiently linear for sinusoidal analysis.   We have frequently varied the amplitude of the stimulating current, bracketing the strength used for further analysis (much stronger currents were avoided for fear of damaging the labyrinth).   There was no systematic change in gain or phase with these changes in intensity.

a) EMG responses to superimposed sine waves.   Modulation of neck muscle EMGs was studied in nine cats.   The electrode was near the horizontal canal nerve in five, near the anterior nerve in three, and clearly stimulated both nerves in one; currents ranged amplitude from 5–80 μA.   There was no obvious difference between responses obtained in these different stimulating situations, and the data were pooled.   At frequencies of 0.08–0.76 Hz mean phase lag ranged from 21°–35°.   Phase advanced with further increases in frequency; at 6.1 Hz the mean phase lead was 23°.   At frequencies of 0.04 Hz and below the results were variable.   In some cats (for example, Figure 5) the

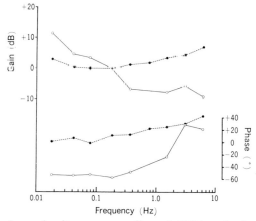

Fig. 5 Bode plot based on simultaneous recording of EMG and of second-order vestibular nucleus neuron. Activity was evoked by multiple sine waves (25 μA). Open circles are data from EMG, filled circles from the second-order neuron. Phase plotted with reference to peak negativity of the stimulus; gain (peak amplitude of response/stimulus amplitude) was normalized at 0.18 Hz.

phase lag was maintained, in others the response was more or less in phase with the stimulus or even showed a small lead.   Gain (response amplitude divided by stimulating current) was highest at the low frequencies and dropped sharply by 0.76 Hz.   Sometimes it increased again, but there were more cases with little or no modulation at the highest frequencies studied (3.1 and 6.1 Hz).

Figure 5 (open circles) illustrates the response to one stimulating sequence.   In this instance (and in other runs in this cat) there was a phase lag close to 60° between 0.018 and 0.18 Hz.   Above 0.18 Hz phase advanced to a 20° lead at 6.1 Hz.   Over the same frequency range gain dropped off.   During the steep part of the drop the slope approached 4 db per octave.

b)   Responses of second-order vestibular neurons to superimposed sine waves. Neurons were studied in three types of preparations: in cats that were paralyzed; in cats that were not paralyzed but in which the reflex showed little or no phase lag; in good preparations in which there was simultaneous recording of EMG and unit activity.   Both single and superimposed sine waves were used.   Under all of these conditions the neuron responses were similar and this typical behavior is illustrated in Figure 5 (filled circles). Unlike the EMG, second order neurons are more or less in phase with the stimulus at low frequencies; a phase lead develops at 0.1 Hz or above, and reaches approximately 40° at 6.1 Hz.   Gain was generally low at the low frequencies and maximal at the highest frequency that we studied.

The neurons that we recorded from were identified solely by their monosynaptic response to stimulation of the canal nerve with single shocks.   Nothing is known about their other properties and the unlikely possibility remains that there are specific groups of second-order neurons projecting to the spinal cord that behave differently.

c)   Central phase lag.   By subtracting the response of second order neurons from that of the EMG we obtain the central phase lag in our preparations.   The lag in one particular cat can be seen from Figure 5, where neuron and EMG recording was simultaneous. The mean phase lag for all the runs in this cat, obtained by subtracting the phase of each second-order neuron from the phase of the EMG measured simultaneously, and then averaging these values, is shown in Figure 6.   It is about 40° at the lowest frequency and

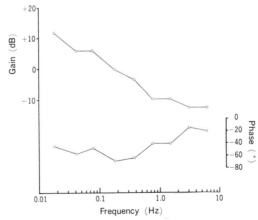

Fig. 6 Phase lag and gain of central vestibulocollic pathways. This Bode plot is based on data from one experiment in which five second-order neurons were studied and the contralateral neck muscle EMG was recorded at the same time. Phase was obtained by averaging the differences between the phase of each unit and that of the EMG . Gain was determined by averaging the individual ratios of muscle gain to neuron gain. Gain normalized at 0.18 Hz.

approaches 70° at 0.18 Hz.   From this frequency the lag decreases, dropping off to 22° by 6.1 Hz.   This curve is very similar to that of Ezure and Sasaki (1978) illustrated in Figure 3A, although the central lag is somewhat smaller.   The calculated curve of Ezure and Sasaki (dashed lines in Figure 3A) predicts decreasing phase lags at higher frequencies, and this is precisely what we saw.   When the results from all cats, rather than this particular preparation, are averaged, the central phase lag is smaller at low frequencies because of the variable behavior of our preparations.   In any case our result, like Ezure and Sasaki's (1978), differs from that of Anderson et al. (1977) who show a phase lag that is still increasing at 1.0 Hz (their Figure 7).   As pointed out earlier this may reflect a difference between vestibular reflexes of neck and forelimb muscles.

Figure 6 also shows, with a curve normalized at 0.18 Hz, the average gain of the central pathways in this same cat (average of gain of muscle/gain of second order neurons). This gain drops steadily from the lowest frequency; between 0.08 and 0.76 Hz the slope of the drop approaches 6 db per octave.

From our results we can conclude the following.   1) Sinusoidal current modulation of single ampullary nerves activates the neural "integrator" and produces in the vestibulocollic reflex a central phase lag which, over a broad frequency range, is of the same order of magnitude as that produced by natural stimulation.   2) Considering the small size of our sample, there was no obvious difference between the results obtained with electrodes near the horizontal and anterior canal nerves, suggesting that the dynamics of the horizontal and vertical systems are similar.   This supports the conclusion made by Soechting et al. (1977) on the basis of less direct evidence.   3) Our technique is suitable as a tool to search for the brain stem neurons relaying the integrated signal to the spinal cord and to study the role of the direct vestibulospinal tracts in the vestibulocollic reflex.

d)   Section of the MVST.   We tested the influence of section of the MLF just rostral to the obex on modulation of the EMG in several cats with single and superimposed sine wave stimulation, particularly with the latter.   Since Ezure et al. (1978) had already shown that such cuts had no obvious effects at frequencies of 0.4 Hz and below, we were especially interested in testing the hypothesis that the MVST plays a more significant role at higher frequencies.   Our results do not support this view.

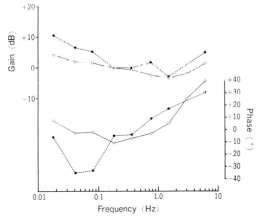

Fig. 7 Effect of MLF cut on phase and gain of vestibulocollic reflex. Open circles show phase and gain before the cut (three runs averaged). MLF transection at first abolished the short-latency EMG evoked by pulse stimulation of the contralateral horizontal canal nerve; the EMG was again present about 2½ hours later, but the latency had increased by 1–2 msec. Filled circles show phase and gain 2½ hours after the MLF cut (two runs averaged).

Figure 7 illustrates a case in which the MLF was transected on the side of the muscle from which we recorded. Three hours after the cut an EMG response to pulse stimulation of the ampullary nerve was visible, but the latency was 5–5.8 msec, as compared to 4 msec before the cut (average latency in cats with intact MLF, 4.3 msec). Control runs (open circles), made rather soon after the start of recording, showed relatively little central phase lag: with reference to the mean firing properties of second-order neurons the lag was no more than 20° or so at 0.2–1.0 Hz and it essentially disappeared at higher frequencies. The normalized gain dropped from 0.018 to 1.5 Hz, then increased. After the cut (filled circles) integration was better at low frequencies, but there was no obvious loss of phase at the higher frequencies. Nor was there any indication that gain was selectively affected at high frequencies, although actual gain dropped over the whole range by a factor of 5. Similar results were obtained in other experiments. In addition, there were typically good phasic responses to square waves delivered at 1, 2, 5 Hz before and after the cut.

CONCLUDING REMARKS

It can be predicted that the substantial phase lag in the vestibulocollic reflex cannot be produced by a disynaptic pathway unless the firing of second-order neurons themselves shows such a phase lag. There is no evidence for such firing behavior in decerebrate cats either in previous work, or in our results. As repeatedly postulated by others the integration in such preparations is produced elsewhere, perhaps by higher-order vestibular neurons or by circuits in the reticular formation. To what extent does the disynaptic pathway contribute to the decrease in central phase lag at higher frequencies? Our results strongly suggest that in the excitable decerebrate cat with the head immobilized the medial vestibulospinal tract does not play a prominent role. At least its interruption causes neither marked changes in phase nor selective loss of gain at higher frequencies. This result suggests that a significant pathway carrying activity whose phase is close to that of second-order neurons is present outside the MLF; it may consist of reticulospinal fibers.

What then is the role of the medial vestibulospinal tracts, which in the vestibulocollic reflex produce a pattern of activity which is so precisely and appropriately organized? We cannot rule out that loss of the MVST contributes to the generalized gain loss that frequently occurs when the MLF is cut, although this loss is very likely due to brain stem trauma. The tract may play a more obvious role in preparations other than hyperexcitable decerebrate animals: when motoneurons are at a lower level of excitability a fast pathway may provide an important priming function. More generally, results obtained in decerebrates do not necessarily predict the role of the tract in behaving animals. For example, a change in central bias may enhance the importance of the direct pathway relative to that of the integrator or to fast reticular pathways. These various possibilities suggest some directions for future studies.

ACKNOWLEDGEMENTS

I am grateful to Drs. B. W. Peterson, K. Fukushima, N. Hirai and Y. Uchino for letting me discuss some of our unpublished results.

REFERENCES

ABZUG, C., MAEDA, M., PETERSON, B. W. and WILSON, V. J.: Cervical branching of lumbar vestibulospinal axons. *J. Physiol.*, *243*: 499–522 (1974)

AKAIKE, T., FANARDIJIAN, V. V., ITO, M., KUMADA, M. and NAKAJIMA, H.: Electrophysiological analysis of the vestibulospinal reflex pathway of rabbit. I. Classification of tract cells. *Exp. Brain Res. 17*: 477–496 (1973a)

AKAIKE, T., FANARDJIAN, V. V., ITO, M. and OHNO, T.: Electrophysiological analysis of the vestibulospinal reflex pathway of rabbit. II. Synaptic actions upon spinal neurones. *Exp. Brain Res.*, *17*: 497–515 (1973b)

ANDERSON, J. H., SOECHTING, J. F. and TERZUOLO, C. A.: Dynamic relations between natural vestibular inputs and activity of forelimb extensor muscles in the decerebrate cat. II. Motor output during rotations in the horizontal plane. *Brain Res.*, *120*: 17–34 (1977)

BERTHOZ, A. and ANDERSON, J. H.: Frequency analysis of vestibular influence on extensor motoneurons. I. Response to tilt in forelimb extensors. *Brain Res.*, *34*: 370–375 (1971a)

BERTHOZ, A. and ANDERSON, J. H.: Frequency analysis of vestibular influence on extensor motoneurons. II. Relationship between neck and forelimb extensors. *Brain Res.*, *31*: 376–380 (1971b)

BRODAL, A.: Anatomy of the vestibular nuclei and their connections. *In* KORNHUBER, H. H. (ed.): *Handbook of Sensory Physiology*, Vol. 6/1, Vestibular System, pp. 239–352. Springer, Berlin (1974)

BRODAL, A. and POMPEIANO, O.: The vestibular nuclei in the cat. *J. Anat.*, *91*: 438–454 (1957)

BRODAL, A., POMPEIANO, O. and WALBERG, F.: *The Vestibular Nuclei and their Connections*. Oliver and Boyd, Edinburgh and London (1962)

COHEN, B.: The vestibulo-ocular reflex arc. *In* KORNHUBER, H. H. (ed.): *Handbook of Sensory Physiology*, Vol. 6/1, Vestibular System, pp. 477–540, Springer, Berlin (1974)

CURTHOYS, I. S. and MARKHAM, C. H.: Convergence of labyrinthine influences on units in the vestibular nuclei of the cat. I. Natural stimulation. *Brain Res.*, *35*: 469–490 (1971)

DUENSING, F. and SCHAEFFER, K. P.: Die Aktivität einzelner Neurone der Formatio reticularis des nicht gefesselten Kaninchens bei Kopfwendungen und vestibulären Reizen. *Arch. Psychiat. Nervenkr.*, *201*: 97–122 (1960)

ENGBERG, I., LUNDBERG, A. and RYALL, R. W.: Reticulospinal inhibition of transmission in reflex pathways. *J. Physiol.*, *194*: 201–223 (1968)

EZURE, K. and SASAKI, S.: Frequency-response analysis of vestibular-induced neck reflex in cat. I. Characteristics of neural transmission from the horizontal semicircular canal to neck motoneurons. *J. Neurophysiol.*, *41*: 445–458 (1978)

EZURE, K., SASAKI, S., UCHINO, Y. and WILSON, V. J.: Frequency-response analysis of vestibular-induced neck reflex in cat. II. Functional significance of cervical afferents and polysynaptic descending pathways. *J. Neurophysiol.*, *41*: 459–471 (1978)

FERNANDEZ, C., GOLDBERG, J. and ABEND, W. K.: Response to static tilts of peripheral neurons innervating otolith organs of the squirrel monkey. *J. Neurophysiol.*, *35*: 978–997 (1972)

GACEK, R. R · The course and central termination of first order neurons supplying vestibular end organs in the cat. *Acta Oto-Laryngol.*, Suppl. *254*. 1 66 (1969)

GRILLNER, S., HONGO, T. and LUND, S.: The vestibulospinal tract. Effects on alpha motoneurones in the lumbosacral spinal cord in the cat. *Exp. Brain Res.*, *10*: 94–120 (1970)

GRILLNER, S., HONGO, T. and LUND, S.: Convergent effects on alpha motoneurones from the vestibulospinal tract and a pathway descending in the medial longitudinal fasciculus. *Exp. Brain Res.*, *12*: 457–479 (1971)

GRILLNER, S. and LUND, S.: The origin of a descending pathway with monosynaptic action on flexor motoneurones. *Acta physiol. scand.*, *74*: 274–284 (1968)

HONGO, T., KUDO, N. and TANAKA, R.: The vestibulospinal tract: crossed and uncrossed effects on hindlimb motoneurones in the cat. *Exp. Brain Res.*, *24*: 37–55 (1975)

HWANG, J. C. and POON, W. F.: An electrophysiological study of the sacculoocular pathways in cats. *Japan J. Physiol.*, *25*: 241–251 (1975)

ITO, M., HONGO, T. and OKADA, Y.: Vestibular-evoked postsynaptic potentials in Deiters' neurones. *Exp. Brain Res.*, *7*: 214–230 (1969)

JANKOWSKA, E., LUND, S., LUNDBERG, A. and POMPEIANO, O.: Inhibitory effects evoked through ventral reticulospinal pathways. *Arch. ital Biol.*, *106*: 124–140 (1968)

JANKOWSKA, E. and ROBERTS, W. J.: Synaptic actions of single interneurones mediating reciprocal Ia inhibition of motoneurones. *J. Physiol. 222*: 623–642 (1972)

KORNHUBER, H. H. (ed.): *Handbook of Sensory Physiology*, Vol. 6, Vestibular System. Springer, Berlin (1974)

LLOYD, D. P. C.: Activity in neurons of the bulbospinal correlation system. *J. Neurophysiol.*, *4*: 115–134 (1941)

LORENTE DE NÓ, R.: Anatomy of the eight nerve. *Laryngoscope*, *43*: 1–38 (1933a)

LORENTE DE NÓ, R.: Vestibulo-ocular reflex arc. *Arch. Neurol. Psychiat.*, *30*: 245–291 (1933b)

LUND, S. and POMPEIANO, O.: Monosynaptic excitation of alpha motoneurones from supraspinal structures in the cat. *Acta physiol. scand.*, *73*: 1–21 (1968)

MAEDA, M., MAUNZ, R. A. and WILSON, V. J.: Labyrinthine influence on cat forelimb motoneurons. *Exp. Brain Res.*, *22*: 69–86 (1975)

MELVILL JONES, G. and MILSUM, J. H.: Characteristics of neural transmission from the semicircular canal to the vestibular nuclei of cats. *J. Physiol.*, *209*: 295–316 (1970)

MELVILL JONES, G. and MILSUM, J. H.: Frequency-response analysis of central vestibular unit activity resulting from rotational stimulation of the semicircular canals. *J. Physiol.*, *219*: 191–215 (1971)

PARTRIDGE, L. D. and KIM, J. H.: Dynamic characteristics of response in a vestibulomotor reflex. *J. Neurophysiol.*, *32*: 485–495 (1969)

PETERSON, B. W., FILION, M., FELPEL, L. P. and ABZUG, C.: Responses of medial reticular neurons to stimulation of the vestibular nerve. *Exp. Brain Res.*, *22*: 335–350 (1975)

PETERSON, B. W., PITTS, N. G., MACKEL, R. and FUKUSHIMA, K.: Monosynaptic excitation and inhibition of neck motoneurons by a reticulospinal pathway. *Neuroscience Abst.*, *2*: 528 (1976)

RAPOPORT, S., SUSSWEIN, A., UCHINO, Y. and WILSON, V. J.: Properties of vestibular neurons projecting to neck segments of the cat spinal cord. *J. Physiol.*, *268*: 493–510 (1977a)

RAPOPORT, S., SUSSWEIN, A., UCHINO, Y. and WILSON, V. J.: Synaptic actions of individual vestibular neurons on cat neck motoneurons. *J. Physiol.*, *272*: 367–382 (1977b)

REIGHARD, J. and JENNINGS, H. S.: *Anatomy of the Cat*. 3rd. ed. Holt, New York, N. Y. (1935)

RICHMOND, F. J. R. and ABRAHAMS, V. C.: Morphology and enzyme histochemistry of dorsal muscles of the cat neck. *J. Neurophysiol.*, *38*: 1312–1321 (1975)

SHIMAZU, H. and PRECHT, W.: Inhibition of central vestibular neurons from the contralateral labyrinth and its mediating pathway. *J. Neurophysiol.*, *29*: 467–492 (1966)

SHINODA, Y. and YOSHIDA, K.: Dynamic characteristics of responses to horizontal head angular acceleration in vestibuloocular pathway in the cat. *J. Neurophysiol.*, *37*: 653–673 (1974)

SKAVENSKI, A. A. and ROBINSON, D. A.: Role of the abducens nucleus in vestibulo-ocular reflex. *J. Neurophysiol.*, *36*: 724–738 (1975)

SOECHTING, J. F., ANDERSON, J. H. and BERTHOZ, A.: Dynamic relations between natural vestibular inputs and activity of forelimb extensor muscles in the decerebrate cat. III. Motor output during rotations in the vertical plane. *Brain Res.*, *120*: 35–48 (1977)

STEIN, B. M. and CARPENTER, M. B.: Central projections of portions of the vestibular ganglia innervating specific parts of the labyrinth in the Rhesus monkey. *Amer. J. Anat.*, *120*: 281–318 (1967)

SUZUKI, J.-I. and COHEN, B.: Head, eye, body and limb movements from semicircular canal nerves. *Exp. Neurol.*, *10*: 393–405 (1964)

SUZUKI, J.-I., GOTO, K., TOKUMASU, K. and COHEN, B.: Implantation of electrodes near individual vestibular nerve branches in mammals. *Ann. Otol. Rhin. Laryngol.*, *78*: 815–826 (1969a)

SUZUKI, J.-I., TOKUMASU, K. and GOTO, K.: Eye movements from single utricular nerve stimulation in the cat. *Acta oto-laryngol.*, *68*: 350–362 (1969b)

VICTOR, J. D., SHAPLEY, R. M. and KNIGHT, B. W.: Nonlinear analysis of cat retinal ganglion cells in the frequency domain. *Proc. Natl. Acad. Sci.*, *74*: 3068–3072 (1977)

WALBERG, F., BOWSHER, D. and BRODAL, A.: The termination of primary vestibular fibers in the vestibular nuclei in the cat. An experimental study with silver methods. *J. Comp. Neurol.*, *110*: 391–419 (1958)

WILSON, V. J.:   Physiological pathways through the vestibular nuclei.   *Int. Rev. Neurobiol.*, *15*: 27–81 (1972)

WILSON, V. J., GACEK, R. R., MAEDA, M. and UCHINO, Y.:   Saccular and utricular input to cat neck motoneurons.   *J. Neurophysiol.*, *40*: 63–73 (1977)

WILSON, V. J., KATO, M., PETERSON, B. W. and WYLIE, R. M.:   A single-unit analysis of the organization of Deiters' nucleus.   *J. Neurophysiol.*, *30*: 603–619 (1967)

WILSON, V. J. and MAEDA, M.:   Connections between semicircular canals and neck motoneurons in the cat.   *J. Neurophysiol.*, *37*: 346–357 (1974)

WILSON, V. J. and MELVILL JONES, C.:   *Mammalian Vestibular Physiology*, Plenum, New York (1979)

WILSON, V. J. and PETERSON, B. W.:   Peripheral and central substrates of vestibulospinal reflexes.   *Physiol. Rev.*, *58*: 80–115 (1978)

WILSON, V. J., WYLIE, R. M. and MARCO, L. A.:   Synaptic inputs to cells in the medial vestibular nucleus.   *J. Neurophysiol.*, *31*: 176–186 (1968)

WILSON, V. J. and YOSHIDA, M.:   Comparison of effects of stimulation of Deiters' nucleus and medial longitudinal fasciculus on neck, forelimb and hindlimb motoneurons.   *J. Neurophysiol.*, *32*: 743–758 (1969a)

WILSON, V. J. and YOSHIDA, M.: Moxosynaptic inhibition of neck motoneurons by the medial vestibular nucleus.   *Exp. Brain Res.*, *9*: 365–380 (1969b)

WILSON, V. J., YOSHIDA, M. and SCHOR, R. H.:   Supraspinal monosynaptic excitation and inhibition of thoracic back motoneurons.   *Exp. Brain Res.*, *11*: 282–295 (1970)

DISCUSSION PERIOD

HIGHSTEIN: What happens to an alert animal when you make a lesion in this pathway? What does its behavior look like?

WILSON: This is something that we haven't done.   If such a lesion is made it will interrupt a variety of fibers, and it would be difficult to ascribe any effects just to interruption of the vestibular pathways.

MARCUS: I saw in your slides a response to the sum of sinusoids.   I wonder if you analyzed second order interactions between the sinusoids.   Could you reproduce from the response you have to the simple sinusoids, the response to square waves?

WILSON: Not yet.   We haven't gotten into this.

MARCUS: There is a second thing I wanted to ask you.   You stimulated one ampullary nerve?

WILSON: Yes.

MARCUS: Did you try to stimulate two to see the summation, the interaction between them?

WILSON: The only time we stimulated two is when we did it inadvertently.   Once we realized that the anterior and horizontal canals systems behaved similarly, we did not worry if in an occasional animal we obviously stimulated both.   But we have not really tried to stimulate separately and sum.

COHEN: Your stimulus bypasses the cupula.   You lose one integration, and your stimulus is related to head velocity, rather than to head acceleration.

WILSON: My stimulus is an electric current applied to the nerve.

COHEN: You had an increase in gain at the lower frequencies of stimulation.   Do you think that bypassing the cupula is the cause for it?

WILSON: I don't want to compare what I get with the behavior of the whole system. I think that's very risky.   All I am prepared to do is to compare the behavior of the central circuitry in vestibular-neck or vestibulo-ocular reflexes, by whatever means they are activated.   I realize that in bypassing the receptor we are missing a big part of the system, but for our purposes it doesn't matter.

RETICULO-MOTOR PATHWAYS: THEIR CONNECTIONS AND POSSIBLE ROLES IN MOTOR BEHAVIOR*

Barry W. PETERSON

The Rockefeller University
New York, NY

INTRODUCTION

Electrophysiological analysis of the descending pathways linking the brainstem reticular formation with spinal motor centers (reticulo-motor pathways) began with the work of Lloyd (1941). His analysis indicated that stimulation of the medullary reticular formation produced powerful indirect activation of hindlimb motoneurons and suggested that there might also be a weak direct excitatory connection between reticulospinal neurons and motoneurons. The topography of the brainstem region from which facilitation of hindlimb motor activity could be evoked was described a few years later by Rhines and Magoun (1946). According to the nomenclature of Brodal (1957), this region begins in the rostro-dorsal part of *nucleus reticularis* (*n. r.*) *gigantocellularis* and extends anteriorly through *n. r. pontis caudalis* and *oralis* into the mesencephalic reticular formation and midline thalamic nuclei. In the same year Magon and Rhines (1946) described another reticular region corresponding to *n. r. ventralis* and the caudo-ventral part of *n. r. gigantocellularis* which when stimulated produced a profound depression of hindlimb motoneurons. Thus by 1946 it was clear that reticulo-motor pathways had a strong influence on motoneurons supplying the muscles of the hindlimb.

In the years following the early work of Lloyd and of Magoun and Rhines a variety of anatomical and electrophysiological approaches have been employed to investigate the properties of reticulospinal neurons and to explore their action on spinal motoneurons. While this work has greatly expanded our knowledge of reticulo-motor pathways, it has not as yet led to a clear understanding of the role of these pathways in motor behavior. This review will attempt to bring together and examine information about reticular actions on motoneurons and about the inputs that reach reticulospinal neurons from sensory and motor systems in the hope that such an examination will lead to useful hypotheses about possible functions of reticulo-motor pathways. It will begin with an analysis of the anatomy and physiology of reticular projections to spinal motor centers and of the types of movements with which these projections are associated. Following this initial section, the remainder of the review will be devoted to examining three classes of inputs that reach reticulospinal neurons: inputs from somatic receptors, inputs from the vestibular system and inputs from motor-related structures such as motor cortex, cerebellar nuclei or superior colliculus. Each input will be discussed in the light of possible functional roles of reticulo-motor pathways in motor behavior.

* Work in the author's laboratory supported by: NSF grant BMS 75 00487 and NIH grants NS 02619 and EY 02249.

RETICULOSPINAL ACTION ON SPINAL MOTONEURONS

Anatomical studies have shown that there are several reticulospinal pathways. Lesions made in the medial pontine reticular formation lead to degeneration of reticulospinal fibers running in the ventromedial funiculi whereas lesions made more caudally, in the medullary reticular formation, cause degeneration not only in the ventromedial funiculi but also in the ventrolateral funiculi on both sides of the spinal cord (NYBERG-HANSEN, 1966; PETRAS, 1967). In this review the reticulospinal projection in the ventromedial funiculi will be referred to as the medial reticulospinal pathway while the projections in the lateral funiculi will be referred to as the lateral reticulospinal pathway. While each of these pathways is likely to contain a variety of functionally diverse elements, studies of reticular action on spinal motoneurons have indicated that the medial and lateral reticulospinal pathways have different patterns of action on the motor apparatus.

Medial reticulospinal pathway. Electrophysiological studies (ITO et al., 1970; PETERSON et al., 1975b) have shown that the neurons of origin of medial reticulospinal fibers are located primarily in *n. r. pontis oralis* and *caudalis* and in the dorsorostral part of *n. r. gigantocellularis*. Most of these neurons project at least as far as the upper lumbar spinal cord but this does not indicate that they have no action at higher spinal levels. PETERSON et al. (1975b) have shown that many reticulospinal neurons send axon branches to more than one level of the spinal cord so that lumbar-projecting medial reticulospinal neurons are likely to have an action upon neurons in the cervical or thoracic spinal cord as well.

The reticular region from which medial reticulospinal fibers originate lies entirely within the region from which RHINES and MAGOUN (1946) obtained facilitation of hindlimb reflexes. It is therefore reasonable to expect that the medial reticulospinal system should have a predominantly excitatory action on motoneurons. Several groups of investigators have explored the synaptic basis of this reticulo-motor excitation by recording synaptic potentials evoked in motoneurons by a stimulus applied to the reticular formation. Electrical stimuli applied to the medial longitudinal fasciculus (MLF), through which many medial reticulospinal fibers run on their way to the spinal cord, have been shown to evoke both direct, monosynaptic and indirect, polysynaptic excitation of motoneurons supplying muscles of the neck, back, forelimbs and hindlimbs (GRILLNER and LUND, 1968; WILSON and YOSHIDA, 1969a; WILSON et al., 1970; GRILLNER et al., 1971). Thus, as originally suggested by LLOYD (1941), part of the reticulospinal excitation of motoneurons is produced by direct excitatory connections between reticulospinal neurons and motoneurons.

In addition to stimulating the MLF, GRILLNER and LUND (1968) stimulated points throughout the pontomedullary reticular formation and found that monosynaptic excitation of hindlimb motoneurons was evoked only when stimuli were applied within a region corresponding to *n. r. pontis caudalis* and the dorsorostral part of *n. r. gigantocellularis*. My colleagues and I (PITTS et al., 1977; PETERSON et al., 1978) have recently extended these observations by examining the responses of motoneurons at different spinal cord levels to stimuli applied to a variety of sites within the pontomedullary reticular formation. The region from which we obtained monosynaptic excitation of hindlimb motoneurons is shown in Figure 1D and corresponds quite well to that described by GRILLNER and LUND (1968). Both this region and the region from which we obtained direct excitation of forelimb motoneurons lie entirely within the caudal portion of the medial reticulospinal projection area, which is located anterior and dorsal to the dotted line in Figure 1D. It therefore appears that the medial reticulospinal system plays the primary role in producing direct reticulospinal excitation of motoneurons supplying muscles of the fore- and hindlimbs. Participation of lateral reticulospinal neurons in such excitation cannot be ruled out, however, because JANKOWSKA et al. (1974) have reported that monosynaptic reticulospinal excitation can still be observed in some hindlimb motoneurons following destruction of the ventromedial funiculi.

As shown in Figure 1, stimuli applied within the region of origin of medial reticulospinal fibers produce direct excitation not only of limb motoneurons but also of motoneurons supplying muscles of the neck and back. Comparison of the frequency of occurrence and amplitude of monosynaptic reticulospinal EPSPs in different groups of motoneurons indicated that the direct excitatory action of the medial reticulospinal pathway was strongest in neck motoneurons, of intermediate intensity in back motoneurons and weakest in limb motoneurons. Among limb motoneurons GRILLNER and LUND (1968) and GRILLNER et al. (1971) found the strongest reticulospinal excitation in flexor motoneurons whereas WILSON and YOSHIDA (1969) and PITTS et al. (1977) found equivalent amounts of excitation in both flexors and extensors. All investigators agree, however, that direct reticulospinal excitation can be found in a wide variety of motoneurons supplying both proximal

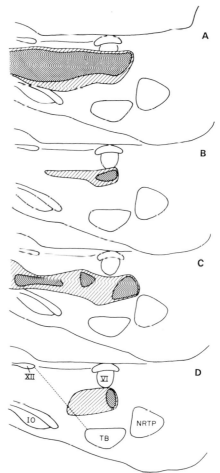

Fig. 1 Reticular regions from which monosynaptic excitation of spinal motoneurons could be evoked. The effectiveness of 100 μA stimuli applied at points located 1–2 mm from the midline in evoking monosynaptic excitation of ipsilateral neck (A), forelimb (B), back (C) and hindlimb (D) motoneurons is indicated by shaded areas in each schematic parasagital section. Light shading indicates regions which contained a few effective points (i.e. points at which a 100 μA stimulus produced monosynaptic excitation in more than 10 per cent of the motoneurons tested). Dark shading indicates areas within which more than half of the points were effective. The dotted line in D separates zones 1 and 2 as defined by PETERSON et al. (1975b). Zone 1, which lies anterior and dorsal to this line, contains primarily medial reticulospinal neurons while lateral reticulospinal neurons projecting beyond the neck are clustered in zone 2, which lies posterior and ventral to the line. Abbreviations: IO, inferior olive; NRTP, nucleus reticularis tegmeneti pontis; TB, trapezoid body; VI, abducens nucleus; XII, hypoglossal nucleus.

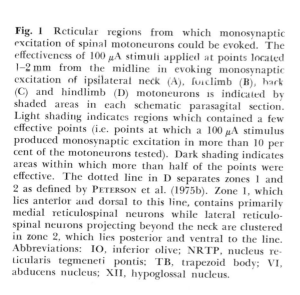

and distal limb muscles.   Thus the medial reticulo-motor pathway has direct excitatory access to motoneurons supplying muscles throughout the body with a preferential action on axial (neck and back) motoneurons.

Our data also indicate that the rostral part of the medial reticulospinal projection zone, corresponding to *n. r. pontis oralis* is not part of the region from which direct excitation of motoneurons can be evoked.   Stimulation of this reticular nucleus produced only less direct, di- or polysynaptic EPSPs in motoneurons.   Such later EPSPs were also produced when stimuli were applied to the more caudal part of the medial reticulospinal projection zone and they were often larger than the direct EPSPs produced by the same stimuli, especially when trains of stimulus pulses were applied.

Lateral reticulospinal pathway.   The motor action of the lateral reticulospinal pathway is quite different from that of the medial reticulospinal pathway.   Neurons that give rise to lateral reticulospinal fibers extending beyond the C_4 segment are clustered in the caudo-ventral portion of *n. r. gigantocellularis* (PETERSON et al., 1975b), a region that overlaps very little with the region from which most medial reticulospinal fibers originate. Although neurons in the caudo-ventral part of *n. r. gigantocellularis* send axon branches to the ventral horn at all spinal levels (NYBERG-HANSEN, 1966; PETRAS, 1967; PETERSON et al., 1975b), electrical stimuli applied to this region do not produce the widely divergent direct motor action that is seen when regions containing medial reticulospinal neurons are stimulated.   Stimuli applied ventrally and caudally within the reticular formation never evoke monosynaptic PSPs in limb motoneurons while they do evoke direct excitation of motoneurons supplying the dorsal muscles of the neck and back as illustrated in Figure 1 (PITTS et al., 1977; PETERSON et al., 1978).

Lateral reticulospinal projections to the upper cervical (neck) segments of the spinal cord differ in several ways from long lateral reticulospinal projections.   While the neck segments probably receive inputs from axon collaterals of long lateral reticulospinal neurons located in the caudo-ventral part of *n. r. gigantocellularis*, they also receive inputs from a population of lateral reticulospinal neurons whose axons do not extend beyond C_4 (N cells).   Although some N cells are found in the caudo-ventral part of *n. r. gigantocellularis*, many others are found in the rostro-dorsal region of that nucleus just posterior to the abducens nucleus (PETERSON et al., 1975b).   This latter region overlaps extensively the zone of origin of medial reticulospinal fibers.

Figure 1 shows that neck motoneurons can be directly excited by stimuli applied throughout a wide area that includes all but the most anterior regions that give rise to reticulospinal fibers.   As stimulus sites are shifted more caudally, the monosynaptic EPSPs recorded in neck motoneurons become progressively larger indicating that neurons distributed along the entire length of the effective area shown in the diagram contribute to the direct reticulospinal excitation of neck motoneurons (PETERSON et al., 1978).   After midline lesions that interrupt medial reticulospinal and vestibulospinal fibers, direct excitation of neck motoneurons can still be obtained by stimulation of both the rostro-dorsal and caudo-ventral parts of *n. r. gigantocellularis*, which suggests that N cells projecting via the lateral reticulospinal pathway are in part responsible for the direct excitation of neck motoneurons obtained when stimuli are applied to the region just behind the abducens nucleus. The lateral reticulospinal neurons located in this region, which project only to the neck, are likely to carry specialized signals related to head movements.

Lateral reticulospinal pathways projecting to the neck also include neurons that establish direct, inhibitory connections with neck motoneurons (PETERSON et al., 1978).   Mapping of the reticular sites from which such inhibition can be evoked indicates that it is produced by neurons located in the dorsal part of *n. r. gigantocellularis* and in *n. r. ventralis*.

Electrophysiological studies (PETERSON et al., 1975b) and data obtained with retrograde labelling of reticulospinal neurons with horseradish peroxidase (PETERSON and COULTER, unpublished observations) indicate that both of these regions contain a substantial number of N cells some of which may be responsible for the monosynaptic inhibition of neck motoneurons since such inhibition is not present in motoneurons in spinal segments below C_4 (LLINÁS and TERZUOLO, 1964; JANKOWSKA et al., 1968; PITTS et al., 1977).

The available data thus suggest that lateral reticulo-motor pathways include at least three distinct components, one consisting of long projection neurons that excite axial motoneurons at many spinal levels, a second which specifically excites neck motoneurons and a third which is responsible for direct inhibiton of neck motoneurons. These three components together with the widely divergent, excitatory medial reticulo-motor pathway provide a variety of routes via which the medial pontomedullary reticular formation can directly modulate the excitability of spinal motoneurons. These direct reticulo-motor connections are of interest because their action on motoneurons is relatively invariant and hence easier to understand than the action of polysynaptic reticulo-motor connections which have a stronger but far more variable action on motoneurons. Having learned something about the topography and connections of direct reticulo-motorpathways, we are in a position to attempt to determine how these pathways are involved in motor behaviors elicited by somatic, vestibular or other stimuli. On the other hand, we are still a long way from understanding the function of polysynaptic motor pathways where the ultimate action upon motoneurons depends upon many factors controlling the excitability of each interneuron in the chain linking the reticular formation with motor nuclei.

Patterns of movement associated with the activity of reticulospinal neurons

Following the work of LLOYD (1941) and MAGOUN and RHINES (1946), the motor role of reticulospinal pathways has been studied in a number of investigations employing stimulation or lesions of the reticular formation and recording of the behavior of reticular neurons. The early work with electrical stimulation (MAGOUN and RHINES, 1946; RHINES and MAGOUN, 1946) gave the impression that activation of reticular neurons led to an overall facilitation or depression of motoneurons supplying muscles throughout the body. A follow-up study by SPRAGUE and CHAMBERS (1954), however, showed that such global effects were only seen when strong stimuli were applied. With weaker stimuli a variety of more discrete patterns of motor activity could be evoked. A commonly observed response was deflection of the head toward the stimulated side together with flexion of the limbs on that side and extension of the opposite limbs. With juxtathreshold stimuli even more restricted responses, such as flexion of a single limb, were sometimes observed. It thus appears that activation of reticular elements can lead to a varied repetoire of movements that might form components of many motor behaviors.

As a result of observations of fiber degeneration and behavioral deficits following lesions interrupting fibers coursing through the medial medulla, KUYPERS (1964) concluded that reticulospinal pathways belong to the class of medial descending systems. The axons of these systems terminate preferentially in the ventromedial part of the spinal ventral horn (NYBERG-HANSEN, 1966; PETRAS, 1967) a region that is associated with the control of axial and proximal muscles (STERLING and KUYPERS, 1968). Behaviorally, lesions interrupting the medial systems lead to deficits in righting and control of postural muscles but have little effect on fine movements performed by distal muscles. While there have been no observations of deficits in the control of skeletal muscles following lesions interrupting only reticulospinal fibers, KUYPERS' observations suggest that reticulospinal pathways should be especially important in behaviors that involve control of the axial and proximal musculature.

Medial descending systems are predominantly uncrossed, a feature which differentiates them from the corticospinal and rubrospinal tracts, which are predominantly crossed. BRINKMAN and KUYPERS (1973) made use of this difference in their analysis of visually guided movements in split brained, chiasm-sectioned monkeys. When one eye was blindfolded, these animals were able to reach for and retrieve food from small holes in a board in front of them when they were allowed to use the arm contralateral to their seeing eye. When forced to use the arm ipsilateral to that eye, however, they could still make accurate reaching movements but could not perform the precise movements of the digits required to extract food from the holes. The movements in this latter case are likely to depend upon neurons of one or more of the medial descending systems to relay motor signals originating in the cerebral cortex to ipsilateral spinal motor nuclei. Likely candidates for such a relay are reticulospinal neurons, which receive strong, direct inputs from the sensorimotor cortex (MAGNI and WILLIS, 1964a; PETERSON et al., 1974). It appears from BRINKMAN and KUYPERS' (1973) observations that these relay neurons are able to mediate controlled movements of the arm but do not have sufficiently precise connections with motoneurons supplying distal muscles to mediate independent digital movements. The latter require the participation of crossed corticospinal or rubrospinal neurons. Once again, then, lesion studies suggest that reticulospinal and other medial descending pathways are primarily involved in the control of proximal muscles. In this case, however, such control is part of a highly specific voluntary behavior rather than a component of reflexes involved in righting and postural control.

Ultimately one may hope that direct evidence for involvement of reticulospinal neurons in both voluntary and reflex motor behavior will come from observations of the activity of reticulospinal neurons in alert animals. Such evidence does not now exist. While it has been reported that medial pontomedullary reticular neurons exhibit bursts of activity during bodily movements, especially movements of the head (SIEGEL and McGINTY, 1977; VERTES, 1977), these neurons were not identified as reticulospinal neurons and the precise relation of their activity to muscle activation was not determined. There is thus no assurance that the neuronal activity observed played a role in producing the motor activity that accompanied it. Hopefully future experiments with behaving animals will provide evidence for a causal link between reticular activity and voluntary or reflex activation of motoneurons.

SOMATIC AFFERENT ACTIVATION OF RETICULOSPINAL NEURONS

The preceeding sections have reviewed evidence that reticulospinal pathways play an important role in the control of skeletal muscles, especially axial and proximal muscles, and have provided some insight into the types of motor behavior in which these pathways may participate. The present section and those that follow will focus on afferent pathways that control the activity of reticulospinal neurons. An attempt will be made throughout this discussion to interpret the action of these afferent pathways in terms of the possible patterns of motor activity they might elicit by activation of reticulomotor pathways.

Relayed activity from somatic afferent fibers represents a major input to the entire medial pontomedullary reticular formation. Electrophysiological studies (POMPEIANO and SWETT, 1963a, b; CASEY, 1969) have shown that somatic actions on reticular neurons are mediated by both low and higher threshold cutaneous afferent fibers and by higher threshold (i.e. Group II and above) muscle afferent fibers. When natural stimuli are used, some reticular neurons can be activated by hair bending, the majority are activated by touch, pressure or tapping on the skin but the most vigorous responses are elicited by strong, noxious stimuli (SEGUNDO et al., 1967b; BOWSHER et al., 1968; CASEY, 1969). The receptive fields associated with these responses are typically large (ranging from one limb to most of the body surface) and may include complex combinations of excitation and inhibition (SEGUNDO et al., 1967a, b; PETERSON et al., 1975a). The pathways involved in mediating responses of medial reticular neurons to somatic stimuli are invariably oligosynaptic (MAGNI and WILLIS, 1964b; SEGUNDO et al., 1967a; PETERSON et al., 1975a) and are not well understood. They presumably include both direct spinoreticular pathways (ROSSI and BRODAL, 1957; MEHLER et al., 1960) which carry signals related to a variety of somatic afferent inputs (ALBE-FESSARD et al., 1974; FIELDS et al., 1975, 1977; MAUNZ et al., 1978) and other less direct pathways that include relays in other brainstem structures that project to the reticular formation.

While anatomical studies (ROSSI and BRODAL, 1957) have indicated that direct spinoreticular pathways terminate preferentially in *n. r. pontis caudalis* and *ventralis*, physiological studies (PETERSON et al., 1975a; ECCLES et al., 1975, 1976) have indicated that the responses of reticulospinal neurons to somatic stimuli are generally similar throughout the medial pontomedullary reticular formation. Thus somatic inputs should reach both medial and lateral reticulospinal neurons. Also, while there is a general tendency for stimulation of the ipsilateral body surface to produce more excitation than contralateral stimulation, reticulospinal neurons show a wide variety of patterns of response to somatic stimuli and these patterns do not correlate in any detectable manner with the location or level of projection of the neuron concerned (PETERSON et al., 1975a). There is thus no evidence that somato-reticular pathways are organized so that stimulation of a point on the body surface would lead to selective activation of a localized population of reticulospinal neurons.

While somatic afferent inputs to reticulospinal neurons probably play a part in a diverse variety of motor behaviors, there is at present only one clearly defined motor activity identified with somato-reticular input: the spino-bulbo-spinal (SBS) reflex. This reflex is elicited by activation of cutaneous or high threshold muscle afferents and gives rise to a late burst of activation of flexor motoneurons coupled with depression of extensor motoneurons (SHIMAMURA and LIVINGSTON, 1963; SHIMAMURA et al., 1967; DEVANANDAN et al., 1968a, b; MARGHERINI et al., 1971). As illustrated in Figure 2A, the SBS reflex elicited by stimulation of a single nerve or dorsal root appears in motoneurons at different spinal levels at varying times after the stimulus. By extrapolating the latency of the SBS reflex volley against distance between the brainstem and the ventral root in which the volley was recorded (See Fig. 2A), SHIMAMURA and LIVINGSTON (1963) calculated that the reflex had an ascending conduction velocity of 65 m/sec, a descending conduction velocity of 33 m/sec and a central delay of 3–6 msec. In view of LLOYD's (1941) finding that monosynaptic reticulo-motor connections are too weak to elicit motoneuron discharge, it is likely that part of the central delay represents the time required for disynaptic activation of flexor motoneurons. The disynaptic nature of the descending pathway probably also explains its apparent low conduction velocity, which is well below the typical conduction velocity of excitatory reticulo-motor axons (GRILLNER and LUND, 1968; WILSON and YOSHIDA, 1969). The excitatory action of the faster fibers is presumably too weak to activate a sufficient number of excitatory relay neurons to elicit motoneuron discharge so that such discharge is only seen when excitation produced by slower fibers conducting on the order of 35–40 m/sec has converged with excitation produced by the faster fibers.

SHIMAMURA and LIVINGSTON (1963) reported that SBS reflexes in the cat were not markedly diminished following transverse lesions of the medial reticular formation 6 mm anterior to the obex (i.e. in the rostral part of *n. r. gigantocellularis*) but became progressively smaller as the lesion site was shifted posteriorly and disappeared altogether when the lesion was made 2 mm anterior to the obex (in *n. r. ventralis*). SBS reflexes can thus be elicited when only those areas giving rise to lateral reticulospinal fibers are intact but do

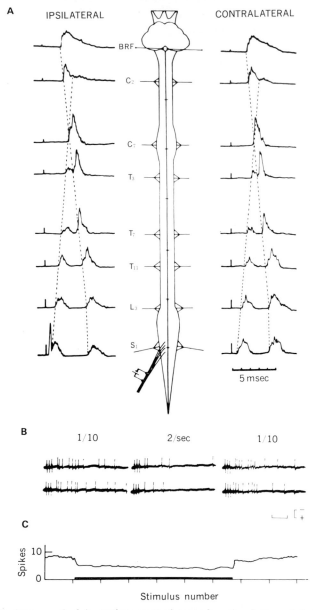

Fig. 2 *A*: Reflex discharge evoked in various ventral roots by stimulation of first sacral dorsal root. SBS reflex appears after segmental and propriospinal reflex volleys in T_3-S_1 roots and before the propriospinal reflex volleys in C_2 and C_7 roots (from SHIMAMURA and LIVINGSTON, 1963). *B, C*: Response of reticular neuron to stimulation of sciatic nerve at 1/10 sec and 2/sec. Oscilloscope records are shown in B. C plots number of spikes evoked by each stimulus (period of 2/sec stimulation is indicated by dark bar) (from PETERSON et al., 1976). Voltage calibration in B 0.5 mv, time calibration 10 msec.

not reach their maximum amplitude until the lesion site is moved far enough anterior to spare at least part of the zone from which medial reticulospinal fibers originate.   In light of these findings and of the fact that many reticulospinal neurons in the medial reticulo-spinal zone are activated by somatic stimulation, it is likely that both systems participate in producing the motor activity that characterizes SBS reflexes.

SBS reflexex are observed in decerebrate and chloralose-anesthetized animals but may have a behavioral counterpart in the widespread motor activation that occurs during startle responses.   One of the defining features of such responses is that they are only gener-ated by a novel sensory stimulus.   When the stimulus is repeated, the response declines or habituates.   Such a decline in output during repetitive activation is also seen in SBS reflexes and in reticular responses to somatic stimuli in general (SHIMAMURA and LIVINGSTON, 1963; SCHEIBEL and SCHEIBEL, 1965; SEGUNDO et al., 1967b; PETERSON et al., 1976).   In our recent study my colleagues and I (PETERSON et al., 1976) showed that the decline in reti-cular responses during repetitive somatic stimulation, an example of which is shown in Figure 2B, C, has many of the parametric features that characterize behavioral habitu-ating systems (THOMPSON and SPENCER, 1966).   Thus the decline in reticular and SBS reflex responses to somatic stimuli is likely to be related to the declining effectiveness of such repeated stimuli in evoking startle responses in behaving animals.

To summarize, the SBS reflex is an example of a pattern of motor activation which is generated by reticulospinal pathways and which may have a behavioral counterpart in the startle response.   The reflex is very non-specific both in the diversity of stimuli that may elicit it and in the global pattern of motor activity it produces.   Its only specificity is in the temporal domain where habituation restricts maximal reflex output to novel or infrequently presented stimuli.   The lack of input or output specificity in the SBS reflex does not imply a similar lack in specificity of reticulo-motor connections, however, since the extensive divergence and convergence that takes place in somato-reticular pathways is probably to a large extent responsible for the widespread motor activation pattern that characterizes the SBS reflex.

VESTIBULAR AFFERENT MODULATION OF RETICULOSPINAL ACTIVITY

A second major source of afferent input to the medial pontomedullary reticular forma-tion is the vestubular labyrinth.   Afferent activity from semicircular canal and macular receptors reaches reticular neurons indirectly via relay neurons in the vestubular nuclei or cerebellum.   Studies involving both natural and electrical stimulation have shown that activation of vestibular afferent fibers can produce both excitation and inhibition of reti-cular neurons (DUENSING and SCHAEFER, 1960; PETERSON et al., 1975a; FUKUSHIMA et al., 1977).

Labyrinth-vestibulo-reticular pathways have been investigated electrophysiologically by PETERSON and ABZUG (1975).   In agreement with the anatomical data of LADPLI and BRODAL (1968), they found that each of the four major vestibular nuclei contains neurons projecting to the medial pontomedullary reticular formation.   These vestibulo-reticular neurons appear likely to carry a diverse variety of signals.   As shown in Figure 3, some of them are directly or indirectly excited by stimulation of labyrinthine afferent fibers and thus presumably act as relay neurons transmitting labyrinthine afferent activity to the reti-cular formation while many others can not be excited by such stimuli and thus are likely to carry more complex signals only indirectly related to labyrinthine input.   Collectively

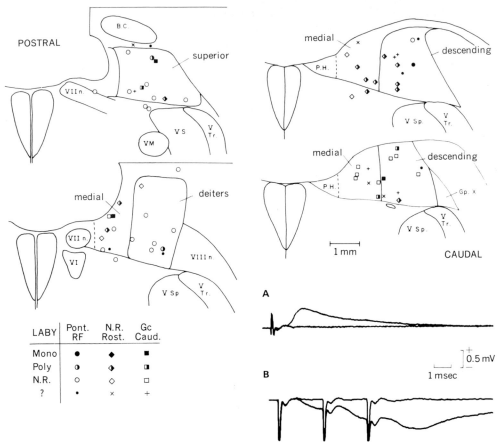

Fig. 3 Vestibulo-reticular projections. Schematic cross sections through vestibular nuclei indicate the locations of neurons that could be driven antidromically from the contralateral medial reticular formation. Symbols shown in key at lower left indicate for each neuron the reticular region from which it was driven and its response to stimulation of the vestibular nerve. Column headings in key indicate: neurons driven from the medial pontine reticular formation, from rostral *n.r. gigantocellularis* and from caudal *n.r. gigantocellularis*. Row headings indicate: monosynaptic, polysynaptic, no response and undetermined response to stimulation of vestibular nerve. Traces in A and B illustrate monosynaptic excitation and inhibition of reticular neurons evoked by stimulation of the contralateral vestibular nuclei.

Abbreviations: Deiters, descending, medial and superior indicate the four main vestibular nuclei; B.C., brachium conjunctivum; Gp. x, vestibular cell group x; P.H., prepositus hypoglossi nucleus; Vm, Vs, V Sp. and V Tr. indicate the trigeminal motor nucleus, sensory nucleus, spinal nucleus and spinal tract respectively; VI, abducens nucleus; VII n., facial nerve; VIII n., vestibular nerve. (from PETERSON and ABZUG, 1975)

vestibulo-reticular projections have an important action on reticulospinal neurons: activation of these projections by stimulation of the vestibular nuclei gives rise to direct excitation and/or inhibition of the great majority of reticulospinal neurons in *n. r. pontis caudalis* and *gigantocellularis* (PETERSON and ABZUG, 1975). These direct synaptic connections between vestibular and reticular neurons must play an important role in producing the di- and polysynaptic responses of reticulospinal neurons to stimulation of labyrinthine afferent fibers (PETERSON et al., 1975a). Labyrinth-cerebello-reticular pathways may also play a role in transmitting labyrinthine signals to reticulospinal neurons but the detailed synaptic connections within such pathways have not been investigated.

Modulation of the activity of reticulospinal neurons by labyrinthine afferent activity is presumably part of the process that converts labyrinthine signals into vestibular reflex activation of the somatic musculature. SPYER et al. (1974) have found that 20–30° roll tilts induce tonic changes in the discharge rates of neurons in the medial pontomedullary reticular formation, suggesting that reticulospinal neurons located in those regions may participate in static vestibular reflexes evoked by tilting.   Only 14 per cent of the neurons studied responded, however, and these exhibited a mixture of response patterns so that further information on tilt-evoked responses of identified reticulospinal neurons is required to evaluate the role of reticulospinal pathways in static vestibular reflexes.

Recent work in our laboratory (PETERSON, et al., 1978) has focused on the role of reticulospinal neurons in the phasic vestibular-neck (vestibulocollic) reflex evoked by activation of semicircular canal afferents. As described by WILSON in the preceeding paper, this reflex is characterized by a 50–80° shift in phase between a sinusoidal vestibular afferent signal and the resulting sinusoidal modulation of neck motoneuron discharge. Medullary reticular neurons of unknown projection had been shown to be modulated in phase with such motoneuron discharge during sinusoidal rotation on the horizontal plane (FUKUSHIMA et al., 1977).   In our experiments we have used electrical activation of horizontal canal afferents to determine whether reticulospinal neurons receive input from the horizontal canals and whether their response to sinusoidal modulation of canal afferent activity is in phase with the vestibulocollic reflex activation of neck motoneuron discharge.

In an initial series of experiments, which were designed to examine responses of a wide variety of reticulospinal neurons to horizontal semicircular canal input, we recorded the responses of antidromically identified reticulospinal neurons in precollicular decerebrate cats to trains of bipolar pulses applied to electrodes implanted close to the horizontal semicircular canal ampulae using the technique of SUZUKI et al. (1969).   Using extracellular recording, we found that many reticulospinal neurons were activated by trains of 9–12 pulses (0.1 msec, 300/sec) applied to the contralateral horizontal canal nerve at 3–7 times the threshold for evoking field potentials in the contralateral vestibular nuclei.   Relatively few reticulospinal neurons were excited by similar stimuli applied to the ipsilateral horizontal canal nerve.   As shown in Figure 4A, B, there was also a difference in the responsiveness of medial (A) and lateral (B) reticulospinal neurons to the contralateral canal stimulus: 47 per cent of medial reticulospinal neurons tested were excited by the stimulus whereas only 15 per cent of the lateral reticulospinal neurons responded.   As indicated by the filled circles, many of the responsive neurons projected beyond the C_4 spinal segment. This finding, plus the fact that most of the responsive neurons were found within the zone from which activation of muscles throughout the body can be evoked (see Fig. 1), suggests that reticulospinal neurons are likely to be involved in vestibular reflex activation of muscle throughout the body.

We have recently begun recording the responses of reticulospinal neurons in decerebrate cats during vestibular reflexes evoked by modulated continuous polarization of semicircular canal nerves.   As described by WILSON (1978) the modulating waveform consisted of nine superimposed sinusoids which were odd, relatively prime multiples of a common base frequency.   In each run the gain and phase of a reticulospinal neuron's response at each of the nine frequencies was compared with the corresponding gain and phase of the rectified EMG response recorded from neck muscles.   Preliminary results indicate that the discharge of some medial reticulospinal neurons is modulated in phase with the activity of neck muscles on the same side.   Figure 4C shows an example of simultaneously recorded activity of a reticulospinal neuron (filled circles) and the biventer cervicis muscle (open circles) on the left side to modulated polarizing current applied to an electrode close to the right horizontal semicircular canal nerve.   As the frequency increased from 0.084 to 0.76 Hz, neuron and muscle activity shifted from a phase lead to phase lag and decreased in amplitude.   At higher frequencies, both neuronal and muscle modulation became too weak to allow quantitative measurements of their phase and gain.   Similar data from other neurons indicate that the medial reticulospinal tract carries signals with the appropriate gain and phase to contribute to the vestibular control of neck and other body muscles. Further work is necessary to assess the importance of this contribution relative to that of other descending pathways.

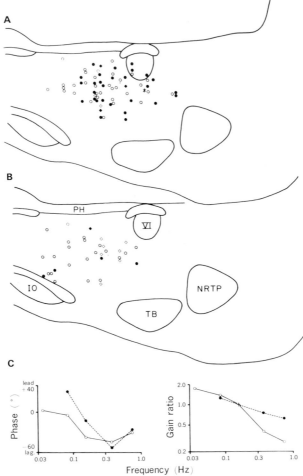

Fig. 4 Semicircular canal input to reticulospinal neurons. *A* and *B* show locations of reticulo-spinal neurons whose responses to trains of pulses applied to the contralateral horizontal semi-circular canal nerve were observed. Neurons projecting in the medial reticulospinal tract are shown in A, those projecting in the ipsilateral lateral reticulospinal tract in B. Filled symbols indicate neurons that responded to the canal stimulus. Diamonds indicate neurons driven anti-dromically from C_1 but not from C_4 segment (neck cells), circles indicate neurons driven from both levels. Asterisk indicates location of neuron whose response is illustrated in C. PH indicates prepositus hypoglossi nucleus; other abbreviations as in Fig. 1. C: Response of medial reticulo-spinal neuron to modulated polarization applied to electrode close to contralateral horizontal semicircular canal ampulla. Modulation consisted of nine superimposed sinusoids which evoked sinusoidal changes in activity of neuron and of neck muscles on the same side. The phase and gain of neuronal (filled circles) and muscle (open circles) activity are plotted against frequency. Phase is relative to maximum negative polarization, gain relative to gain at 0.18 Hz.

To summarize, the modulation of their discharge by vestibular afferent signals suggests that reticulospinal neurons play a role in vestibular reflexes acting on the somatic musculature. The pattern of reticulospinal neuron activity during reflexes elicited by semicircular canal stimulation is more specialized and specific than reticulospinal activity during spino-bulbo-spinal reflexes. A brief train of pulses applied to one horizontal semicircular canal nerve primarily activates reticulospinal neurons located in the contralateral brainstem, and modulation of semicircular canal input produces a rise and fall of reticulospinal neuron activity that is in phase with activity of the ipsilateral musculature. This reticulospinal activity has a pattern which suggests that reticulospinal pathways participate in periodic activation of muscles on one side of the body coupled with relaxation of muscles on the opposite side. This is clearly quite different from the overall, bilateral muscle activation of the SBS reflex.

Other inputs to reticulospinal neurons

While more specific than that accompanying SBS reflexes, the pattern of muscle activity produced by semicircular canal activity is still quite broad. It is therefore possible that this input does not reveal the ultimate levels of specificity present in reticulo-motor pathways. In addition to somatic and vestibular inputs, reticulospinal neurons also receive direct excitatory inputs from the superior colliculi (UDO and MANO, 1970; PETERSON, et al., 1974), cerebral cortex (MAGNI and WILLIS, 1964a; PETERSON et al., 1974) and deep cerebellar nuclei (ECCLES et al., 1975; BANTLI and BLOEDEL, 1975). These inputs, which produce powerful activation of many reticulospinal neurons, are likely to play a significant role in control of somatic muscles by the superior colliculus, cortex or cerebellum. Comparison of data on the responses of motoneurons and reticulospinal neurons to stimulation of the superior colliculi (ANDERSON et al., 1971, 1972; PETERSON et al., 1974) suggests that tecto-reticulospinal connections may in fact represent the major route via which the colliculi act upon the somatic musculature. It is thus possible that the reticulospinal system, under the control of one of these three structures, might participate in movements requiring the activation of a restricted set of muscles such as the reaching movements studied by BRINKMAN and KUYPERS (1973)—see previous section. An alternative possibility is that the primary motor function of reticulospinal pathways may be to produce the changes in tone of axial and postural muscles that accompany voluntary movements in which case specificity of reticulomotor action beyond that observed in vestibular reflex studies may not be required. Experiments involving observation of the activity of reticulospinal neurons during a variety of voluntary movements are required to decide between these two possibilities.

CONCLUSION

Research involving analysis of the function of reticulospinal pathways is in a stage of transition. It has been clearly demonstrated that these pathways have a strong action upon somatic motoneurons and recent anatomical and physiological studies have provided information about the topography and organization of reticulo-motor connections and of reticular afferent systems. Attention is now turning to analysis of the behavior of reticular neurons in the context of a variety of motor activities. The earliest work of this kind involved analysis of SBS reflexes, which unfortunately provided little information about the mode of reticular action on motor centers. At present work is under way recording the activity of reticular neurons in freely moving animals and studying the participation of reticulospinal neurons in vestibular reflexes. This review has considered the problem of the degree of specificity of reticulo-motor connections, which is one of the central questions that must be addressed in these studies.   Other important questions are whether reticulo-spinal neurons participate in phasic or tonic control of muscle activity, or in both and how reticular activity relates to the various parameters of movement such as limb position or muscle force and their derivitives.   Hopefully the next several years will see a resolution of these questions and a resulting increase in our appreciation of the function of reticulo-motor pathways.

REFERENCES

Albe-Fessard, D., Levante, A. and Lamour, Y.:   Origin of spinothalamic and spinoreticular pathways in cat and monkeys. In Bonica, J. J. (ed.):   Advances in Neurology, Vol. 4, International Symposium on Pain, pp. 157–166, Raven Press, New York (1974)

Anderson, M. E., Yoshida, M. and Wilson, V. J.:   Influence of the superior colliculus on cat neck motoneurons. J. Neurophysiol., 34: 898–907 (1971)

Anderson, M. E., Yoshida, M. and Wilson, V. J.:   Tectal and tegmental influences on cat forelimb and hindlimb motoneurons.   J. Neurophysiol., 35: 462–470 (1972)

Bantli, H. and Bloedel, J. R.:   Monosynaptic activation of a direct reticulospinal pathway by the dentate nucleus. Pflügers Arch., 357: 237–242 (1975)

Bowsher, D., Mallart, A. and Albe-Fessard, D.:   A bular relay to centre median.   J. Neurophysiol., 31: 288–300 (1968)

Brinkman, J. and Kuypers, H. G. J. M.:   Cerebral control of contralateral and ipsilateral arm, hand and finger movements in the split-brain Rhesus monkey. Brain, 96: 653–674 (1973)

Brodal, A.:   The Reticular Formation of the Brain Stem.   Oliver and Boyd, Edinburgh (1957)

Casey, K.:   Somatic stimuli, spinal pathways and size of cutaneous fibers influencing unit activity in the medial medullary reticular formation. Exp. Neurol., 25: 35–56 (1969)

Devanandan, M. S., Eccles, R. M., Lewis, D. M. and Stenhouse, D.:   Responses of flexor alpha motoneurons in cats anesthetized with chloralose. Exp. Brain Res., 8: 163–176 (1969a)

Devanandan, M. S., Eccles, R. M., Lewis, D. M. and Stenhouse, D.:   Responses of extensor alpha motoneurons in cats anesthetized with chloralose. Exp. Brain Res., 8: 177–189 (1969b)

Duensing, F. and Schaefer, K. P.:   Die Aktivatät einzelner Neurone der Formatio reticularis des nicht gefesselten kaninchens bei kopfwendungen und vestibulären Reizen. Arch. Psychiat. Nervenkr., 201: 97–122 (1960)

Eccles, J. C., Nicoll, R. A., Rantucci, T., Taborikova, H. and Willey, T. J.:   Topographic studies on medial reticular nucleus. J. Neurophysiol., 39: 109–118 (1976)

Eccles, J. C., Nicoll, R. A., Schwarz, W. F., Taborikova, H. and Willey, T. J.:   Reticulospinal neurons with and without monosynaptic inputs from cerebellar nuclei. J. Neurophysiol., 38: 513–530 (1975)

Fields, H. L., Clanton, C. H. and Anderson, S. D.:   Somatosensory properties of spinoreticular neurons in the cat. Brain Res., 120: 49–66 (1977)

Fields, H. L., Wagner, G. M. and Anderson, S. D.:   Some properties of spinal neurons projecting to the medial brain-stem reticular formation. Exp. Neurol., 47: 118–134 (1975)

Fukushima, Y., Igusa, Y. and Yoshida, K.:   Characteristics of responses of medial brain stem neurons to horizontal head angular acceleration and electrical stimulation of the labyrinth in the cat. Brain Res., 120: 564–570 (1977)

Grillner, S., Hongo, T. and Lund, S.:   Convergent effects on alpha motoneurones from the vestibulospinal tract and a pathway descending in the medial longitudinal fasciculus. Exp. Brain Res., 12: 457–479 (1971)

Grillner, S. and Lund, S.:   The origin of a descending pathway with monosynaptic action on flexor motoneurones. Acta physiol. scand., 74: 274–284 (1968)

Ito, M., Udo, M. and Mano, N.:   Long inhibitory and excitatory pathways converging onto cat's reticular and Deiters' neurons, and their relevance to the reticulofugal axons. J. Neurophysiol., 33: 210–226 (1970)

Jankowska, E., Lund, S., Lundberg, A. and Pompeiano, O.:   Inhibitory effects evoked through ventral reticulospinal pathways. Arch. ital. Biol., 106: 124–140 (1968)

JANKOWSKA, E., LUNDBERG, A., ROBERTS, W. J. and STUART, D.: A long propriospinal system with direct effect on motoneurones and interneurones in the cat lumbosacral cord. *Exp. Brain Res.,* *21*: 169–194 (1974)

KUYPERS, H. G. J. M.: The descending pathways to the spinal cord, their anatomy and function. In ECCLES, J. C. and SCHADE, J. (eds.): *Organization of the Spinal Cord.* pp. 178–200, Elsevier, New York (1964)

LADPLI, R. and BRODAL, A.: Experimental studies of commissural and reticular formation projections from the vestibular nuclei in the cat. *Brain Res.,* *8*: 65–96 (1968)

LLINÁS, R. and TERZUOLO, C. A.: Mechanisms of supraspinal actions upon spinal cord activities. Reticular inhibitory mechanisms on alpha-extensor motoneurons. *J. Neurophysiol.,* *27*: 579–591 (1964)

LLOYD, D. P. C.: Activity in neurons of the bulbospinal correlation system. *J. Neurophysiol.,* *4*: 115–134 (1941)

MAGNI, F. and WILLIS, W. D.: Cortical control of brain stem reticular neurons. *Arch. ital. Biol.,* *102*: 418–433 (1964a)

MAGNI, F. and WILLIS, W. D.: Subcortical and peripheral control of brain stem reticular neurons. *Arch. ital. Biol.,* *102*: 434–448.

MAGOUN, H. W. and RHINES, R.: An inhibitory mechanism in the bulbar reticular formation. *J. Neurophysiol.,* *9*: 165–171 (1946)

MARGHERINI, P. C., THODEN, U. and POMPEIANO, O.: Spino-bulbospinal reflex inhibition of monosynaptic extensor reflexes of hindlimb in cats. *Arch. ital. Biol.,* *109*: 110–129 (1971)

MEHLER, W. R., FEFERMAN, M. E. and NAUTA, W. J. H.: Ascending axon degeneration following anterolateral cordotomy. An experimental study in the monkey. *Brain,* *83*: 719–750 (1960)

MAUNZ, R. A., PITTS, N. G. and PETERSON, B. W.: Cat spinoreticular neurons: locations, responses and changes in responses during repetitive stimulation. *Brain Res.,* *148*: 365–379 (1978)

NYBERG-HANSEN, R.: Functional organization of descending supraspinal fibre systems to the spinal cord. Anatomical observations and physiological correlations. *Ergebn. Anat. Entwickl.-Gesch.* 30, Heft, 2: 1–48 (1966)

PETERSON, B. W.: Identification of reticulospinal projections that may participate in gaze control. In BERTHOZ, A. and BAKER, R. (eds.): *Control of Gaze by Brain Stem Neurons, Developments in Neuroscience.* Vol. 1, Elsevier/North-Holland Biomedical Press, Amsterdam (1977)

PETERSON, B. W. and ABZUG, C.: Properties of projections from vestibular nuclei to medial reticular formation in the cat. *J. Neurophysiol.,* *38*: 1421–1435 (1975)

PETERSON, B. W., ANDERSON, M. E. and FILION, M.: Responses of ponto-medullary reticular neurons to cortical, tectal and cutaneous stimuli. *Exp. Brain Res.,* *21*: 19–44 (1974)

PETERSON, B. W., FILION, M., FELPEL, L. P. and ABZUG, C.: Responses of medial reticular neurons to stimulation of the vestibular nerve. *Exp. Brain Res.,* *22*: 335–350 (1975a)

PETERSON, B. W., FRANCK, J. I., PITTS, N. G. and DAUNTON, N. G.: Changes in responses of medial pontomedullary reticular neurons during repetitive cutaneous, vestibular, cortical and tectal stimulation. *J. Neurophysiol.,* *39*: 564–581 (1976)

PETERSON, B. W., FUKUSHIMA, K., HIRAI, N., SCHOR, R. H. and WILSON, V. J.: Activation of vestibular and reticular neurons during vestibular reflexes induced by sinusoidal polarization of semicircular canal afferents. *Soc. for Neurosci. Abstr.,* *4*: 613 (1978)

PETERSON, B. W., MAUNZ, R. A., PITTS, N. G. and MACKEL, R. G.: Patterns of projection and branching of reticulospinal neurons. *Exp. Brain Res.,* *23*: 333–351 (1975b)

PETERSON, B. W., PITTS, N. G., FUKUSHIMA, K. and MACKEL, R.: Reticulospinal excitation and inhibition of neck motoneurons. *Exp. Brain Res.,* *32*: 471–489 (1978)

PETRAS, J. M.: Cortical, tectal and tegmental fiber connections in the spinal cord of the cat. *Brain Res.,* *6*: 275–324 (1967)

PITTS, N. G., FUKUSHIMA, K. and PETERSON, B. W.: Reticulospinal action on cervical, thoracic and lumbar motoneurons. *Soc. for Neurosci. Abstr.,* *3*: 276 (1977)

POMPEIANO, O. and SWETT, J. E.: Actions of graded cutaneous and muscle afferent volleys on brain stem units in the decerebrate cerebellectomized cat. *Arch. ital. Biol.,* *101*: 552–583 (1963a)

POMPEIANO, O. and SWETT, J. E.: Cerebellar potentials and responses of reticular units evoked by muscle afferent volleys in the decerebrate cat. *Arch ital. Biol.,* *101*: 584–613 (1963b)

RHINES, R. and MAGOUN, H. W.:   Brain stem facilitation of cortical motor response.   *J. Neurophysiol.*, *9*: 219–229 (1946)

ROSSI, G. F. and BRODAL, A.:   Terminal distribution of spinoreticular fibers in the cat.   *Arch. Neurol. Psychiat. (Chic.)*, *78*: 439–453 (1957)

SCHEIBEL, M. E. and SCHEIBEL, A. B.:   The response of reticular units to repetitive stimuli.   *Arch ital. Biol.*, *103*: 279–299 (1965)

SEGUNDO, J. P., TAKENAKA, T. and ENCABO, H.:   Electrophysiology of bulbar reticular neurons.   *J. Neurophysiol.*, *30*: 1194–1220 (1967a)

SEGUNDO, J. P., TAKENAKA, T. and ENCABO, H.:   Somatic sensory properties of bulbar reticular neurons.   *J. Neurophysiol.*, *30*: 1221–1238 (1967b)

SHIMAMURA, M. and LIVINGSTON, R. B.:   Longitudinal conduction systems serving spinal and brain stem coordination.   *J. Neurophysiol.*, *26*: 258–272 (1963)

SHIMAMURA, M., MORI, S. and YAMAUCHI, T.:   Effects of spino-bulbo-spinal reflex volleys on extensor motoneurons of hindlimb in cats.   *J. Neurophysiol.*, *30*: 319–332 (1967)

SIEGEL, J. M. and McGINTY, D. J.:   Pontine reticular formation neurons: relationship of discharge to motor activity.   *Science*, *176*: 678–680 (1977)

SPRAGUE, J. M. and CHAMBERS, W. W.:   Control of posture by reticular formation and cerebellum in the intact, anesthetized and unanesthetized and in the decerebrated cat.   *Amer. J. Physiol.*, *176*: 52–64 (1954)

SPYER, K. M., GHELARDUCCI, B. and POMPEIANO, O.:   Gravity responses of neurons in main reticular formation.   *J. Neurophysiol.*, *37*: 705–721 (1974)

STERLING, P. and KUYPERS, H. G. J. M.:   Anatomical organization of the brachial spinal cord of the cat. III.   The propriospinal connections.   *Brain Res.*, *7*: 419–443 (1968)

SUZUKI, J. I., GOTO, K., TOKUMASU, K. and COHEN, B.:   Implantation of electrodes near individual vestibular nerve branches in mammals.   *Ann. Otol.*, *78*: 815–826 (1969)

THOMPSON, R. F. and SPENCER, W. A.:   Habituation: a model phenominon for the study of neuronal substrates of behavior.   *Psychol. Rev.*, *173*: 16–43 (1966)

UDO, M. and MANO, N.:   Discrimination of different spinal monosynaptic pathways converging onto reticular neurons.   *J. Neurophysiol.*, *33*: 227–238 (1970)

VERTES, R. P.:   Selective firing of rat pontine gigantocellular neurons during movement and REM sleep.   *Brain Res.*, *128*: 146–152 (1977)

WILSON, V. J.:   Electrophysiological and dynamic studies of vestibulospinal reflexes.   *In* ASANUMA, H, and WILSON, V. J. (eds.):   *Integration in the Nervous System*, Igaku-Shoin Ltd., Tokyo, New York (1978)

WILSON, V. J. and YOSHIDA, M.:   Comparison of effects of stimulation of Deiters' nucleus and medial longitudinal fasciculus on neck, forelimb and hindlimb motoneurons.   *J. Neurophysiol.*, *32*: 743–758 (1969)

WILSON, V. J., YOSHIDA, M. and SCHOR, R. H.:   Supraspinal monosynaptic excitation and inhibition of thoracic back motoneurons.   *Exp. Brain Res.*, *11*: 282–295 (1970)

DISCUSSION PERIOD

SKOGLUND: If I got you right, you said that the projection of the reticulospinal system to axial muscles, mostly to the neck, was characterized by small monosynaptic EPSPs, but that the later PSPs were larger.

PETERSON: In general the indirect effects—this was already shown by LLOYD in 1941—are larger than the direct.   That's true even more so of the limb muscles.   The direct effects are strongest on the neck, next strongest on the back, and least strong on the limb muscles.

SKOGLUND: So you have difficulty getting monosynaptic excitation of the axial muscles?   I put that question because as you know there are reports that people when stimulating Ia afferents saw no monosynaptic reflexes in neck muscles.   We have been doing some work on back muscles and we have also had difficulty in getting monosynaptic activation.

PETERSON: Yes.   The reticulospinal system has just the inverse relationship to the monosynaptic reflexes you've been describing.   It has its strongest action on the axial muscles, and a weaker action on the limb muscles.   In fact, it's entirely possible that looped reflexes going through the brainstem may be involved in activation of the axial musculature, whereas local segmental reflexes may be stronger and more prominant in the limb muscles.

CORTICAL AND SUBCORTICAL INTEGRATION (1)

Chairman: H. KEFFER HARTLINE

Editors note that at the beginning of this session a lecture entitled "A General Paradigm for Cortical Function; the Unit Module and the Distributed System" was read by Professor Vernon MOUNTCASTLE, Johns Hopkins University, Baltimore.

MULTIPLE REPRESENTATION IN THE MOTOR CORTEX: A NEW CONCEPT OF INPUT-OUTPUT ORGANIZATION FOR THE FOREARM REPRESENTATION*

Peter L. STRICK and James B. PRESTON

Research Service, Veterans Administration, and Departments of Neurosurgery and Physiology, Upstate Medical Center
Syracuse, NY

INTRODUCTION

Much of our present understanding of the motor representation of the body in the cerebral cortex has developed from studies employing electrical stimulation. These studies have shown that it is possible to evoke relatively localized movements of individual body parts by stimulating a variety of cytoarchitectural areas (e. g., Fritsch and Hitzig, 1870; Leyton and Sherrington, 1917; Penfield and Boldrey, 1937; Chang et al., 1947; Woolsey et al., 1952; Welker et al., 1957; Landgren et al., 1962; Asanuma and Rosén, 1972; Kwan et al., 1978). The lowest threshold region for evoking movements of limb musculature consistently lies within area 4.

Maps of motor responses have been constructed from studies in which the surface of the primary motor cortex was stimulated. The results of these mapping experiments have been summarized by projecting a diagram of the body onto the cerebral cortex. The location of each body part in the diagram indicates the region of cortex where stimulation evoked movement of that part. Figure 1 is an example of a diagram constructed in this manner by Penfield and his associates from their studies in man (Penfield and Rasmussen, 1950). The diagram illustrates that each body part is represented in an orderly sequence and each part is represented only once in the motor cortex. Also illustrated is the observation that movements of distal limb parts are elicited from a larger area of cortex than are movements of proximal body parts.

Similar motor maps and body image diagrams have been constructed from stimulation studies in other animals (e. g., Woolsey et al., 1952; Welker et al., 1957). The same general relationships as illustrated in Figure 1 have been found. Woolsey et al. (1952) also summarized their studies in the rhesus monkey (Figure 2) by portraying the representation in the primary motor cortex as a distorted drawing of the body parts in which each had a single representation. Furthermore, Figure 2 illustrates the rostro-caudal gradient in the representation of the limbs. For example, the digits of the forelimbs are represented caudally in the bank of the central sulcus while wrist, elbow, and shoulder are represented at successively more rostral sites in the motor cortex.

Using the somatotopic maps developed in these earlier studies, current research has focused on the fine structure of the organization of motor cortex output (Asanuma and Sakata, 1967; Evarts, 1967; Phillips, 1969; Asanuma and Rosén, 1972; Andersen et al., 1975; Jankowska et al., 1975b).

In addition to describing the somatotopic organization of the motor cortex, the mapping

* This study was supported in part by funds from the Veterans Administration Research Fund and USPHS Grant NS02957.

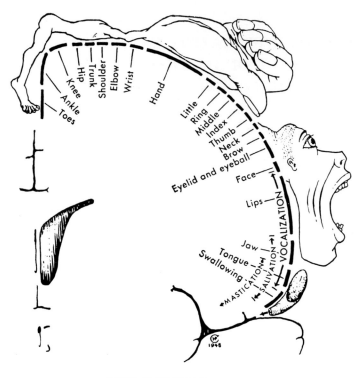

MOTOR HOMUNCULUS

Fig. 1 The drawing indicates the movements which can be elicited upon electrical stimulation of different regions in the human motor cortex. The size of each body part in the drawing is distorted to indicate the proportion of motor cortex devoted to its representation. The length of the thick black lines outlining the cortex also reflects the relative extent of each representation. (from PENFIELD and RASMUSSEN, 1950)

studies led to the development of a number of other concepts. One of these suggested that there is a correlation between the relatively large area allotted to the hand and wrist representation and the highly developed motor capabilities of these parts. This concept has been further supported by behavioral studies which show that, of all movements, those of hand and wrist are most severely affected by lesions of the motor cortex or its output (LAWRENCE and KUYPERS, 1968; KUYPERS, 1973).

Increased area of representation alone may not be sufficient to account for the specialized abilities of the hand and wrist. In addition to having a larger area of cortex, a unique pattern of organization also might be required to deal with the complexities of hand and wrist movements. One such pattern of organization might be to have multiple representations of the hand and wrist. Each representation could then be designed to deal with selected aspects of hand and wrist motor behavior. WOOLSEY et al. (1952) clearly emphasized that "successive overlap" of body parts is a characteristic feature of cortical representation. It occurred to us that multiple representations could be buried within the "successive overlap" observed in earlier work. The idea of multiple representations of body parts finds support in studies on the primary somatosensory cortex (PAUL et al., 1972; SUR et al., 1978).

In order to explore the possibility that multiple representations exist within area 4, we mapped the forearm area of primary motor cortex in the squirrel monkey. This animal was chosen because none of the arm or hand motor representation is buried within a sulcus

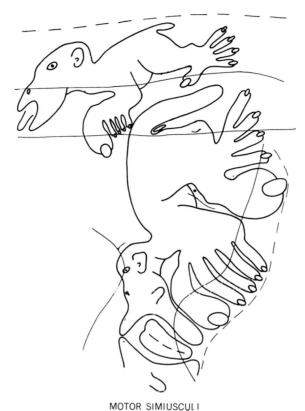

MOTOR SIMIUSCULI

Fig. 2 The two drawings indicate the body representation and location of the primary (vertically oriented figurine) and supplementary (horizontally oriented figurine) motor areas in the Rhesus monkey. As in Fig. 1, the size and location of the body parts in the two drawings reflect the extent and location of cortex devoted to the motor representation of those parts. The vertical dashed line is the bottom of the central sulcus. (from WOOLSEY et al., 1952, Used by permission of ARNMD)

(WELKER et al., 1957; SANIDES, 1968).   In our studies microstimulation showed that there are two anatomically separate hand-wrist representations in area 4.   Furthermore, natural stimulation of the forelimb during unit recording demonstrated that different patterns of afferent input project to these two representations.

We suggest that the two motor representations reflect two separate control systems within the hand-wrist area of the motor cortex.   Furthermore, we suggest that the two systems deal with different components of motor behavior.

Some of these results have been presented briefly elsewhere (PAPPAS and STRICK, 1979; STRICK and PRESTON, 1978a, b).

METHODS

Experiments were performed on squirrel monkeys (Saimiri Sciureus) weighing 0.75–1.2 kg.   The animals were anesthetized with 10 mg/kg of Ketamine HCl given intramuscularly and 25 mg/kg of pentobarbital sodium given intraperitoneally.   During the course of experiments, supplemental IM doses of Ketamine HCl were given as needed to maintain anesthesia.   Our results were obtained when the animal was not making spontaneous movements and when little or no withdrawal reflexes could be demonstrated. Hydration was maintained by intravenous drip of sterile ringer-lactate solution. The rectal temperature of animals was maintained between 37 and 38 degrees.

Each animal's head was rigidly held by a large bolt which was secured to the skull with dental acrylic. Using the coronal suture as a landmark, the calvarium was removed in the area surrounding the central fissure. A plastic cylinder was fixed to the skull with low melting point wax. The cylinder was filled with warm mineral oil and formed the base of a closed chamber system (DAVIES, 1956).

Glass coated, platinum-iridium microelectrodes with impedances of 0.7 to 1.5 megohms were used for both microstimulation and single neuron recording. The microelectrodes were tapered so that they measured approximately 10 μm wide at 15 μm from the tip and 80 μm at 1 mm from the tip. These microelectrodes were driven into the motor cortex approximately perpendicular to its surface by means of a hydraulic microdrive clamped to the top of the plastic cylinder.

The sites of microelectrode penetrations were determined during the experiment with the aid of a dissecting microscope and each point marked on an enlarged photograph of the exposed cortex.

Microstimulation consisted of a 50–60 msec cathodal pulse train delivered at a frequency of 300–400 Hz with a pulse duration of 0.2 msec (ASANUMA and SAKATA, 1967; ASANUMA and ROSÉN, 1972). The indifferent electrode for both microstimulation and unit recording was a screw fixed to the skull. Current intensity was monitored continuously. Thresholds for evoking movements varied between 1.0 and 25 μA (in most cases below 10 μA). As others have noted (ASANUMA and ARNOLD, 1975), current intensities in this range did not appear to produce cellular damage. We could record from a single neuron before and after stimulation and discern no changes in the discharge characteristics of the unit. The effects of microstimulation were determined by muscle palpation, visual inspection and in some cases verified by EMG recording.

Single units were recorded using conventional methods of amplification. Units which were activated by non-noxious natural stimulation of the contralateral forearm were searched for as the electrode was slowly advanced into the cortex. The adequate stimulus and receptive field of an isolated unit were determined by stroking or gently tapping skin and hair, and by bending joints. For display purposes the receptive field of some units was stimulated by a probe attached to a Ling vibrator. The probe was arranged to produce single small displacements of skin, hair or joints.

At the termination of each experiment the animal was deeply anesthetized and perfused with a solution containing 1 % paraformaldehyde and 1.25 % glutaraldehyde in a 0.1 M phosphate buffer. The brain was removed, and a tissue block containing the motor cortex was later frozen sectioned at 50 μm intervals. These sections were stained with cresyl violet. The location of penetrations found in the tissue sections was correlated with the surface photograph and with small electrolytic lesions placed at selected points.

RESULTS

The physical arrangement of the squirrel monkey's primary sensory and motor cortices is well suited for mapping experiments. This is illustrated in Figures 3 and 4 which are adapted from the cytoarchitectural study of SANIDES (1968). An outline of a lateral view of the cerebral cortex of the squirrel monkey is shown in Figure 3. The presumed analogue of the central sulcus of other primates is the central fissure, labeled CF in this figure. Anterior to the central fissure lies part of the somatosensory cortex, area 3a and part of area

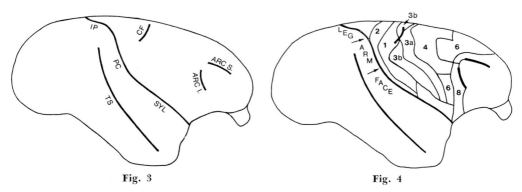

Fig. 3   Fig. 4

Fig. 3 Outline of the right hemisphere of the squirrel monkey cerebral cortex. The major sulci are labeled. ARC I.: inferior arcuate sulcus; ARC S.: superior arcuate sulcus; CF: central fissure; IP: intraperietal sulcus; PC: postcentral sulcus; SYL: sylvian sulcus; TS: temporal sulcus.
Fig. 4 The cytoarchitectural zones of the motor and somatosensory areas are indicated by the thin lines and numbers (Both Fig. 3 and Fig. 4 are adapted from SANIDES, 1968)

3b (see Figure 4).   As in other primates area 4 lies anterior to area 3a.   Thus, area 4 in this primate is completely exposed on the surface of the cortex.

Microstimulation in area 4, in the region just rostral to area 3a, evoked movements of the hand (thumb and fingers).   A zone in which predominately wrist and radio-ulnar joint movements were evoked (wrist flexion and extension, wrist ulnar and radial deviation, and forearm supination and pronation) was found just rostral to the hand zone.   Rostral to this wrist zone there was an abrupt transition to a zone from which thumb and finger movements were once again evoked   Both the thresholds for evoking movements and the movements evoked here are the same as for those movements evoked in the region of area 4 just rostral to area 3a.

The presence of this second zone of hand representation in area 4 does not conform to the classical viewpoint of motor cortex representation; namely, movements of more proximal portions of the limb are evoked from points rostral to a single area of hand representation (WOOLSEY et al., 1952).   Furthermore, immediately rostral to the second hand zone lies another zone in which movements of the wrist and radio-ulnar joint are again evoked. As with the hand zones the movements evoked and their thresholds were similar in the two wrist zones.   Microstimulation did not evoke additional hand movements rostral to this second wrist representation.

We have called the hand and wrist zones nearest the central fissure the caudal motor representation and the second hand and wrist zones, which are more remote from the central fissure, the rostral motor representation.   Histological analysis of the sites of lesions marking both caudal and rostral representations demonstrated that both were located in area 4.

Figure 5 illustrates some of these findings.   Figure 5A shows an oblique view of the left hemisphere of the squirrel monkey.   The parallelogram outlined on the cortical surface (labeled B) is a segment of area 4 located at the center of the hand-wrist region.   Figure 5B is an enlarged view of the parallelogram labeled B in Figure 5A.   Each symbol shows the site of one microelectrode penetration made in this 2×2 mm area.   The relatively large spaces where penetrations were not made were regions occupied by surface blood vessels.   The filled circles represent sites from which thumb or finger movements were evoked and the open circles are sites where stimulation elicited movements of the wrist or

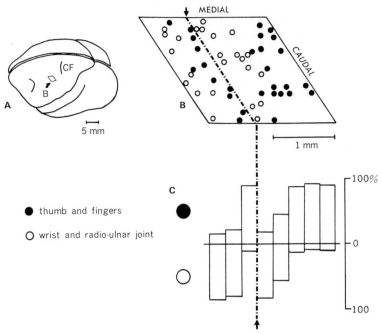

● thumb and fingers

○ wrist and radio-ulnar joint

Fig. 5

A: Oblique view of squirrel monkel left hemisphere. Parallelogram (labeled B) represents a 2×2 mm segment of area 4 at the center of the hand-wrist representation. CF: central fissure.
B: Enlarged view of parallelogram in Fig. 5A. Symbols indicate sites of microelectrode penetrations. Filled circles are sites where thumb and finger movements were evoked. Open circles are sites where wrist or radio-ulnar movements were evoked. The dashed line indicates the border between the two motor representations.
C: Graph of results from three animals. Comparable 2×2 mm parallelograms from three animals were divided into 8 equal mediolateral bands. Parallelograms were aligned on the border between the two representations (dashed line). Each bar represents the percentage of hand (above) and wrist (below) responses seen in each band. See text. (from STRICK and PRESTON, 1978a)

radio-ulnar joint. Note the clustering of like responses which tend to orient in mediolateral bands, and the alternation of the hand and wrist bands. The dashed line was placed by eye and represents the straight line which best divides the caudal and rostral motor representations in this animal. The transition between the rostral and caudal representations occurred 4 mm from the central fissure in the animal illustrated in Figure 5A and 5B. In four other animals the line of transition was located from 3.7 to 4.2 mm rostral to the central fissure.

Figure 5C is an attempt to represent the results from several experiments in a semi-quantitative fashion. In order to summarize results from different animals, the border between the rostral and caudal representations was used to align maps from three animals. In these animals a sufficient number of penetrations were made around the border region to define it. In each animal stimulation sites near the center of the forelimb representation and within a 2×2 mm area containing the border between the rostral and caudal representations were used in constructing the graph in Figure 5C. In all, 134 stimulation sites were contained within these three 2×2 mm areas of cortex. For each of the three animals the 2×2 mm area was divided into eight 250 μm medio-lateral bands. The number of sites from which we elicited movements of thumb-fingers and wrist-radioulnar joint were separately summed for each band in each animal. The sums from comparable bands in the three animals were then totaled and the results presented in Figure 5C. Each verti-

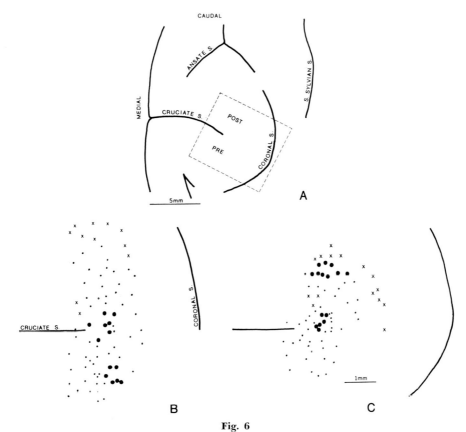

Fig. 6

A: A portion of the cat left hemisphere with relevant sulci and gyri labeled. Dotted rectangle indicates the area explored with intracortical microstimulation. This area appears enlarged in Fig. 6B and 6C.

B, C: Enlarged view of area outlined in Fig. 6A. The last two millimeters of the cruciate sulcus and portions of the coronal sulcus are included for orientation. Each map is from an individual animal. Small dots indicate sites where microstimulation evoked movements in joints other than digit (e.g., wrist, elbow, shoulder). Large filled circles indicate sites where digit movements were evoked. Crosses indicate sites where no movement was evoked. (from PAPPAS and STRICK, 1979)

cal bar in this figure represents the totals of one of the eight bands. The length of a bar above the horizontal "0" line represents the percentage of thumb-finger responses and the length below represents the percentage of wrist-radioulnar joint responses.

Although there is some overlap of hand and wrist representations, this overlap is not sufficient to mask a clearly defined double representation even when the results from three animals are lumped together. Therefore, the size of the representations must be rather constant from animal to animal. It also is apparent that the thumb-finger zone in the caudal representation occupies a larger area than it does in the rostral representation.

The demonstration of a double representation in area 4 of the squirrel monkey raises several questions. One of these is whether the pattern of multiple representation is species specific or is a general feature of motor cortex organization. Results from microstimulation in the cat motor cortex demonstrate that a double motor representation of the forelimb also exists in area 4 of this species (PAPPAS and STRICK, 1979). The double representation is most clearly seen in the distribution of digit responses. Maps of two animals illustrating the two digit representations are shown in Figure 6. The area within the dashed lines in Figure 6A indicates the region of cortex which was explored with microstimulation. This region is enlarged in Figures 6B and C. The location of all penetrations where stimulation below 50 μA evoked movement are indicated by dots. The crosses indicate penetrations where microstimulation below 50 μA failed to evoke movements. Digit movements were elicited at sites indicated by large filled circles. Note that digit responses could be evoked from two separate regions in both animals (Figures 6B and C). The two areas of digit representation were separated by a 1.5–2.0 mm field in which responses at more proximal joints were evoked. Histological analysis showed that both digit representations were confined to area 4 γ of the cortex (HASSLER and MUHS-CLEMENT, 1964). Thus, a double representation of the distal forelimb can be demonstrated in area 4 in a primate and in a carnivore.

Another question raised by the demonstration of two hand-wrist representations in the squirrel monkey motor cortex is whether the two representations have similar or different afferent inputs. The results from experiments in which we recorded from single neurons in area 4 demonstrate that the caudal and rostral motor representations receive different concentrations of cutaneous and deep (joint and/or muscle) inputs.

Ninety-five units responded to natural stimulation of the contralateral forelimb. These responsive units were classified into three categories; cutaneous, deep, or mixed. Cutaneous units were those whose response was limited to activation of skin and hair. Deep units were those whose activation was restricted to passive manipulation of joints. Most units could be placed confidently in one of these two categories although three units, classified as mixed, responded to cutaneous and deep type inputs.

Fifty-three of the ninety-five responsive neurons were classified as cutaneous, thirty-nine classified as deep, and three as mixed. In each experiment the boundary between the caudal and rostral motor representations was determined by observing the motor responses evoked by microstimulation through the recording electrodes. Only one of fifty-three cutaneous units was located in the rostral motor representation while seven of the thirty-nine deep units were located in the caudal motor representation. Therefore, single units activated by cutaneous input were clearly concentrated in the caudal hand-wrist representation while neurons responding to deep inputs were concentrated in the rostral hand-wrist representation.

Figure 7 illustrates the differences in the distribution of cutaneous and deep units within the rostral and caudal hand-wrist representations. The symbols in the diagram indicate the location of forty-two electrode penetrations within the motor cortex. Those penetrations in which only cutaneous units were recorded are indicated by filled circles, those containing only deep units are indicated by open circles, and those with both cutaneous and deep units by crosses. The dashed line indicates the border between the rostral and the caudal motor representations. Note the concentration of cutaneous tracks in the caudal representation to the right of the dashed line and deep tracks in the rostral representation to the left of the line.

Several different response patterns were observed for both deep and cutaneous units. The most common response patterns for deep units were: (1) a brief burst during joint movements, (2) a response limited to the extremes of joint movement, and (3) a continuous response during joint rotation. Neurons 1 and 2 in Figure 7 were classified as deep units and were located in the rostral representation. The figurine below each response indicates the contralateral joint movement which caused the neuron to discharge (1.–elbow flexion; 2.–thumb abduction).

The majority of the cutaneous units were rapidly adapting and responded with a brief burst to stimulation within their receptive fields. Only a few units gave a tonic discharge

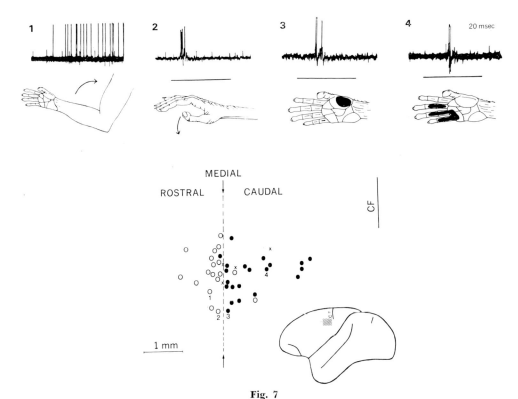

Fig. 7

Top: 4 examples of representative unit responses. Tracts from which units were recorded are indicated by numbered symbols in bottom half of figure. The figurine below each response indicates the receptive field for the neuron. The stimulus for: 1.–elbow flexion; 2.–thumb abduction; 3. and 4.–light touch to shaded areas on the figurines. The lines below traces 2, 3, and 4 indicate the duration of probe displacement used to trigger responses.

Bottom: Map of electrode penetrations. The shaded rectangle in the brain drawing in lower right corner indicates area explored. The region is enlarged in bottom center of figure. Dashed line indicates border between rostral and caudal motor representations. Penetrations recording only cutaneous units indicated by filled circles, those recording only deep units by open circles, and mixed penetrations by crosses. C.F.=central fissure. (from STRICK and PRESTON, 1978b)

to sustained stimulation.   Furthermore, the receptive fields for many cutaneous units were located on the glabrous skin of the hand although some units responded exclusively to movement of hairs on the back of the hand.   Neurons 3 and 4 in Figure 7 were classified as cutaneous units and were located in the caudal representation.   The shaded area on the figurine shown below each response indicates the location of the receptive field.

Thus, we have observed that the cutaneous and deep inputs are not randomly intermingled in the motor cortex but are differentially distributed in the rostral and caudal motor representations.   Although the separation is not complete, neurons driven by cutaneous inputs are concentrated in the caudal motor representation.   Neurons driven by deep input are concentrated in the rostral motor representation.

The data in Figure 8 summarizes some of the results of microstimulation and unit recording.   We have chosen four closely spaced tracks from one animal.   The location of these tracks is illustrated in the bottom of Figure 8.   The motor response evoked by microstimulation in each track is indicated by the horizontal row of figurines labeled motor. The receptive field and unit discharge of a representative neuron recorded in each track are shown in the horizontal rows labeled sensory.

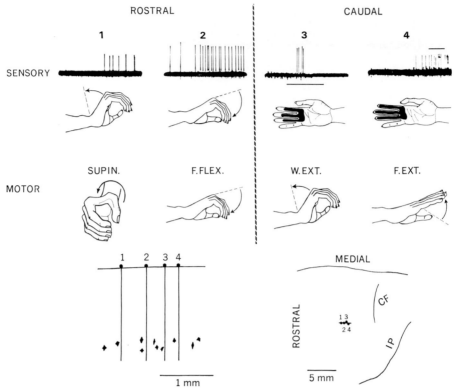

Fig. 8 Results of microstimulation and unit recording in four closely-spaced, microelectrode penetrations.
Top: Sensory: Receptive field and unit discharge of a representative unit recorded in each track. Rostral representation, 1 and 2, 1: wrist extension; 2: finger flexion. Caudal representation, 3 and 4, cutaneous receptive fields indicated by darkened area on figurines.
Motor: The motor response evoked by microstimulation in each track. 1: supination; 2: finger flexion; 3: wrist extension; 4: finger extension.
Bottom: *Left*: The rostro-caudal spacing of the microelectrode penetrations.
        Right: The sites of entry on the cortical surface. CF: central fissure; IP: intraparietal sulcus.

The microelectrode was placed initially in the rostral wrist representation.   For each subsequent penetration the microelectrode was moved caudally by a small increment. Microstimulation evoked supination in track 1, finger flexion in track 2, wrist extension in track 3, and finger extension in track 4.   The discharge of single neurons in the rostral representation (1 and 2) was evoked by joint movements.   The discharge of single neurons in the caudal representation (3 and 4) was evoked by stimulation of the skin on the volar surface of the hand.

In summary, this figure illustrates our two major observations.   First, there are two hand-wrist motor representations in area 4.   This is indicated by the alternation of hand and wrist motor responses.   Second, the rostral and caudal motor representations receive different concentrations of cutaneous and deep inputs.

DISCUSSION

Motor representation

Although the question may be one of semantics, there has been a long-standing and as yet unresolved debate on whether movements or muscles are represented in the motor cortex (e. g., JACKSON, 1931; WALSHE, 1943; MURPHY and GELLHORN, 1945; RUCH et al., 1948; FULTON, 1949; EVARTS, 1967; ASANUMA and ROSÉN, 1972; PHILLIPS, 1975). From this debate another controversy has developed; namely, whether electrical stimulation of the motor cortex demonstrates the existence of a non-overlapping mosaic in which each muscle has a discrete representation. Recently, in an attempt to resolve the issue of discrete localization, the technique of intracortical microstimulation, developed by ASANUMA and his colleagues (ASANUMA, 1975) has been employed. In spite of the elegance of this technique, some disagreement concerning the degree of overlap in the cortical representation of single muscles remains (ASANUMA and ROSÉN, 1972; ANDERSEN et al., 1975; JANKOWSKA et al., 1975a; ASANUMA et al., 1976; SHINODA et al., 1976). This is in part due to differences in the interpretation of results from surface and intracortical stimulation (see JANKOWSKA et al., 1975 a and b; ANDERSEN et al., 1975; ASANUMA et al., 1976 for a more complete discussion). However, there seems to be a consensus that the motor cortex contains sites where output neurons which project to the same spinal motoneuron pool occur in high densities. These high density sites in the primate have been termed "cortical efferent zones" by ASANUMA and ROSÉN (1972) and "aggregations of colonies" by ANDERSEN, et al. (1975).

In our study we have not attempted to re-examine the size of these high density sites. Rather, we have employed the technique of intracortical microstimulation to determine the muscle contraction or movement which is *most represented* at each stimulation site. We defined *most represented* as that muscle contraction or movement evoked at the lowest stimulus intensity. With this criterion we employed microstimulation to re-investigate the patterns of motor representation within the forearm region of area 4. Our results indicate that the concentration of points from which we evoked hand movements peak in two spatially separated zones within area 4. The same is true for wrist movements. These observations most likely reflect similar peaks in the spatial distribution of output neurons.

As noted earlier, we have labeled the hand and wrist zones nearest the central fissure, the caudal motor representation, and the second more anterior hand and wrist zones, the rostral motor representation. This pattern of hand and wrist motor representation is summarized by the caricatures shown in Figure 9. The size of the hands and wrists in the figure indicate the relative size of the hand and the wrist zones in the two motor representations.

The existence of a double representation in area 4 is further supported by the results of the unit recording experiments. These experiments demonstrated marked differences in the distribution of somatosensory afferent input to each representation. Neurons driven by cutaneous input are concentrated in the caudal motor representation while neurons driven by deep input are concentrated in the rostral representation.

The double hand-wrist representation which we have demonstrated is a clear departure from the classical scheme of body representation previously described for primate area 4. Recently another modification of the classical scheme of body representation has been proposed for motor cortex (WONG et al., 1977; KWAN et al., 1978). The authors concluded that the representation of the forelimb in the stump-tailed monkey can be described as concentric overlapping rings of shoulder, elbow, and wrist fields surrounding a central

AREA 4 MOTOR REPRESENTATION

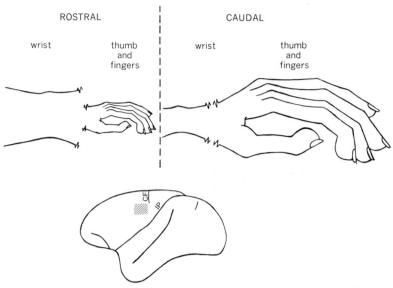

Fig. 9 Diagram of the double representation in area 4 of the squirrel monkey. The relative size and location of the hands and wrists roughly reflect the extent and location of cortex allotted to the representation of these parts. The shaded area in the brain outline at the bottom of the figure indicates the location of the two motor representations in relation to major sulci. CF: central fissure; IP: intraparietal sulcus.

core of finger representation. The rings of shoulder and elbow representation are incomplete and have an opening at the central sulcus. The opening is occupied by finger and wrist motor points. Our findings of a localized specialization within the hand-wrist representation differ from those of Kwan et al. (1978) in that they did not report the double representation which we have found in the squirrel monkey. The difficulty in reconstructing the topography within the depths of the central sulcus in the stump-tailed monkey may account for this difference.

Although we made no attempt to systematically explore the representation of proximal musculature, we do have observations which suggest that a concentric arrangement may exist for this representation in the squirrel monkey. There were experiments in which elbow and shoulder movements were evoked both medial and lateral to the two hand-wrist representations. These observations are just what one would predict if the double representation we found in the squirrel monkey was surrounded by rings of elbow and shoulder representations.

Afferent input

It is clear from our results that the motor cortex of the squirrel monkey receives input not only from cutaneous (Zimmerman, 1968) but also from deep somatosensory afferents as does the motor cortex of other primates (e.g., Albe-Fessard and Liebeskind, 1966; Fetz and Baker, 1969; Rosén and Asanuma, 1972; Wiesendanger, 1973; Hore et al., 1976; Lemon and Porter, 1976; Wong et al., 1977). Our results demonstrated that neurons driven by cutaneous input are concentrated posteriorly in area 4 within the caudal motor representation. In contrast, neurons driven by deep inputs are concentrated anteriorly in area 4 within the rostral motor representation. This pattern in the distribution of somatosensory inputs to the motor cortex has not been described previously. However, LEMON and PORTER (1976) did state that units driven by cutaneous input in the arm area of the cynomolgus motor cortex were located entirely in the central sulcus. This location is where our caudal motor representation would most likely be found in primates with a deep central sulcus.   Units responding to deep inputs apparently had a wider distribution in their experiments.   Furthermore, FETZ (personal communication) has also noted that motor cortex neurons driven by cutaneous input are concentrated deep in the anterior bank of the central sulcus.

GOLDRING and RATCHESON (1972) investigated the afferent input to the hand area of human motor cortex.   They isolated 30 cells of which 16 responded to peripheral somatosensory input.   All of their responsive cells were activated by kinesthetic input and none by cutaneous input.   These observations led to the conclusion that human motor cortex differs from that of other primates in that it lacks cutaneous input.   Although this interpretation may be correct, in light of our results, another possibility exists.   If the pattern of organization found in the forearm area of the squirrel monkey motor cortex also occurs in man, then the caudal representation, where cutaneous input is most concentrated, would be buried within the human central sulcus.   The rostral representation, where deep input is most concentrated, would most likely be located on the exposed surface of the precentral gyrus.   Although the information was not given, it is unlikely that GOLDRING and RATCHESON recorded their units from the depths of the central sulcus.   If this supposition is correct, their sample would have been taken from a region where units are dirven primarily by deep inputs.

Functional implications

Prior studies of sensory input to the motor cortex and the discharge patterns of pyramidal tract neurons during movements strongly suggest the involvement of the motor cortex in a number of reflex-like motor responses (e. g., WOOLSEY and BARD, 1936; DENNY-BROWN, 1960; PHILLIPS, 1969; ROSÉN and ASANUMA, 1972; EVARTS, 1973; CONRAD et al., 1975). Our results suggest that these cortically dependent responses of the forearm may not be mediated by a common population of motor cortex neurons.   Two observations lead us to this suggestion.   First, there are two spatially separate hand-wrist representations in area 4.   Second, these two representations receive different concentrations of deep and cutaneous inputs.

The concentration of cutaneous input to the caudal motor representation suggests it may be designed to control movements which use tactile input for their execution and guidance as, for example, in the tactile grasping reaction (DENNY-BROWN, 1960; ROSÉN and ASANUMA, 1972).   On the other hand, the concentration of deep input to the rostral motor representation suggests a different function for it.   This representation may be designed to control movements which use kinesthestic input for their execution and guidance as, for example, in load compensation (PHILLIPS, 1969; EVARTS, 1973; CONRAD, et al., 1975).   Thus, our hypothesis is that the double representation reflects two motor control systems within area 4 that deal with different components of motor behavior. While it would be surprising if these systems are completely independent, they may have been anatomically separated to facilitate differential control over their input and/or output. The reasons why this strategy for differential control would be selected over others, such as gating inputs to common output neurons, are unclear.

Whether the unique pattern of organization which we have demonstrated for the forearm region of area 4 in the squirrel monkey also exists in the representation of other body parts and in other primate species remains to be investigated.

ACKNOWLEDGEMENTS

The authors wish to acknowledge the expert assistance of Ms. Cathryn SKRETCH and Ms. Agnes HELCZ in the conduct of this research and in the preparation of the figures for this manuscript.

REFERENCES

ALBE-FESSARD D. et LIEBESKIND, J.: Origine des messages somato-sensitifs activant les cellules du cortex moteur chez le singe. *Exp. Brain Res., 1*: 127–146 (1966)

ANDERSEN, P., HAGAN, P. J., PHILLIPS, C. G. and POWELL, T. P. S.: Mapping by microstimulation of overlapping projections from area 4 to motor units of the baboon's hand. *Proc. R. Soc. Lond. B, 188*: 31–60 (1975)

ASANUMA, H.: Recent developments in the study of the columnar arrangement of neurons within the motor cortex. *Physiol. Rev., 55*: 143–156 (1975)

ASANUMA, H. and SAKATA, H.: Functional organization of a cortical efferent system examined with focal depth stimulation in cats. *J. Neurophysiol., 30*: 35–54 (1967)

ASANUMA, H. and ROSÉN, I.: Topographical organization of cortical efferent zones projecting to distal forelimb muscles in the monkey. *Exp. Brain Res., 14*: 243–256 (1972)

ASANUMA, H. and ARNOLD, A. P.: Noxious effects of excessive currents used for intracortical microstimulation. *Brain Res., 96*: 103–107 (1975)

ASANUMA, H. ARNOLD, A. and ZARZECIKI, P.: Further study on the excitation of pyramidal tract cells by intracortical microstimulation. *Exp. Brain Res., 26*: 443–461 (1976)

CHANG, H.-T., RUCH, T. C. and WARD, A. A.: Topographical representation of muscles in motor cortex of monkeys. *J. Neurophysiol., 10*: 39–56 (1947)

CONRAD, B., MEYER-LOHMANN, J., MATSUNAMI, K. and BROOKS, V. B.: Precentral unit activity following torque pulse injections into elbow movements. *Brain Res., 94*: 219–236 (1975)

DAVIES, P. W.: Chamber for microelectrode studies in the cerebral cortex. *Science, 124*: 179–180 (1956)

DENNY-BROWN, D.: Motor mechanisms—Introduction: The general principles of motor integration. *In: Handbook of Physiology.* Section 1 Neurophysiology Vol. 2. pp. 781–796. Williams and Wilkins, Baltimore, (1960)

EVARTS, E. V.: Representation of movements and muscles by pyramidal tract neurons of the precentral motor cortex. *In* YAHR, M. D. and PURPURA, D. P. (eds.): *Neurophysiological Basis of Normal and Abnormal Motor Activities.* pp. 215–254, Raven Press, New York (1967)

EVARTS, E. V.: Motor cortex reflexes associated with learned movement. *Science, 179*: 501–503 (1973)

FETZ, E. E. and BAKER, M. A.: Response properties of precentral neurons in awake monkeys. *The Physiologist, 12*: 223 (1969)

FRITSCH, G. and HITZIG, E.: Über die elektrische Erregbarkeit des Grosshirns. *Arch. Anat. Physiol. wiss Med., 37*: 300–332 (1870)

FULTON, J. F.: Cerebral Cortex: The motor areas and pyramidal system. *In: Physiology of the Nervous System.* 3rd ed. pp. 392–420, Oxford Univ. Press, (1949)

GOLDRING, S. and RATCHESON, R.: Human motor cortex: Sensory input data from single neuron recording. *Science, 175*: 1493–1495 (1972)

HASSLER, R. und MUHS-CLEMENT, K.: Architektonischer Aufbau des sensomotorischen und parietalen cortex der Katze. *J. Hirnforsch., 6*: 377–420 (1964)

HORE, J., PRESTON, J. B., DURKOVIC, R. G. and CHENEY, P. D.: Responses of cortical neurons (areas 3 and 4) to ramps tretch of hindlimb muscles in the baboon. *J. Neurophysiol., 39*: 484–500 (1976)

JACKSON, J. H.: TAYLOR, J. (ed.) *Selected writings of John Hughlings Jackson.* Vol. I. Hodder and Stoughton, London (1931)

JANKOWSKA, E.. PADEL, Y. and TANAKA, R.: The mode of activation of pyramidal tract cells by intracortical stimuli. *J. Physiol., 249*: 617–636 (1975a)

JANKOWSKA, E., PADEL, Y. and TANAKA, R.: Projections of pyramidal tract cells to α-motoneurones innervating hindlimb muscles in the monkey. *J. Psyiol., 249*: 637–667 (1975b)

KUYPERS, H. G. J. M.: The anatomical organization of the descending pathways and their contributions to motor control especially in primates. *In* DESMEDT, J. E. (ed.): *New Developments in Electromyography and Clinical Neurophysiology,* Vol. 3, pp. 38–68, Karger, Basel, (1973)

KWAN, H. C., MACKAY, W. A., MURPHY, J. T. and WONG, Y. C.:   An intracortical microstimulation study of output organization in precentral cortex of awake primates.   *J. Physiol. (Paris)*, (1978 in press)

LANDGREN, S., PHILLIPS, C. G. and PORTER, R.:   Cortical fields of origin of the monosynaptic pyramidal pathways to some alpha motoneurons of the baboon's hand and forearm.   *J. Physiol. Lond., 161*: 112–125 (1962)

LAWRENCE, D. G. and KUYPERS, H. G. J. M.:   The functional organization of the motor system in the monkey.   I. The effects of bilateral pyramidal lesions.   *Brain, 91*: 1–14 (1968)

LEMON, R. N. and PORTER, R.:   Afferent input to movement-related precentral neurones in conscious monkeys.   *Proc. R. Soc. Lond. B., 194*: 313–339 (1976)

LEYTON, A. S. F. and SHERRINGTON, C. S.:   Observations on the excitable cortex of the chimpanzee, orang-utan and gorilla.   *Quart. J. Exp. Physiol., 11*: 135–222 (1917)

MURPHY, J. B. and GELLHORN, E.:   Multiplicity of representation versus punctate localization in the motor cortex.   *Arch. Neurol. Psychiat. (Chicago), 54*: 256–273 (1945)

PAPPAS, C. L. and STRICK, P. L.:   Double representation of the distal forelimb in cat motor cortex.   *Brain Res.*, (1979 in press)

PAUL, R. L., MERZENICH, M. and GOODMAN, H.:   Representation of slowly and rapidly adapting cutaneous mechanoreceptors of the hand in Brodmann's areas 3 and 1 of macaca mulatta.   *Brain Res., 36*: 229–249 (1972)

PENFIELD, W. and BOLDREY, E.:   Somatic motor and sensory representation in the cerebral cortex of man as studied by electrical stimulation.   *Brain, 60*: 389–443 (1937)

PENFIELD, W. and RASMUSSEN, T.:   The Cerebral Cortex of Man.   Chapter II, pp. 11 65, The Macmillan Co., New York (1950)

PHILLIPS, C. G.:   The Ferrier Lecture.   Motor apparatus of the baboon's hand.   *Proc. R. Soc. B, Lond., 173*: 141–174 (1969)

PHILLIPS, C. G.:   Laying the ghost of muscles versus movements.   *Canadian J. Neurol. Sci., 2*: 209–218 (1975)

ROSÉN, I. and ASANUMA, H.:   Peripheral afferent inputs to the forelimb area of the monkey motor cortex: Input-output relations.   *Exp. Brain Res., 14*: 257–273 (1972)

RUCH, T. C., CHANG, H.-T. and WARD, A. A.:   The pattern of muscular response to evoked cortical discharge.   *Res. Publ. Ass. Nerv. Ment. Dis., 26*: 61–83 (1948)

SANIDES, F.:   The architecture of the cortical taste nerve areas in squirrel monkey (Saimiri Sciureus) and their relationships to insular, sensorimotor and prefrontal regions.   *Brain Res., 8*: 97–124 (1968)

SHINODA, Y., ARNOLD, A. P. and ASANUMA, H.:   Spinal branching of corticospinal axons in the cat.   *Exp. Brain Res., 26*: 215–234 (1976)

STRICK, P. L. and PRESTON, J. B.:   Multiple representation in the primate motor cortex.   *Brain Res., 154*: 366–370 (1978)

STRICK, P. L. and PRESTON, J. B.:   Sorting of somatosensory afferent information in primate motor cortex.   *Brain Res., 156*: 364–368 (1978)

SUR, M., NELSON, R. J. and KAAS, J. H.:   The representation of the body surface in somatosensory area I of the grey squirrel.   *J. Comp. Neurol., 179*: 425–450 (1978)

WALSHE, F. M. R.:   On the mode of representation of movements in the motor cortex with special reference to "convulsions beginning unilaterally" (Jackson).   *Brain, 66*: 104–139 (1943)

WELKER, W. I., BENJAMIN, R. M., MILES, R. C. and WOOLSEY, C. N.:   Motor effects of stimulation of cerebral cortex of squirrel monkey (Saimiri Sciureus).   *J. Neurophysiol., 20*: 347–364 (1957)

WIESENDANGER, M.:   Input from muscle and cutaneous nerves of the hand and forearm to neurones of the precentral gyrus of baboons and monkeys.   *J. Physiol., 228*: 203–219 (1973)

WONG, Y. C., KWAN, H. C., MACKAY, W. A. and MURPHY, J. T.:   Topographic organization of afferent inputs in monkey precentral cortex.   *Brain Res., 138*: 166–168 (1977)

WOOLSEY, C. N. and BARD, P.:   Cortical control of placing and hopping reactions in macaca mulatta.   *Am. J. Physiol., 116*: 165 (1936)

WOOLSEY, C. N., SETTLAGE, P. H., MEYER, D. R., SENCER, W., PINTO-HAMUY, T. and TRAVIS, A. M.:   Patterns of localization in precentral and "supplementary" motor areas and their relation to the concept of a premotor area.   *Res. Publ. Ass. Nerv. Ment. Dis., 30*: 238–264 (1952)

ZIMMERMAN, I. D.:   A triple representation of the body surface in the sensorimotor cortex of the squirrel monkey.   *Exp. Neurol., 20*: 415–431 (1968)

DISCUSSION PERIOD

HENNEMAN: Dr. STRICK, in your representation of the caudal and rostral zones of the thumb and wrist, I noticed that a column of rostral points are rather high, and that those of the distal part are rather low, and vice versa—if it's high, it's distal, if it's low it's rostral. So that the total length of the columns seems to be roughly the same. Does that have any particular significance to your findings?

STRICK: I am not entirely certain that I understand your question. I believe you are referring to Figure 5C. In this figure, the bars do not represent cortical columns. They represent the distribution of hand and wrist points within a 250 μM mediolateral strip of cortex. The length of the bar above and below the zero line indicates the percentage of hand and wrist responses respectively. The total length of the bar will equal 100 % and thus be the same total length for each strip.

LARSEN: You didn't very carefully explain to us your stimulation parameters. You have a large number of tracks in a small area, so that you must have thoroughly activated everything in the two by two mm area. Could this many penetrations damage the area?

STRICK: No, we've used very fine electrodes, which have a very long taper and avoided blood vessels very carefully. Because of these precautions there was very little swelling during these experiments, and no compromise to the blood supply. (See text for complete description of stimulus parameters.)

LARSEN: There are a large number of muscles in the forearm and more than one can cause flexion of the wrist.

STRICK: If by this comment you are asking whether the same muscles are activated by stimulation in the two representations, the answer is yes, at least for the superficial wrist flexor and extensors and for the long flexors and extensors of the hand. We have not studied the individual intrinsic hand muscles in sufficient detail to make a confident statement about their representation.

LARSEN: You have demonstrated localization of different sensory inputs to different parts of cortex. I recall from other data in cats and monkeys that within a penetration in the motor cortex there are both skin and deep receptive fields, and single cells with mixed modality.

STRICK: One of the major advantages of using the squirrel monkey is that the motor cortex is completely exposed on the surface and none of the arm area is buried in a sulcus. In other primates where the receptive fields of motor cortex neurons have been examined most of the penetrations were made into the rostral bank of the central sulcus or very near it, where the cortex is curving. Even in those studies, some authors namely LEMON and PORTER, as well as FETZ, have reported that cutaneous units were concentrated deep in the sulcus, where you might expect our caudal representation to be.

BURKE: PETER, when you talk about finger movements, were there any detected differences between activation of long finger muscles vs. the intrinsic hand muscles for these two areas?

STRICK: We don't think so. However, I can't be all that confident about the intrinsic representation. You can be quite confident about those muscles which are superficial and can be visually or electrically recorded easily.

QUESTION: Many of the finger points, then are the long muscles?

STRICK: Yes.

LAPORTE: Have you any idea about the type of motor units which cause the contraction?

STRICK: No.   The EMG monitoring that we did was fairly gross, using large EMG electrodes.   Therefore, we cannot say anything about the type of motor units activated.

DIRECT SENSORY PATHWAYS TO THE MOTOR CORTEX IN THE MONKEY: A BASIS OF CORTICAL REFLEXES*

HIROSHI ASANUMA, KENNETH D. LARSEN and HARUHIDE YUMIYA

The Rockefeller University
New York, NY

INTRODUCTION

It has been a continuing question whether a small area of the motor cortex controls contraction of a muscle or a group of muscles.   In previous experiments, we have shown that weak intracortical microstimulation (ICMS) can produce contraction of individual muscles from a small area within the depth of the cortex (ASANUMA, 1975).   Based on these experiments, we have proposed that these low threshold areas (cortical efferent zones) have the highest concentration of neurons which project to a particular motoneuron pool although the same area also projects to other motor nuclei with lesser concentration. Furthermore, it has been shown that these efferent zones receive peripheral inputs related to the contraction of the target muscles constituting loop circuits between the cortex and the periphery.   The present experiments were designed to further clarify the characteristics of these circuits so that they can be used as a tool for the exploration of the interaction between various areas of the central nervous system and the motor cortex.   Since the present experiments are based on our previous conclusion that a given cortical efferent zone projects, primarily, to a given motoneuron pool, we want to start by reviewing the historical background on the localization of cortical motor function.

Cortical surface stimulation

It was little more than a century ago when FRITSCH and HITZIG (1870) convincingly demonstrated that there is localization of motor function within the mammalian cerebral cortex.   The dominant view at that time was that the cerebral cortex functions exclusively for mentation, although there were reports by J. Hughlings JACKSON (1868, 1875) which inferred the possibility of the existence of motor function in the cerebral cortex based on his clinical observations.   Since the demonstration by FRITSCH and HITZIG was so sensational that a great number of the contemporary neurologists and neurophysiologists were fascinated in further elucidating the mechanisms underlying cortical motor function.   The question put forward was whether the motor cortex controls contraction of individual muscles or a pattern of contractions, i. e., movements.   JACKSON, deeply influenced by his contemporary evolutionists, favored the idea that there is a widespread overlapping of the representation of muscle groups within the motor cortex (WALSHE, 1943).   This idea was based on the interpretation that neural function is characterized by a hierarchy in which successive levels re-represent movements controlled by lower levels, but with progressively greater refinement, complexity and spontaneity.   This interpretation of so called "minute representation" was also supported by many investigators who repeated stimulation experiments following FRITSCH and HITZIG (1870).   They found it was

---

* This research was supported by the NIH Grant NS–10705.

difficult to produce contraction of individual muscles by cortical stimulation and the combination of muscles activated was always in a reciprocal fashion (SHERRINGTON, 1906).

However, the notion that the motor cortex is organized as a simple "mosaic", each component containing the nervous mechanism subserving a single restricted movement could never be explicitly excluded (WALSHE, 1943). FULTON (1949b) argued that "the controversy would seem clearly to be the one which can be resolved more readily by recourse to experiment than by philosophical reflection" supported by his colleagues CHANG, RUCH and WARD. Aided by the improved electrical technique, they (CHANG et al., 1947) could produce contraction of single muscles by cortical stimulation, although it was occasionally. They concluded that the "Betz cells for a particular muscle are distributed over a contiguous area of the cortex with the highest cell concentration located at a particular focus." The results of their experiments were discussed repeatedly and are still being discussed, especially in relation to the Jacksonian conception. EVARTS (1967) argued that "the fact that threshold electrical stimulation excites motoneuron of one and only one muscle indicates that the tissue in the vicinity of the stimulating electrode has a stronger association with this muscle than with any other muscle, but JACKSON never proposed that the unit in the corpus striatum (motor cortex) represented all muscles equally." He concluded that CHANG, RUCH and WARD do not refute JACKSON's theories of motor representation that "the motor cortex is to be conceived of, not as a mosaic of abrupt localizations, but as a complex pattern of overlapping and graded representations." PHILLIPS (1975) argued that (JACKSON's) famous statement that "the central nervous system knows nothing of muscles, it only knows movements" has so often been quoted without its essential qualification "to speak figuratively" that his real position has been all but universally misunderstood. He also proposed to lay down the question of muscle vs. movement because the answer does not solve the real problem of how the motor cortex controls movement. Although the question of whether the cortex thinks in terms of movements or muscles has been asked frequently (RUCH, 1965), this question did not exist in a true sense. It is obvious, especially after the establishment of neuron doctrine at the turn of the century (c. f. FULTON, 1949a), the real question concerning "muscle vs. movement" is how dense is the connection from a particular part of the motor cortex to a particular part of the spinal cord. The question then is whether there is a grouping of neurons in the cortex which have the same destination in the spinal cord. As stated explicitly by CHANG et al. (1947), there is an uneven distribution of corticospinal neurons in the motor cortex which are destined to a particular muscle.

Many questions may arise concerning the mode of projection from a particular part of the cortex to a particular motor nucleus, but one of the most important questions is the distribution of neurons within the motor cortex projecting to a given motor nucleus. There are many problems in answering the question. In the feline, the pyramidal tract does not make direct connection with motoneurons. In the primate, some pyramidal tract fibers make synapses with motoneurons, but still the majority terminate at interneurons (BRODAL, 1969). It is difficult to trace, anatomically, the course of projection beyond the synapse. Electrophysiological methods also have limitations. With the cortical surface stimulation, it is difficult to restrict the spread of current to within a limited area and still produce measurable effects. While stimulation on the surface can produce contraction of a single muscle (CHANG et al., 1947), a slight increase in the stimulating current recruits the contraction of other muscles. It is known that threshold current for evoking muscle contraction is higher than that for exciting corticospinal cells (HERN et al., 1962). It is also known that a given PT cell could be activated from over a wide area of the cortex (2.0 to 3.0 mm) with threshold currents of similar intensity (ASANUMA et al., 1976).

Under these technical limitations, it is practically impossible to determine, accurately, the distribution of PT neurons projecting to a particular motor nucleus. Furthermore, cortical surface stimulation produces not only direct, but also indirect (synaptic) activation of PT cells (PATTON and AMASSIAN, 1954). The spread of synaptic activation is rather difficult to delineate. The last problem, however, was solved by the effort of PHILLIPS and his collaborators (HERN et al., 1962) who found that monopolar surface anodal stimulation excites corticofugal neurons directly, but not synaptically. Utilizing this technique, LANDGREN et al. (1962), again, tried to solve the question. Instead of a motor nucleus, they chose a motoneuron representing the nucleus. Instead of measuring the lowest threshold areas to elicit EPSPs in a given motoneuron, threshold changes along the transcortical distances were measured and then the focal areas were calculated. They concluded that in about half the cases, the cortical neuron colonies projecting to a particular motoneuron could be confined within a narrow focus of 1 mm of the cortex, but in the rest of the cases, the colonies were more widespread, the largest example measured being 8×2.5 mm. Similar experiments were repeated by JANKOWSKA et al. (1975), in this case, simply measuring the low threshold areas on the surface. They could not find confined small foci and reported extensive overlap of low threshold areas for various motoneuron species. The results are in good accord with the repeated observation that with surface stimulation it is very difficult to produce solitary contractions of muscles. The results from surface stimulation, after 100 years effort, are thus inconclusive. They could be interpreted as supporting either a specific or a non-specific mode of projection from the motor cortex to the spinal cord, depending on the selection of the results from a vast number of experiments performed under various conditions.

Cortical depth stimulation

The technical difficulty in defining the localization of motor function is that the corticofugal neurons are located deep in the cortex whereas the stimulation was delivered on the surface of the cortex. This difficulty was partly overcome by stimulating the depth of the cortex directly through a microelectrode (ASANUMA et al., 1967, 1968). Utilizing this method, we found that the threshold current for eliciting cortical motor effects was far less than that required for the surface. Stimulation at around the threshold intensity commonly produced contraction of single muscles. Then low threshold points for a particular muscle were located within a small area of the motor cortex, i. e., the cortical efferent zone as shown in Figure 1B. At the edge of the efferent zone, the thresholds increased sharply (A) and the fringe overlapped with the fringes of other zones and the zones as a whole formed an overlapping mosaic within the motor cortex. Subsequent electroanatomical studies on the projection of PT cells to the spinal cord in the cat (SHINODA et al., 1976) and the monkey (SHINODA et al., 1978; ASANUMA et al., 1978) revealed further details. They demonstrated that although a considerable fraction of PT cells send branches to separate levels of the spinal cord, the majority send branches only to a limited area of the spinal cord (SHINODA et al., 1976, 1978). In the primate, each PT cell sends branches to various motor nuclei within a given area suggesting that a given PT cell synapses to motoneurons innervating various muscles (ASANUMA et al., 1978). However, in both species, a group of PT cells located close together in the cortex have a common target area in the spinal cord in addition to wide distribution of branches by their constituting member of PT cells. The organization of projection revealed by these studies suggest that corticofugal effects from a given area of the cortex (cortical efferent zone) appear most strongly in a small area in the spinal cord, most likely, in a particular motoneuron pool. In addition, the effects from the same area appear in various parts of the

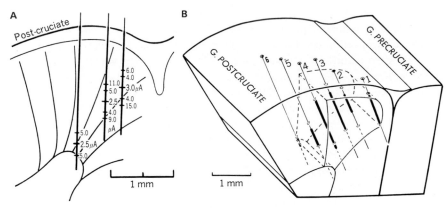

Fig. 1 Restricted small cortical areas which project to a given motoneuron pool—cortical efferent zones. *A*: Threshold changes along the microelectrode penetrations for facilitation of a particular monosynaptic reflex. *B*: An example of cortical efferent zones. Stimulation with a fixed intensity produced the effect only from the thickened part of the penetrations. These effective regions are confined in a small area within the motor cortex (Modified from Asanuma and Sakata, 1967).

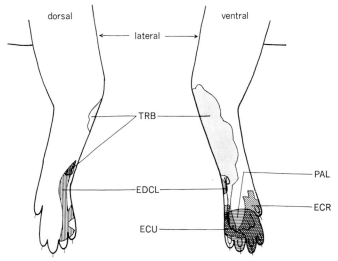

Fig. 2 Afferent inputs converging to the cortical efferent zones. Critical efferent zone which produce contraction of Extensor Carpi Radialis (wrist adductor) receives inputs from ventro-medial paw. Efferent zone for Extensor Digitorum Communis et Lateralis (wrist dorsiflexor) receives inputs from dorsal paw. Efferent zone for Extensor Carpi Ulnaris (wrist abductor) receives inputs from ventrolateral paw. Efferent zone for Palmaris (wrist ventroflexor) receives inputs from ventral paw. Efferent zone for Triceps Brachii (elbow extensor) receives inputs from lateral forearm (Modified from Asanuma et al., 1968).

spinal cord, the combination of which is not yet known. This organization may explain the difficulty of eliciting solitary contraction of muscles by surface stimulation.

Studies about the afferent inputs to the motor cortex (Asanuma et al., 1968; Rosén and Asanuma, 1972) have shown that these efferent zones receive peripheral inputs which are related to the contraction of muscle to which the zones project. A typical example of this relationship in the cat is shown in Figure 2. The results altogether revealed that there is a closed loop circuit between the cortical efferent zone and the periphery which, by itself, can circulate nerve impulses.

A natural question concerning this loop is what would be the function of this circuit?

This circuit may contribute to the tactile grasping reaction in which a tactile stimulus applied to the hand elicits persistent grasping of the manipulandum (DENNY-BROWN, 1965). On the other hand, the activity of this circuit seems to be suppressed, at least during the initial period, of another cortical reflex, i. e., the placing reaction (BARD, 1938). The typical initial movement of this reflex is withdrawal of the limb from the stimulus. We were puzzled by the complexity of these cortical reflexes especially in view of the existence of the cortico-peripheral loop circuit. If this loop plays an important role in such cortical reflexes, then the response should be a fixed movement depending on the site and the nature of the stimulus. It is already known that both placing and grasping reactions disappear after ablation of the sensory cortex. Therefore, we have asked a question of whether the cortico-peripheral loop involves the sensory cortex or not. If these peripheral inputs arrive from the thalamus directly to the motor cortex, then the cortico-peripheral loop is not directly involved in these cortical reflexes. Instead it could constitute a more basic and simpler cortical reflex pathway.

EXPERIMENTS WITH CATS

In this section, we want to summarize the results that we reported recently (ASANUMA et al., 1979 a, b; LARSEN and ASANUMA, 1979). Since it is already known that input-output organization of cortical efferent zones is similar in the cat (ASANUMA et al., 1968) and the monkey (ROSÉN and ASANUMA, 1972), we started the experiments using the cat. The motor cortex receives its major inputs from the nucleus ventralis lateralis (VL) of the thalamus, but neurons in VL do not receive somesthetic inputs from the periphery (MASSION and ALBE-FESSARD, 1965 a, b; ASANUMA et al., 1974). We first examined whether the VL is the only source of projection from the thalamus by injecting horseradish peroxidase (HRP) into the area of the motor cortex where the potentials evoked by stimulation of the superficial and deep radial nerves were the largest (LARSEN and ASANUMA, 1979). This area was consistently located lateral to the cruciate sulcus although there was a small variation of the location from animal to animal (OSCARSSON and ROSÉN, 1966). To avoid the spread of HRP to the white substance, a small amount (0.15 μl) of HRP solution (50 %) was divided into three parts and they were injected into three adjacent spots located within 1.0 mm of each other and all at the depth of 0.8 mm. As expected, the labeled cells were found most densely in VL, but in addition, cells located at the border area between VL and VPL were also labeled by the HRP. As shown in Figure 3, B and C, these cells formed a shell surrounding the rostral portion of VPL. However, the labeled cells were never found in the center of VPL.

It has been reported that the neurons in the rostral region of VPL receive inputs from the spino-cervical tract (LANDGREN et al., 1965). This tract carries somesthetic information arising from the periphery (MORIN, 1955; BROWN, 1973). Therefore, it became likely that neurons located at the border area between VL and VPL convey somesthetic information directly to the motor cortex. This possibility was examined in the following ways. The first was to identify projection neurons in the VL-VPL border area by antidromic activation from the motor cortex. For this purpose, several microelectrodes were implanted into the pericruciate cortex and intracortical microstimulation (ICMS) was delivered while inserting another microelectrode into the thalamus. The intensity of ICMS was weak enough so that the effect of stimulation current never spread in to the underlying white matter (cf. ASANUMA et al., 1976). Whenever a cell was activated antidromically, a microlesion was made to reconstruct the site of the neuron histologically. The distribution of thalamic neurons located in the VL-VPL border area and activated

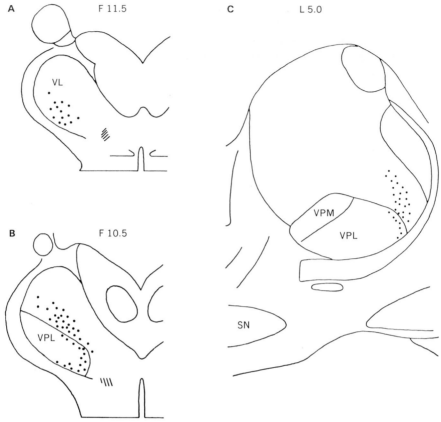

Fig. 3 Location of thalamic cells stained by horseradish peroxidase injected into the motor cortex. *A and B*: Frontal section. Cells in VL (A) and in border area between VL and PVL are stained by HRP. *C*: Distribution of stained cells in sagittal section. VL: n. ventralis lateralis; VPL: n. ventralis postero-lateralis; VPM: n. ventralis postero-medianus. (Modified from LARSEN and ASANUMA, 1979).

antidromically from the motor cortex was strikingly similar to the distribution of HRP-labeled cells shown in Figure 3. After identifying the antidromic nature of the spikes, the receptive field of each neuron was examined by naturally stimulating the periphery. As reported previously (ASANUMA et al., 1974), none of the neurons located in VL had clear receptive fields. Altogether, 32 neurons could be activated antidromically from the motor cortex and also from the periphery. Twelve of them responded to stimulation of small areas on the skin and twenty responded to stimulation of deep structures, such as passive movement of a joint or pressure to a particular area. These antidromically activated neurons were intermixed with other VPL neurons which received specific inputs from the periphery. As previously reported (POGGIO and MOUNTCASTLE, 1963), neurons with similar receptive fields were grouped together in a small area and the receptive fields shifted gradually as the electrode moved gradually. Figure 4 illustrates a typical example of the results. Four penetrations were made in this experiment and altogether 53 neurons were isolated from around the VL-VPL border area. Of these 53 neurons, 31 were driven by natural stimulation somewhere on the contralateral forelimb and the rest of the neurons could not be driven at all from the periphery. Of these 53 neurons, 3 could be activated antidromically from the motor cortex and are shown by arrows in Figure 4. All of these

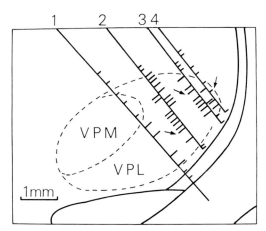

Fig. 4 Location of thalamic neurons activated antidromically by stimulation of the motor cortex (indicated by arrows). Numbers indicate electrode tracks. Short bars on the tracks indicate location of neurons which had no receptive fields in the periphery. Longer bars on the tracks show location of neurons activated by natural peripheral stimuli. Long bars on the left side of the tracks are cells driven by skin stimulation and right side are cells driven by stimulation of deep receptors. Further details are in the text (Modified from Asanuma et al., 1979).

3 neurons were located at the border area and 2 of them were activated by passive movement of the wrist and a digit respectively. The third neuron could not be driven from the periphery. The driven cells on track No. 2 appear to be located in the center of VPL, but this is because of the direction of the histological section. They were actually located at the medial border between VL and VPL.

EXPERIMENTS WITH MONKEYS

The results so far revealed that neurons in the border area between VL and VPL send somesthetic information arising from the periphery directly to the motor cortex in the cat. These results raised the possibility that the peripheral inputs observed in the primate motor cortex (ROSÉN and ASANUMA, 1972) also arrive directly from the thalamus. It is known that neurons in the n. ventralis posterolateralis pars oralis (VPLo) of the thalamus which is located caudal to the VL send axons directly to the motor cortex in the primate (STRICK, 1975), but it is not known whether cells in VPLo receive peripheral inputs. To examine whether these cells transfer peripheral inputs to the motor cortex, experiments were carried out using 6 rhesus monkeys (*Maccaca mulatta*). Aseptic operations were performed under a mixture of phencyclidine hydrochloride (1 mg/kg, Sernylan; Bio-ceutic Lab., Inc.) and pentobarbital sodium (25 mg/kg, Nembutal) anesthesia. Two closed chambers were installed on the skull, one directed toward VPLo of the thalamus and the other over the motor cortex. In addition, several bolts were attached to the skull to anchor the head-holders which restrained head movement. The experiments were carried out on the following 2 days. Each morning, 8 tungsten in pipette electrodes (STONEY et al., 1968), separated by 1.5 mm distances and aligned in 2 rows 1.5 mm apart, were implanted around the forelimb area of one of the motor cortices. While delivering intracortical microstimulation (ICMS) of 30 μa simultaneously or individually through each of the electrodes, a recording electrode was inserted into the VPLo area of the thalamus. Whenever the recording electrode picked up spikes responding to ICMS, the antidromic nature was ascertained as already described (ASANUMA et al., 1979b). Figure 5 shows typical

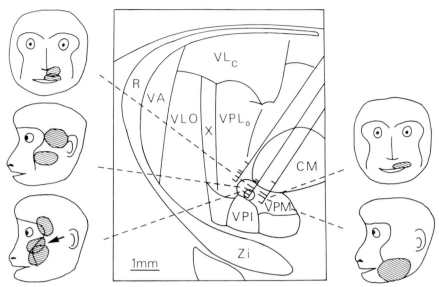

Fig. 5 Location of a thalamic neuron activated antidromically from the motor cortex (marked by a circle). Long and short bars on the tracks indicate driven and undriven cells from the periphery. All the cells driven had skin receptive fields on the contralateral face which are shown by respective figurines. Multiple receptive fields in single figurine means stimultaneous recordings from the same electrode. Arrow indicates receptive field of the cell activated from the motor cortex. VPM: n. ventralis posterior medialis; VPLo: n. ventralis posterior lateralis pars oralis; VPLc: n. ventralis posterior pars caudalis; CM: n. centralis medianus; VPI: n. ventralis posterior inferior.

examples.   Three penetrations were made into the area around the border between VPM and VPLo.   A total of 15 cells could be isolated in this area and 5 of them could be driven by light touch and/or hair bending of the contralateral face.   These driven cells were clustered in a small area and the receptive fields were also located in a similar area of the contralateral face.   It was a general observation that a group of cells located close together in this border region had similar receptive fields as in the case of neurons in VPL (POGGIO and MOUNTCASTLE, 1963).   Out of these 5 neurons, one neuron marked by an arrow (Fig. 5) could be activated antidromically from the motor cortex with a threshold strength of 20 μa.   A train of ICMS (15 pulses of 0.2 msec duration and 3.0 msec interval) delivered through the same electrode produced eyeblink at a threshold strength of 10 μa.

Altogether 35 neurons located around the VPLo area could be activated antidromically from the motor cortex, and after necessary examination, lesions were made at all the recording sites by passing negative currents of 10 μa for 10 sec.   Figure 6 summarizes the location of these lesions according to the map of OLSZEWSKI (1935).   Since the section was made sagittally, the nuclear boundaries defined by OLSZEWSKI were transferred from the original frontal planes to the corresponding sagittal planes by reconstructing three dimensional maps.   Because of the difficulty in defining the boundaries in actual slides, there are some uncertainties in the accuracy of the locations, but we believe the errors are not as great as to obscure the general configuration.   Out of 35 neurons activated from the motor cortex, 18 could also be driven by peripheral stimulation.   These driven cells were located at around the VPLo area as shown in Figure 6, although some of them were scat-tred in the neighboring areas.   Of these driven cells, the majority (14 cells) were driven by passive movement of finger, hand, elbow or shoulder joint, 2 responded to pressure to

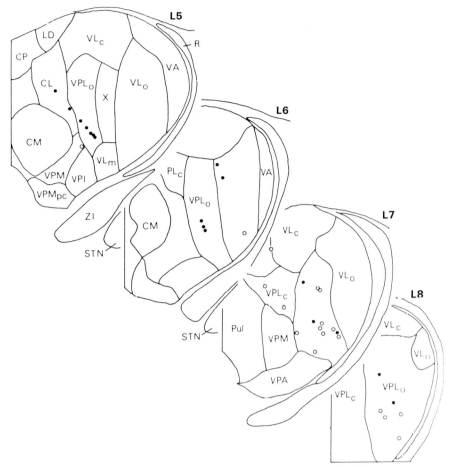

Fig. 6 Distribution of thalamic neurons activated antidromically from the motor cortex. Open circles are the locations of cells activated from both the motor cortex and the periphery. Filled circles are those which were not driven from the periphery. Abbreviations are the same as in Fig. 5.

deep structures and 2 were driven by light touch on non- or lightly-haired portion of the contralateral face.

The results so far demonstrate that there are, in the primate thalamus, neurons which transfer peripheral somesthetic information directly to the motor cortex, and they are located at around the VPLo area. A question still remains as to whether these direct inputs are playing an important role in determining the receptive fields of neurons in the motor cortex. It has been shown, by evoked potential studies, that the primate motor cortex receives peripheral inputs independently of the sensory cortex (MALIS et al., 1953; ROSÉN and ASANUMA, 1972). However, WIESENDANGER (1973), from his latency studies, concluded that somesthetic inputs to the motor cortex are transferred from the sensory cortex. If the latter is the case, then removal of the sensory cortex should abolish the receptive fields of neurons in the motor cortex. This has been examined in 2 monkeys by comparing the receptive fields of neurons in the motor cortex before and after the ablation of the sensory cortex. Figure 7 illustrates the results. Pairs of penetrations were made from the same surface points into the cortex before and after the sensory cortex removal.

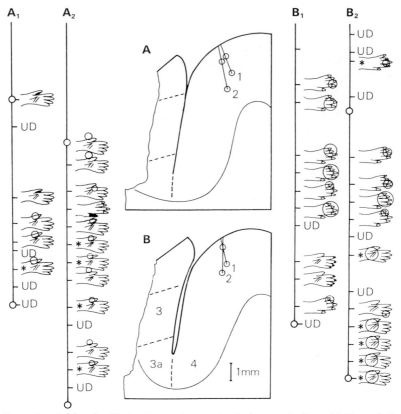

Fig. 7 Receptive fields of cells in the motor cortex before and after ablation of the sensory cortex. A_1 and B_1: Before ablation. A_2 and B_2: After ablation. The direction of the second penetration is different because of the distortion resulting from the ablation of the sensory cortex. Circles on the tracks show locations of lesions made during the penetrations. Circles on the figurines show locations of the joints, the passive movement of which activated the cells. Asterisks mean that these cells were driven by pressure to the respective joint area. Small blackened areas in A_1 and A_2 are receptive fields of respective skin cells. UD: undriven cells.

In A, penetrations were made into the thumb area and ICMS during both penetrations produced thumb movement with weak currents ($<10 \mu a$). Before the ablation, 5 neurons could be driven from the periphery during penetration No. 1. Two received inputs from the ventromedial surface of the thumb, 3 were driven by passive movement of the thumb. After ablation of the sensory cortex, cells responding to superficial stimuli were not found

Table 1 Afferent inputs to thumb and finger areas of the motor cortex before and after ablation of the sensory cortex.

Monkey	Skin cells	Deep cells	Undriven cells
No. 1			
Before	4	12	5
After	1	21	8
No. 2			
Before	2	3	2
After	3	8	12

except for the one in penetration A-2 which were driven by touch of the thumb but not as clearly as typical examples of this type.   Five neurons were driven by passive movement of the thumb and 5 other, marked by asterisks, were driven by pressure to the thumb in addition to passive movement.   Figure 7B shows another example of the results when the penetrations were made into finger area.   Table 1 summarizes the results obtained from 2 monkeys.   In both experiments, penetrations were made exclusively into the thumb and the finger areas.   In the second experiment, 3 cells were driven clearly by stimulation of the volar surface of thumb or finger after sensory cortex ablation.   However, in this case, the ablation was not as complete as the case shown in Figure 7.   The ablation removed areas 1, 2, 3 and 5 completely, but the major portion of 3a was not removed.

CONSIDERATIONS

It has been shown in the cat (ASANUMA et al., 1979b) that the receptive fields of neurons in the motor cortex do not change significantly after the removal of the sensory cortex suggesting that the major portion of peripheral somesthetic inputs to the motor cortex arrive directly from the thalamus and not through the sensory cortex.   The study with the monkey revealed similar results.   Neurons around VPLo received information about passive movement of a particular joint, light touch, pressure on a particular part of body surface or pressure to a joint.   These neurons send axons directly to the areas of the motor cortex where ICMS produced contraction of a muscle related to the peripheral inputs. Furthermore, it has been shown that the topographically organized peripheral inputs, especially the proprioceptive inputs, did not disappear after ablation of the sensory cortex. Although evidence is not as clear as the proprioceptive inputs (Table 1), there are suggestions that the exteroceptive inputs from the limb also arrive directly from the thalamus. In our sample of 18 VPLo neurons which sent axons to the motor cortex, none could be driven from the skin of the limb although two were activated by light touch to the contralateral face.   In one of the ablation experiments in which the sensory cortex was nearly totally removed, none could be driven by exteroceptive inputs after the ablation except for one which was rather unclearly driven by touch of the thumb.   In the other experiment, 3 cells were clearly driven touch of the thumb or finger after ablation of the sensory cortex, but in this case, area 3a was not removed.   Thus, a possibility still exists that exteroceptive inputs from the limb to the motor cortex arrvie through the sensory cortex. However, the possibility is small for the following reasons.   First, there were clear exteroceptive inputs from the face to the face area of the motor cortex.   Since the input-output relationship is the same between the limb area (ROSÉN and ASANUMA, 1972) and the face area (McGUINNESS and ALLMAN, 1977), the basic character of the pathways is likely to be the same.   Second, although we could not find clear skin inputs in one of the ablation experiments, it could be due to the scarcity of the skin inputs to the motor cortex even in the normal brain.   The exteroceptive inputs are seen only in the thumb and finger area of the cortex constituting only a small fraction of inputs to the motor cortex in primates. Third, although area 3a was left intact in one experiment in which skin cells were recorded after the ablation, it is unlikely that area 3a played an important role in transferring the finely grained exteroceptive inputs to the motor cortex because the main inputs to this area are from the muscle whereas the information from the skin goes primarily to areas 1, 2 and 3 (POWELL and MOUNTCASTLE, 1959).   Because of the technical limitation, only one or two cortical electrodes could be inserted into the thumb or finger zones in each experiment, and because the ICMS was limited to 30 μA to restrict the current spread to within a limited area (a radius of 200 μm; ASANUMA et al., 1976), the chance of finding thalamic neurons transferring skin inputs was limited in our trials.   We consider that the structure which constitues the basis of input-output relations in the motor cortex is similar in the cat and the monkey (ASANUMA, 1975).   In the cat, an abundance of thalamic neurons transfers skin inputs directly to the motor cortex (ASANUMA et al., 1979b).   From these, it is concluded that in the primate, as well as in the cat, the finely grained somesthetic inputs to neurons in the motor cortex arrive directly from the thalamus although we do not know whether these inputs also arrive through the sensory cortex.

A natural question then is what would be the functional significance of these inputs arriving independently of the sensory cortex?   It has previously been suggested that these cortico-peripheral loops may serve as a neuronal basis of the grasping reaction, especially of the instinctive grasping reaction (ROSÉN and ASANUMA, 1972).   However, since it is known that the grasping reaction disappears after ablation of the sensory cortex (DENNY-BROWN, 1965), it became clear that this direct loop circuit is not playing an important role in this reaction.   Another way of interpreting the function of this circuit is to assume that the direct inputs to the motor cortex serve as positive feedback information related to the cortically induced movements rather than to assume serving as a part of a particular reflex.   By circulating impulses through this loop circuit, it may be possible to increase the excitability of efferent and afferent relay nuclei in this circuit to prepare for the efficient adaptation of this loop to other inputs to the cortex to achieve purposeful movements. It is known that the motor cortex has multiple loop circuits with multiple sites of the central nervous system such as with various parts of the cerebral cortex, subcortical nuclei, the cerebellum, in addition to the direct loop with the periphery that we have described. It seems reasonable to think that the movement of the animal results from the interaction of the activities of these interwined loop circuits.   It is known that somesthetic inputs such as touch to the paw can produce movement of the animal (placing reaction), but only under particular circumstances, for example, when the animal is suspended in the air. Under normal circumstances such as when an animal is sitting quietly, the same tactile stimulation usually does not produce movements.   It is known that these tactile stimuli always produce discharges of cortical neurons including PT cells (ASANUMA et al., 1968; ROSÉN and ASANUMA, 1972).   Evidently, the tactile inputs to the motor cortex, by themselves, are not powerful enough to produce movement of the animal, but when other inputs, such as those related to the suspension in the air converge in the sensory and the motor cortices, then the same stimulus can produce a movement, i. e., the tactile placing reaction. The interaction of multiple loop circuits may result in a complex pattern of movements. For example, the initial movement of the tactile placing is the withdrawal of the limb from the source of stimulus.   This is the opposite direction of movement that can be predicted by the direct cortico-peripheral loop which is forwarding the limb toward the manipulandum.   It is highly likely that the activity of the direct loop which leads to forward movement is inhibited by the activity of other loops during the initial phase of the reaction. On the other hand, the activity of the same loop circuit seems to be enhanced during the initial phase of the tactile grasping reaction which is another representative of the cortical reflexes.   If we assume that the activity of the motor cortex is dependent on the interaction of multiple loop circuits, then the direct cortical loop circuit may be able to serve as an ideal indicator of the excitability of individual efferent zones because this circuit is not involved in the other loop circuits and still each loop is specific to each cortical efferent zone.

SHERRINGTON (1906) demonstrated the stretch reflex as the simplest loop circuit between the spinal cord and the periphery.   He also demonstrated that each loop is specific to the individual muscle (LIDDELL and SHERRINGTON, 1924).   LLOYD (1943) elaborated on the neuronal mechanisms of the stretch reflex and demonstrated that this reflex consists of the simplest network, i. e., the monosynaptic reflex. Needless to say, the discovery of the monosynaptic reflex made it possible to examine the excitability of a particular moto-neuron pool by conditioning this reflex with various stimuli and opened new fields in the study of the central nervous system. Based on the recent progress of the electrical tech-niques, we believe we have come to the stage that we can extrapolate this method to the study of the higher central nervous system.

SUMMARY

A question of whether the topographically organized peripheral inputs to neurons in the motor cortex are transferred from the sensory cortex or arrive directly from the thalamus was examined using slightly sedated monkeys. There were neurons which received somesthetic inputs from the periphery and projected to the motor cortex and they were located at VPLo area of the thalamus. They received localized proprioceptive as well as exteroceptive inputs similar to those received by the neurons in the motor cortex. Acute ablation of the sensory cortex did not abolish the peripheral receptive fields in neurons in the motor cortex. It is concluded that, at least, some of the afferent impulses which carry somesthetic information from the periphery arrive in the motor cortex directly from the thalamus and not through the sensory cortex. Functional significance of this direct pathway was discussed in relation to the known cortical reflexes.

ACKNOWLEDGEMENTS

The authors would like to express their gratitude to Ms. K. ALEXIEVA for her technica lassistance, Mrs. A. JEAN-MARIE for preparing for the experiments and Ms. N. MARMOR for her assistance in pre-paring the histology and the manuscript.

REFERENCES

ASANUMA, H.: Recent development in the study of the columnar arrangement of neurons within the motor cortex. *Physiol. Rev.*, *55*: 143–156 (1975)

ASANUMA, H., ARNOLD, A., ZARZECKI, P.: Further study on the excitation of pyramidal tract cells by intracortical microstimulation. *Exp. Brain Res.*, *26*: 443–461 (1976)

ASANUMA, H., FERNANDEZ, J., SCHEIBEL, M. E. and SCHEIBEL, A. B.: Characteristics of projections from the nucleus ventralis lateralis to the motor cortex in the cats: an anatomical and physiological study. *Exp. Brain Res.*, *20*; 315–330 (1974)

ASANUMA, H., JANKOWSKA, E., ZARZECKI, P., HONGO, T. and MARCUS, S.: Projection of individual pyramidal tract neurons to lumbar motoneuron pools of the monkey. *Exp. Brain Res.* (1978 in press)

ASANUMA, H., LARSEN, K. D. and ZARZECKI, P.: Peripheral input pathways projecting to the motor cortex in the cat. *Brain Res.* (1979a in press)

ASANUMA, H., LARSEN, K. D. and YUMIYA, H.: Somatosensory inputs from the thalamus to the motor cortex in the cat. *Brain Res.* (1979b in press)

ASANUMA, H. and SAKATA, H.: Functional organization of a cortical efferent system examined with focal depth stimulation in cats. *J. Neurophysiol.*, *30*: 35–54 (1967)

ASANUMA, H., STONEY, S. D. Jr. and ABZUG, C.: Relationship between afferent input and motor outflow in cat motorsensory cortex. *J. Neurophysiol.*, *31*: 670–681 (1968)

BARD, P.: Studies on the cortical representation of somatic sensibility. *Bull. New York Acad. Med.*, *14*: 585–607 (1938)

BRODAL, A.: *Neurological Anatomy in Relation to Clinical Medicine.* 2d edition, Oxford University Press, New York (1969)

BROWN, A. G.:   Ascending long spinal pathways: dorsal columns, spinocervical tract and spinotha-lamic tract.   *In* IGGO, A. (ed.):   *Handbook of Sensory Physiology*, Vol. II, Somatosensory System pp. 315–338, Springer Verlag, New York (1973)

CHANG, H.-T., RUCH, T. C. and WARD, A. A.:   Topographical representation of muscles in motor cortex of monkeys.   *J. Neurophysiol.*, *10*: 39–56 (1947)

DENNY-BROWN, D.:   *The Cerebral Control of Movement.*   Charles C Thomas, Spripgfield, Ill. (1966)

EVARTS, E. V.:   Representation of movements and muscles by pyramidal tract neurons of the pre-central motor cortex.   *In* PURPURA, D. P. and YAHR, M. D. (eds.):   Symposium on "Neurophy-sical Basis of Normal and Abnormal Motor Activities," pp. 215–251, Raven Press, New York (1967)

FRITSCH, G. and HITZIG, E.:   Über die elektrische Erregvarkeit des Grosshirns.   *Arch. Anat. Phy-siol. Wiss. Med.*, *37*: 300–332 (1870)

FULTON, J. F.:   *Physiology of the Nervous System*, 3d ed., Oxford University Press, New York (1949a)

FULTON, J. F.:   *Functional Localization in the Frontal Lobes and Cerebellum.*   Oxford University Press, Oxford (1949b)

HERN, J. E. C., LANDGREN, S., PHILLIPS, C. G. and PORTER, R.:   Selective excitation of corticofugal neurones by surface-anodal stimulation of the baboon's motor cortex.   *J. Physiol. (Lond.)*, *161*: 73–90 (1962)

JACKSON, J. H.:   Note on localization of convulsive seizure.   Med. Times and GAZETTE, 1868.   *In* TAYLOR, J. (ed.):   *Selected Writings of John Hughlings Jackson*, Vol. 1, pp. 38, Hodder and Stoughton Limited, London (993)

JACKSON, J. H.:   Observations on the localization of movements in the cerebral hemisphere, as re-vealed in cases of convulsion, chorea, and "aphasia".   *In* TAYLOR, J. (ed.):   *Selected Writing of John Hughling Jackson*, Vol. 1, pp. 37–76, Hodder and Stoughton Limited, London (1931)

JANKOWSKA, E., PADEL, Y. and TANAKA, R.:   Projections of pyramidal tract cells to α-motoneurons innervating hind-limb muscles in the monkey.   *J. Physiol. (Lond.)*, *249*: 637–669 (1975)

LANDGREN, S., NORDWALL, A. and WENGSTROM, C.:   The location of the thalamic relay in the spino-cervico-lemniscal path.   *Acta Physiol. Scand.*, *65*: 164–175 (1965)

LANDGREN, S., PHILLIPS, C. G. and PORTER, R.:   Cortical fields of origin of the monosynaptic pyr-amidal pathways to some alpha motoneurones of the baboon's hand and forearm.   *J. Physiol. (Lond.)*, *161*: 112–125 (1962)

LARSEN, K. D. and ASANUMA, H.:   Thalamic projections to the feline motor cortex studied with horseradish peroxidase.   *Brain Res.* (1979 in press)

LIDDELL, E. G. T. and SHERRINGTON, C. S.:   Reflexes in response to stretch (myotatic reflexes).   *Proc. R. Soc. Lond. (Biol.)*, *97*: 267–283 (1924)

LLOYD, D. P. C.:   Conduction and synaptic transmission in the reflex response to stretch in spinal cats.   *J. Neurophysiol.*, *6*: 317–326 (1943)

MALIS, L. I., PRIBRAM, K. H. and KRUGER, L.:   Action potentials in motor cortex evoked by peri-pheral nerve stimulation.   *J. Neurophysiol.*, *16*: 161–167 (1953)

MASSION, J. and ALBE-FESSARD, P. A.:   Activités évoquées chez le chat dans la région du nucleus ventralis lateralis par diverses stimulations sensorielles.   I. étude macrophysiologique.   *Electro-enceph. clin. Neurophysiol.*, *19*: 433–451 (1965a)

MASSION, J. and ALBE-FESSARD, P. A.:   Activités évoquées chez le chat dans la région du nucleus ventralis lateralis par diverses stimulations sensorielles.   II. étude microphysiologique.   *Electro-enceph. clin. Neurophysiol.*, *19*: 452–469 (1956b)

MC GUINNESS, E. and ALLMAN, J.:   Organization of the face area of motor cortex in macaque mon-keys.   *Soc. Neurosci. Abstr.*, *3*: 274 (1977)

MORIN, F.:   A new spinal pathway for cutaneous impulses.   *Amer. J. Physiol.*, *183*: 245–252 (1955)

OLSZEWSKI, J.:   *The Thalamus of the Macaca Mulatta.*   Karger, Basel (1952)

OSCARSSON, O. and ROSEN, I.:   Short-latency projections to the cat's cerebral cortex from skin and muscle afferents in the contralateral forelimb.   *J. Physiol.*, *182*: 164–184 (1966)

PATTON, H. D. and AMASSIAN, V. E.:   Single- and multiple-unit analysis of cortical stage of pyra-midal tract activation.   *J. Neurophysiol.*, *17*: 345–363 (1954)

PHILLIPS, C. G.:   Laying the ghost of 'muscles versus movements'.   *Can. J. Neurol. Sci.*, *2*: 209–218 (1975)

POGGIO, G. F. and MOUNTCASTLE, V. B.:   The functional properties of ventrobasal thalamic neurons studied in unanesthetized monkeys.   *J. Neurophysiol.*, *26*: 775–806 (1963)

POWELL, T. P. S., MOUNTCASTLE, V. B.: Some aspects of the functional organization of the cortex of the postcentral gyrus of the monkey: a correlatiop of findings obtained in a single unit analysis with cytoarchitecture. *Johns Hopk. Hosp. Bull.*, *105*: 133–162 (1959)

ROSÉN, I. and ASANUMA, H.: Peripheral afferent inputs to the forelimb area of the monkey motor cortex: input-output relations. *Exp. Brain Res.*, *14*: 257–273 (1972)

RUCH, T. C.: The cerebral cortex: its structure and motor function. *In* RUCH, T. C. and PATTON, H. D. (eds.): *Physiology and Biophysics*, pp. 252–273, Saunders, Philadelphia (1965)

SHERRINGTON, C.: *The Integrative Action of the Nervous System*, Yale University Press, New Haven (1906)

SHINODA, Y., ARNOLD, A. P. and ASANUMA, H.: Spinal branching of corticospinal axons in the cat. *Exp. Brain Res.*, *26*: 215–234 (1976)

SHINODA, Y., ZARZECKI, P. and ASANUMA, H.: Spinal branching of pyramidal tract neurons in the monkey. *Exp. Brain Res.*, (1978 in press)

STONEY, S. D. Jr., THOMPSON, W. D. and ASANUMA, H.: Excitation of pyramidal tract cells by intracortical microstimulation: effective extent of stimulating current. *J. Neurophysiol.*, *31*: 659–669 (1968)

STRICK, P. L.: Multiple source of thalamic input to the primate motor cortex. *Brain Res.*, *88*: 372–377 (1975)

WALSHE, F. M. R.: The mode of representation of movements in the motor cortex, with special reference to 'convulsions beginning unilaterally'. *Brain*, *66*: 104–139 (1943)

WIESENDANGER, M.: Input from muscle and cutaneous nerves of the hand and forearm to neurones of the precentral gyrus of baboons and monkeys. *J. Physiol.*, *228*: 203–219 (1973)

DISCUSSION PERIOD

AMASSIAN: Your very nice results remided me of the distinction WEINER and I made some time ago between the obligatorily polysynaptic projection from VP to PT neurons and the projection from VL-VA which could be either monosynaptic or polysnaptic. There are two points I would like to inquire about: First, in the cortical ablation you showed, you left S II behind. Now S II is a powerful activator of PT neurons and moreover, it is known from the work of SHARPLESS and TEITELBAUM that S II is important in the transfer of a learned tactile habit, that is, the pathway from S II to PT neurons is not just an electrophysiological curiosity. Secondly, removing completely Somatosensory area I in the cat is surely a little difficult because so much is buried in the banks of the coronal sulcus.

Some results of ours that are consistent with some of your findings include the demonstration that VP projects polysynaptically to PT neurons by at least two pathways; a long interneuron located, for example, posteriorly in S I and a short interneuron located anteriorly much closer to the VL projections to the large PT neurons.

ASANUMA: For the first question, what we were interested in were somatotopically organized finely grained receptive fields. And neurons in S2, although I haven't studied myself, but judging from the others' results, do not have finely grained somatotopically organized receptive fields which are the properties of S1 and 4γ neurons. Therefore, S2 is unlikely to be transferring the fine receptive fields to the motor cortex. Concerning the second question, it was very difficult to take all the coronal gyrus which is located in the depth. Therefore, the deep part was left intact. We don't know whether the part that was left contributed to the input to the motor cortex or not, but we think it's unlikely, because the blood supply to the depth comes from the surface and we sucked out the surface area. From this, we think that the possibility that this remnant of coronal gyrus contributed to the receptive fields in the motor cortex is small.

LAPORTE: Dr. ASANUMA, you mentioned that only Group 2 fibers did activate thalamic neurons...

ASANUMA: Yes. Group I inputs have already been studied extensively. First of all, evoked potential studies clearly show that the Group I fibers project primarily to 3a. Our analysis of sectioning the pathways also showed that the input from Group I to the motor cortex is indirect.

MASSION: Do the thalamic sensory cells projecting to motor cortex also project to the sensory cortex?

ASANUMA: That we don't know, but during our experiments, we never encountered a thalamic neuron which was activated from more than one cortical area in the motor cortex. All the cells were activated by stimulation of a particular part of the motor cortex. And, as I mentioned, stimulation of that area of the cortex frequently produced contraction of a muscle related to the receptive field of the thalamic neuron.

ROLE OF MOTOR CORTEX IN POSTURAL ADJUSTMENTS ASSOCIATED WITH MOVEMENT*

Jean MASSION

Départment de Neurophysiologie générale, I.N.P.-C.N.R.S.
Marseille, France

MOTOR CORTEX AND ADJUSTMENT OF POSTURE

Starting with the work of Sherrington (1947), Magnus (1924) and Rademaker (1931) in the first part of the century it has been demonstrated that decorticate dogs and cats are able to walk and run in a fairly normal fashion (Bard, 1933) and that most reactions which are involved in the regulation of posture persist in the decerebrate animal. As mentioned by Bard (1933), these observations have naturally created the impression that quadrupedal locomotion and posture depend only on the brain stem, cerebellum and spinal cord.

Nevertheless, there is no doubt that the posture and gait of decorticate animals are far from normal. As stressed by Bard (1933), Bard and Rioch (1937) and Villablanca and Marcus (1972), the positioning of the limbs is deficient, as is that of the head, whereas walking is often performed with an enlarged stance. Two important postural reactions, the placing and hopping reactions, are abolished or deeply depressed. Both are dependent on the integrity of sensorimotor cortex (Bard, 1933; Amassian et al., 1972; Villablanca et al., 1976). Other postural reactions are abolished after lesions of area 5, such as the facilitatory influence exerted by neck muscle afferents through propriospinal pathways (Lloyd, 1942) on lumbar motoneurones (Abrahams, 1970).

The fact that several postural reactions considered as elementary depend on the integrity of cortex was originally a matter of surprise (Bard, 1933) and the question was raised as to whether the cortex exerted a tonic function, which could gate the functioning of subcortical circuits responsible for the postural reaction or whether it was included in a phasic reflex responsible for limb positioning. Recent ontogenetic data suggest that placing is organized at the bulbospinal level (Hicks and D'Amato, 1970; Forssberg et al., 1974; Amassian et al., 1972; Amassian and Ross, 1978 a, b) and the possible role of the lateral reticular nucleus has been suggested (Corjava et al., 1977). These data seem to indicate that an important function of the cortex is in the gating of subcortical circuits although a more direct phasic component is also apparent.

Among the neocortical structures which intervene in the control of posture, the sensorimotor cortex plays an important role. Ablation of areas 4 and 6 in the cat produces several motor deficits on the contralateral side. After the cortical lesion, the contralateral limbs are extended when the animal is suspended. This effect depends mainly on lesioning the precruciate area (Adkins et al., 1971). Is limb extension due to a muscle hypotonia, resulting from a fusimotor depression comparable to the hypotonia observed after section of the pyramid (Wiesendanger, 1969; Gilman and Marco, 1971; Gilman et al., 1971), or is it a true extensor rigidity as noticed by Gilman et al. (1974) in monkey? Does the rigidity depend on the lesion being extended towards the supplementary motor area (see Gilman et al., 1974)? These questions are still under discussion. Besides contra-

* Part of this work was supported by contract n° A 659 7304 from INSERM.

lateral limb extension, sensorimotor cortical lesion produces an abolition of contralateral tactile and visual placing, a diminution of proprioceptive placing and hopping
(BARD, 1933; GLASSMAN, 1971, 1973). These postural defects are provoked by a cortical
lesion extending to area 4 and 6, but sparing entirely or almost entirely sensory cortex.
When lesion of SI is added, crossed placing, by which tactile stimulation of one side produces a placing of the contralateral limb also disappears (BARD, 1933; AMASSIAN et al.,
1972).

Several authors have inquired about the respective role of area 4 and 6 in postural
reflexes. A lesion restricted to area 4, including its postcruciate part provokes, besides
the loss of placing reflexes, a tendency of the contralateral forelimb to slide away on the
supporting surface when it is sliding (STEPIEN et al., 1960 a, b). This sign might be
considered as a deficit of the positive supporting reaction in that there is an inability to
adapt to the terrain. It has a tendency to disappear within a short time after a cortical
lesion. A lesion restricted to the medial part of the precruciate area, which includes
mainly area 6 does not produce specific postural defects in the limbs (BARD, 1933). Low
positioning of the head with respect to the body has been described by STEPIEN et al.
(1960 a, b) after bilateral medial precruciate lesion in the dog, whereas a difficulty to maintain the body axis in a given position has been proposed by ROSENKILDE and LAWICKA
(1977) as the mechanism implied in the deficit of time conditioning in the dog which
occurs after a lesion of interhemispherical part of area 6. The role of that part of area 6,
which corresponds to the supplementary motor area has been proposed as being important in postural control in monkey. According to WIESENDANGER et al. (1973), stimulation of that area produces complex synergies of proximal musculature whereas the motor
neglect on the contralateral side (PENFIELD and WELCH, 1951; LAPLANE et al., 1977)
might result from a defect of postural preparation to movement. There is, however, no
doubt that the supplementary motor area has a function which is not limited to simple
postural control, and KONORSKI (1967) mentioned among other troubles that more complex motor integrations such as learned motor sequences are abolished after lesion of that
area and perseverative behaviour is observed (see BRUTKOWSKI, 1965; JEANNEROD et al.,
1968) for extensive lesions.

To conclude, the role of motor cortex in postural control is far from negligeable in
quadrupeds. Area 4 intervenes mainly in the positioning of contralateral limbs as evidenced by the loss of placing and hopping reactions, and area 6 in positioning of head
and trunk.

MOTOR CORTEX AND POSTURAL ADJUSTMENT ASSOCIATED WITH MOVEMENT

Motor cortex is located at the departure of the main pathways which transmit to the
spinal cord the central messages which organize the movement (Fig. 1). According to a
generally accepted view (ALLEN and TSUKAHARA, 1974; BROOKS, 1975), the movement
plan originates at the level of the associative cortex, frontal or parietal. The motor program is elaborated within three different circuits joining the associative cortex to motor
cortex. One is represented by direct cortico-cortical connections, the two others are
indirect, relaying within the neocerebellum or within the basal ganglia. Execution of
movement is initiated from motor cortex, with various internal and external sources of
feedback taking part, together with cerebellum, in the motor performance.

A particular aspect of motor programming hitherto neglected is the postural adjustment
associated with movement i. e. the postural changes which permit the execution of move-

CENTRAL PROGRAM OF MOVEMENT   SUB PROGRAMS

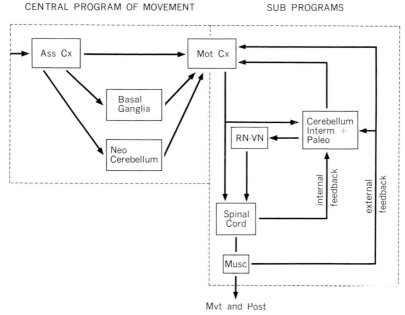

Mvt and Post

Fig. 1 General schema summarizing recent views on central programming of movement. Ass Cx: associative cortex, VN: vestibular nucleus, RN: magnocellular red nucleus (Modified from ALLEN and TSUKAHARA, 1974).

ment without the loss of equilibrium.   Is it part of the central program of movement, and organized on the way to motor cortex, or is it included within the various networks which may be recognized between motor cortex and periphery, or is it initiated at the level of motor cortex itself?

Postural adjustment associated with movement

Under conditions of stable posture, as for example during standing, the distribution of muscle tone keeps the center of gravity of the body within narrow limits.   Several categories of sensory signals are involved in the detection of displacements of the center of gravity and the readjustment of posture.   They are mainly labyrinthine, visual and proprioceptive signals (BROOKHART et al., 1965; BROOKHART and TALBOTT, 1974; NASHNER, 1976, 1977; DICHGANS et al., 1972; GURFINKEL et al., 1974; LESTIENNE et al., 1977; BERTHOZ, 1978).

When a movement is performed, an anticipatory adjustment of posture always takes place, as shown by BELENKIY et al. (1967) and ALEXEIEV and NAIDEL (1973) in man and by BROOKHART et al. (1965) and IOFFE and ANREYEV (1969) in quadrupeds.   The postural adjustment serves two purposes.   First it makes possible the displacement of a limb that was previously supporting a portion of the body weight.   The flexion of a leg while in the standing position needs, as a first step, that the part of the body weight supported by that leg be shifted towards the other leg.   A second reason why there is a need for associated postural adjustment is that each displacement of a body segment is in itself a source of disequilibrium, and an adjustment of posture is needed to maintain the center of gravity within limits compatible with equilibrium.   When the arm is raised forwards, for example, a backwards displacement of the body takes place, which compensates the disequilibrium which the movement would have produced.

Postural adjustments associated with movement have been studied in man by BELENKIY et al. (1967), GURFINKEL et al. (1974) and ALEXEIEV and NAIDEL (1973) and in quadrupeds by BROOKHART et al. (1965), IOFFE and ANDREIEV (1969), IOFFE (1975) and MASSION et al. (1975).   Several general properties of this type of adjustment have been determined.

It appears that, at least in man, the postural adjustment has an *anticipatory* character with respect to the movement with which it is associated, that is, it starts before the onset of the contraction of the muscles which initiate the movement.   Thus, for example, in the standing man, the contraction of biceps which provokes the flexion movement of the arm is preceded by 50–100 msec by the contraction of the contralateral triceps suralis of the leg.   The anticipatory character of the postural adjustment with respect to movement distinguishes this type of adjustment from the postural adjustment elicited by a sensory signal be it visual, proprioceptive or labyrinthine in nature.   The latter responses are reactional, that is, they appear as a consequence of disequilibrium.   There might even appear a temporary conflict between both types of adjustment.   The first type, which is associated with movement tends in a first step to shift the center of gravity before a disequilibrium produced by the movement occurs whereas the second type, elicited by sensory signals, tends to prevent a shift of the center of gravity.   The hypothesis may be put forward that in order to prevent such conflicts the central program of movement includes not only the triggering of the associated postural adjustment but also the temporary exclusion of the reactional postural adjustment.

A second feature of the associated postural adjustment is that its intensity is regulated through *peripheral indices* which might be the pressure on the footpad (GURFINKEL, personal communication).   Thus, the leg's postural adjustment associated with the movement of raising the arm is not present when there is no need for the adjustment as for example when the subject is lying down or when he is leaning against a wall.

The Postural adjustment in the standing cat

In order to study the role of the motor cortex in postural adjustment associated with movement, we have choosen an experimental model which permits the simultaneous analysis of both aspects of motor activity.   The standing quadruped is a particularly good preparation because the animal's weight is approximately equally distributed on four thrust points, the limbs, and every limb movement is necessarily accompanied by a redistribution of weight on the three other limbs by way of a postural adjustment.

In an experimental series made in the standing cat, (MASSION et al., 1975) we have measured the distribution of weight among the limbs, by placing each limb on a strain gauge equiped platform, which permitted the measurement of the weight supported by each limb (HAOUR et al., 1975).   The distribution of weights can be used to compute the projection of the position of the center of gravity on the horizontal plane.   It is generally located slightly frontalwards so that between 50 and 60 per cent of the animal's weight rests on the forelimbs.   A similar observation has been made in dogs by IOFFE and ANDREIEV (1969), and it may be hypothetized that the weight of the head is responsible for this asymmetry.

Under the condition of a stable posture (reinforced using operant procedures) we provoked placing movements of one or the other forelimb (Fig. 2) by means of mobile trays which could contact either limb.   The stimulated limb was pushed backwards by the tray before it performed the placing movement by which the paw came to rest on the moveable tray.   This form of placing reaction, which is of the proprioceptive type described by BARD (1933), is interesting because it is accompanied by an adjustment of posture.   In fact, one may distinguish two phases in this type of placing reaction, one during which adjustment of posture takes place (duration 200–300 msec), the other, the

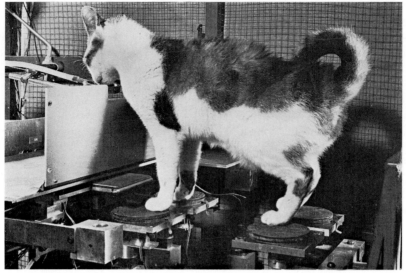

Fig. 2 Cat on the experimental device (for explanation see text).

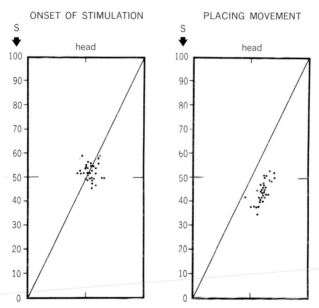

Fig. 3 Distribution of the calculated locations of the center of gravity in a grouped series of trials from one animal. The arrow indicates mechanical stimulation of the left forepaw. The corners of the rectangles represent the position of the animal's paws on the strain-gauge platforms. Each dot represents the center of gravity observed during one trial and is plotted in relation to the scale which indicates the percentage of the animal's weight supported by the forelimbs. The diagram at the left shows that the centers of gravity at stimulus onset were scattered evenly around a relatively central location. The rectangle on the right shows the locations of the calculated center of gravity at the instant the left (stimulated) forepaw was lifted from the platform. The projections of center of gravity were found at this moment to be within a triangular zone defined by the positions of the three weight-bearing limbs.

displacement phase, characterized by the placing movement itself along with the continuing postural adjustment.

During the pre-lift off phase, a change in the position of the center of gravity takes place. As seen in Figure 3, the projection of the center of gravity was sampled at the onset of stimulation (contact of the moving tray with the corresponding forelimb) and at lift off (beginning of placing movement).   At the onset of stimulation, the projection was situated near the center of the rectangle defined by the position of the limbs.   By the end of the pre-lift off phase, the projection of the center of gravity had shifted laterally with respect to the diagonal line joining the contralateral forelimb and the ipsilateral hindlimb.   The same lateral shift was observed for all cats.

Whereas, at the onset of stimulation, the animal's weight is about equally supported by the four limbs, a diagonal postural pattern is apparent at lift-off that is when the weight supported by the stimulated limb reaches zero, in such a way that approximately 90 per cent of the animal's weight is supported by two diagonally opposite limbs, the contralateral forelimb and the ipsilateral hindlimb (Fig. 4).

The first changes in weight which could be observed appear early after the contact of the moving tray with the limb (20–40 msec).   The earlier changes are noticed for most animals on the contralateral forelimb, where an increased weight is seen.   The postural adjustment is thus initiated before a decrease in weight of the limb to be moved is observed. The same anticipatory character of the postural reaction as described in man is thus apparent in the cat.   Other changes are an increased weight of the diagonally opposite hindlimb, whereas the weight on the two other diagonally opposite limbs, the stimulated

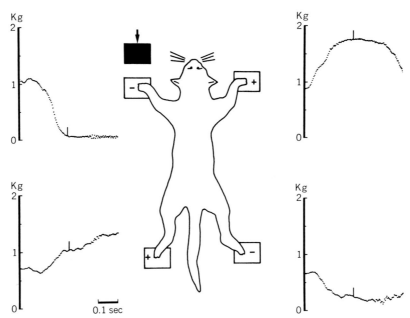

Fig. 4 Forces generated by each of the animal's limbs before and during the placing reaction on the left forepaw. The change in force for each limb is displayed to starting at the instant of mechanical contact of the mobile plate with the paw. This occurs at the intersection of the curve with the ordinate, scaled in kg. The moment of paw lift off for the stimulated forelimb is indicated by the fact that the weight of that limb has dropped down to zero. In this example, nearly 90 per cent of the animal's weight is supported by the diagonally opposed pair of limbs. For most animals studied, the postural reaction occured first in the contralateral forelimb. The (+) sign indicates an increase in weight; (−) denotes decrease in weight.

forelimb and the opposite hindlimb, starts to decrease. At the end of the pre-lift off phase, the animal's weight is thus not equally distributed on three supporting limbs, and a diagonally bipedal stance is apparent.

That the diagonal pattern is not the result of purely mechanical changes, but that active neural mechanism are involved is further indicated by the fact that myographic changes are observed during the changes in weight. During the increased thrust of the contra-lateral supporting limb, a myographic activation of triceps muscle is seen together with a moderate increased activity in biceps.   On the side of the placing limb, activation of biceps and triceps are first detected which are followed by a second activation in biceps and an inhibition in triceps, both occuring at the time of movement.

Furthermore, it was observed that each animal used its own pattern for reaching the diagonal supporting reaction. Individual patterns, indicated by the order in which weight changes for the various limbs were observed, could be noticed.   For example, one cat started changing the weight of both forelimbs, another started with a change in weight of the contralateral limbs earlier, another the contralateral forelimb, and so on. Interestingly, individual patterns were generally symmetrical for left and right placing. The result suggested that the postural adjustment resulted from a central program, triggered by the sensory stimulation, consisting of a diagonal postural support, common for all cats, reached through individual patterns, probably learned during the experi-mental sessions.

Role of motor cortex in associated postural adjustment

Unilateral ablation of motor cortex results in marked deficits in several reflexes involving limb positioning such as visual and tactile placing and hopping.   These effects are contra-lateral.

The placing movement performed in the standing animal under our experimental con-ditions is also markedly depressed after contralateral cortical lesion.   It is almost com-pletely abolished during the first post-operative week, and thereafter is slow and hyper-metric.

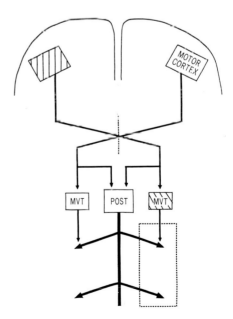

Fig. 5 Schema indicating the ways by which the motor cortex might control the associated postural adjustment. Dashed rectangle contra-lateral to hatched motor cortex (lesioned) sur-rounds the contralateral limbs. MVT: move-ments. POST: postural adjustment.

The diagonal postural adjustment associated with the placing movement begins during the pre-lift off phase of the reaction, and the bipedal stance is maintained during the displacement of the placing limb.   A first interesting question concerning the cortical control of the bipedal stance associated with the placing movement is whether the cortical lesion only affects the placing movement of the limb or whether it also depressed the isometric changes in weight of the four limbs during the pre-lift off phase which are coincident with the associated postural adjustment.   In other words does motor cortex control the contralateral movement alone or together with the postural changes associated with the movement (Fig. 5)?

In a previous experimental series (REGIS et al., 1976 a, b) cortical ablation was performed on cats but only the forelimb weight distribution was measured.   The results obtained indicated that the contralateral placing movement and its associated adjustment were altered.   A new experimental series was performed, with the measure of the weight of the four limbs.   Five cats underwent a cortical ablation.   On three cats, the lesions extended from the pericruciate cortex to the midline inwards, and to the coronal sulcus outwards, the lesion was limited backwards to the dimple and part of the depth of the cruciate sulcus was ablated.   For the two others cats the lesion was restricted to the pericruciate cortex, except for its medial third, whereas the depth of cruciate sulcus was not injured.

A first observation was that after motor cortical ablation, no clear change of projection of center of gravity was observed; the contralateral hypertonia, if it exists, does not result in a change in weight distribution.   The extended lesions abolished visual and tactile placing, and hopping was affected to a lesser extent.

During the placing reaction of the contralateral limb, not only is the placing movement slower and abnormal but also the postural adjustment is deeply depressed during the pre-lift off phase: the latency of change in weight is generally increased, especially for the stimulated limb.   Moreover, marked increase of the duration of the pre-lift off phase is observed, from 200–300 msec to 500–600 msec, which indicates a marked reduction of speed of weight changes in the limbs (Fig. 6).   However, the diagonal supporting pattern is maintained even if it is performed much slower.   The trouble observed persists permanently, though some improvement is observed.   Interestingly, with a more restricted cortical lesion, the same troubles of movement and of postural adjustment are noticed, but they are only transitory.

Unilateral ablation of motor cortex thus depresses the placing movement on the contralateral side, and the accompanying postural adjustment.   This result might be interpreted as indicating that the postural adjustment is controlled by motor cortex concurrently with the movement which it assists.   However, one might object to this interpretation that, in so far as a quantitative link exists between movement and accompanying postural adjustment, just the fact that a contralateral motor paresis exists might have as a consequence a parallel change in the postural adjustment, without the centers responsible for the postural adjustment being depressed.

The motor cortex might influence the postural adjustment in a second way.   One might propose that the result of a unilateral cortical lesion would be a deficit not only of movements involving contralateral limbs but also of the postural adjustments involving these limbs (Fig. 5).   The postural adjustment associated with a placing movement in the standing cat actually involves the four limbs and the diagonal postural pattern is distributed over both halves of the body.   If a motor cortical lesion produces a deficit in the postural adjustments of the contralateral limbs not only would contralateral placing movements be affected, but also ipsilateral placing movements when they require a postural support by the contralateral limbs, as is the case in the standing cat (Fig. 5).

CONTRALATERAL PLACING

BEFORE CORTICAL LESION

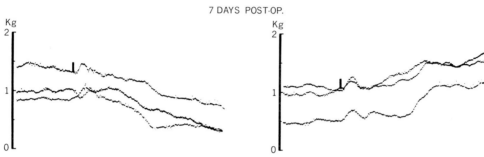

7 DAYS POST-OP.

30 DAYS POST-OP.

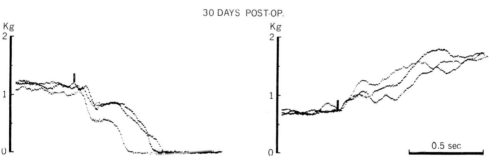

0.5 sec

Fig. 6 Weight changes recorded from both forelimbs during placing by the paw contralateral to the lesion. Three superimposed records are represented. The traces are taken before cortical lesion, seven days after cortical lesion, and 30 days after cortical lesion (small vertical bar indicates time of contact of moving platform with the limb). Notice the increase of the duration of the pre-lift off phase.

In order to check the possibility that cortical ablation influences the postural adjustment of contralateral limbs, an investigation was performed of the adjustment during a placing movement of the ipsilateral side, that is the side under the control of the intact cortex. The placing movement of the ipsilateral limb is entirely normal. The postural adjustment associated with it is similar to what it was before the lesion (Fig. 7). There is no difference in either the latency of the reaction or its amplitude or in its pattern. The adjustment of the limbs contralateral to the lesion is performed as well as that of ipsilateral limbs. These results strongly suggest that there is no specific control by motor cortex of the associated adjustment of contralateral limbs, and that the whole postural pattern depends on the performance of the movement which it assists.

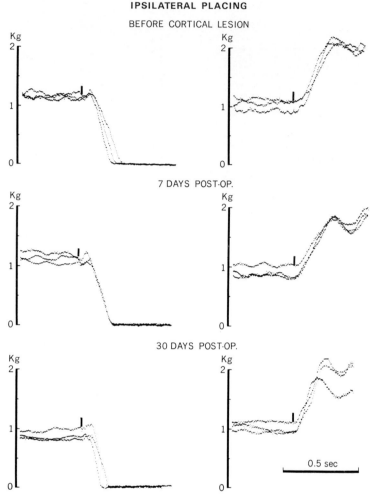

Fig. 7 Weight changes recorded during placement by paw ipsilateral to cortical lesion. As in figure 6, 3 records are superimposed for each time period. Note the lack of deficit of the postural adjustment associated with movement.

Tonic effect and/or phasic effect of motor cortex on postural adjustment associated with movement

The interpretation according to which the placing reaction is organized at a bulbospinal level, and depends on a tonic gating influence of cortical origin is tenable at the present time. In particular, in cat, the motor cortex appears not to be essential for contact placing during the first two postnatal weeks, suggesting the existence of independent subcortical circuits (AMASSIAN et al., 1972, 1978a, b). Recent results (CORJAVA et al., 1977) suggest that the lateral reticular nucleus of the medulla might play an important role not only in the performance of the placing reaction, probably in conjunction with the cerebellum, but also in postural adjustments which might be needed for the performance of the movement. It is thus probable that the effect of motor cortex on the placing movement and on associated postural adjustment might be partly explained by a tonic facilitatory action exerted on the bulbospinal circuits of the placing reaction and of the associated postural adjustment.

There is no doubt, however, that in the placing reaction as in numerous types of flexion movements of the limb, a phasic contribution of motor cortex takes place. Activation of ventrolateral thalamic cells, which are the main relay to motor cortex, and of motor cortical cells, during placing reaction has been described (AMASSIAN et al., 1972, 1978a, b; SMITH et al., 1978). One may thus raise the question of the action of the phasic descending messages, originating in motor cortex during the placing reaction. Do they participate only in the initiation of movement? Or do they also contribute to the postural adjustment? A first hypothesis would be that the descending impulses originating from the forelimb area would provoke only the flexion movement without associated postural adjustment (Fig. 8A). The adjustment would result from either a sensory input as a consequence of movement and/or an external stimulus, such as the moving platform, in the case of placing. A second hypothesis is that impulses from the forelimb area produce a feedforward postural adjustment together with the movement (Fig. 8 B). An interesting method for exploring the problem consists in stimulating the motor cortex topically in order to produce a contralateral flexion movement. In the standing cat, using the measurement of the weight distribution on the platforms, it is possible to see if a postural adjustment takes place and to study its timing with respect to movement.

Previous observations of TARNECKI (1962) indicated that stimulation of motor cortex which provokes a contralateral movement also produces a disequilibrium of the animal; comparable observations were made by WAGNER et al. (1967) and THOMAS (1971). This result was in favor of the hypothesis that the postural adjustment, if present, was late and could not compensate for the disequilibrium produced by limb flexion.

These results contrast with those of NIEOULLON and RISPAL-PADEL (1976). Using the method of stimulation through intracortically implanted electrodes, the authors noticed that moderate stimulation of a cortical site which provoked a contralateral forelimb flexion did not produce a disequilibrium of the cat. The same observation was made for the stimulation of a site which produced flexion of the contralateral hindlimb.

When stimulation of a cortical site corresponding to forelimb flexion is applied in the standing cat, the decreased weight exerted by the contralateral forelimb is accompanied by an increased weight exerted by the other forelimb. The latencies of increases and

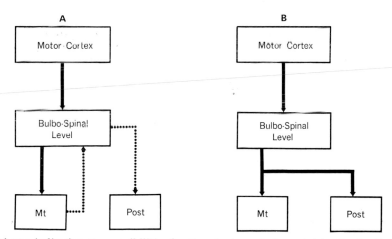

Fig. 8 Schema indicating two possibilities for the phasic control exerted by the forelimb motor area on the movement and on the associated postural adjustment. In A, the postural changes would be secondarily provoked by way of external feedback resulting from the performance of movement, in B, the postural changes would be commanded in a feedforward manner.

decreases in weight are approximately the same (REGIS et al., 1976 a).   This observation
makes improbable the hypothesis by which the increased weight would be secondarily
initiated by afferent signals resulting from flexion of the limb contralateral to the stimulated
cortex.   It suggests, on the contrary, that the weight increases associated with flexion of
the opposite limb are initiated centrally.   This interpretation has received a more precise
experimental support for contralateral hindlimb flexion movements elicited by cortical
stimulation (GAHERY and NIEOULLON, 1978; NIEOULLON and GAHERY, 1978).   Here,
the latency of weight decreases of the stimulated limb is clearly longer that those of the
other limbs.   The weight changes of the forelimbs, in the case of a hindlimb movement,
were preceded by changes in myographic activity of the forelimb triceps muscles which
were obviously initiated primarily by the cortical stimulation because they preceded any
apparent changes in weight distribution (Fig. 9).

It may thus be concluded that cortical stimulation induces a postural adjustment which
is initiated at the same time or even earlier than the movement.   The experiments of
GAHERY and NIEOULLON (1978), also indicated that cortical stimulation produces the same
diagonal supporting pattern as that which is observed during flexion movements of the
limb of other origin (IOFFE and ANDREIEV, 1969).   Thus, forelimb flexion produced by
stimulation of left motor cortex is accompanied by a diagonal support on left forelimb
and right hindlimb, with a moderately decreased thrust of the left hindlimb together with
flexion of the contralateral forelimb.   An interesting observation is that the effect produced
by cortical stimulation appears to be quantitative.   Contralateral decreased upthrust and
ipsilateral increased upthrust covary as a function of increased stimulation (REGIS et al.,
1976 a).

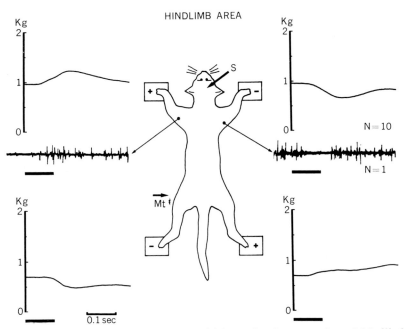

Fig. 9 Stimulation of a site in motor cortex which produced a contralateral hindlimb movement. The stimulus intensity (train of 200 c.s lasting 0.1 sec) was adjusted so that the paw did
not lift off the platform. The changes in weight exerted by each limb are shown besides the
corresponding limb. Myographic records of triceps muscles of both forelimbs are shown. Notice
that increased or decreased triceps activity preceeds the weight changes of the forelimbs. (Modified
from GAHERY and NIEOULLON, 1978).

The role of motor cortex in associated postural adjustment is thus not purely tonic, but it may also intervene in a phasic manner and initiate the postural changes associated with movement.

It is interesting to notice that stimulation of motor cortex is still effective in eliciting the contralateral movement and the associated postural adjustment after pyramidal tract section (NIEOULLON and GAHERY, 1978). Moreover, stimulation of the rubrospinal tract also initiates both the movement and associated postural changes even after ablation of motor cortex in the standing cat. The same occurs after stimulation of the superficial radial nerve which also produces an ipsilateral flexion accompanied by a postural adjustment (REGIS et al., 1976 a). Taken together, the results suggest that central or sensory stimulation always acts simultaneously on the network responsible for the movement and on the network at the origin of the postural adjustment. One explanation of this fact would be that the command pathways are by their wiring able to link the command of movement and the command of associated posture. A first observation of ABZUG et al. (1974) indicated that descending tracts such as vestibulospinal tract may have branching axons terminating at different spinal cord levels. The recent observation that the pyramidal tract fibers have branching axons which may end at distant spinal cord segments may serve as a morphological basis for the postural control of the different limbs (SHINODA et al., 1976). Similar observations were also made for the rubrospinal tract (SHINODA et al., 1977). Another possibility would be that the descending motor fibers act at the same segmental level both on the network for movement and on propriospinal pathways organizing the intersegmental postural adjustment. In this respect there are several examples in the litterature indicating that diagonally opposite limbs have a tendancy to be flexed or extended together (SHERRINGTON, 1947; ROBERTS, 1967). It is suggested by instrumental conditioning experiments. As noticed by DOBRZECKA (1975), conditioned flexion of a forclimb is more quickly acquired when the conditioning tactile stimulus is applied on the contralateral hindlimb. Extension of diagonally opposite limb is also apparent in behavioral situations such as trotting, where forward progression is realized by a succession of

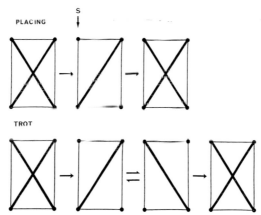

Fig. 10 This figure gives a comparison between the diagonal postural pattern used during placing reaction and during trotting.

In the upper part, the postural events accompanying the placing movement are represented. The postural support is equally distributed on four limbs before placing, then becomes predominantly diagonal during placing and finally returns to an equal distribution on the four limbs after the movement.

On the lower part, the succession of events appears to be comparable during trotting, except that alternate diagonal support recurs rhythmically as long as trotting takes place.

extension of diagonally opposite limbs (ROBERTS, 1967; GRILLNER, 1975). Postural adjustment associated with movement probably partly utilizes the propriospinal circuits which are used in locomotion (see GRILLNER, 1975) and the central command might act on these propriospinal circuits (Fig. 10).

CENTRAL CONTRIBUTION TO POSTURAL ADJUSTMENT ASSOCIATED WITH MOVEMENT

The question which was raised concerning the postural adjustments associated with movement is the level at which they are programmed. In particular, are they part of the central program of movement and does the motor cortex or the higher central structures actively participate in their organization, or are the postural adjustments a result of a subprogram whose circuitry lies between motor cortex and periphery?

The answer to that question is not a simple one because it depends on the type of associated postural adjustments which takes place.

Central contribution to the diagonal postural adjustment

The postural adjustment of the diagonal type, which accompanies the placing movement is one type of adjustment which serves to facilitate movements performed along the major body axis. Flexion movements and locomotion are other examples of movements using the same postural pattern. This type of adjustment is most probably organized at the bulbospinal level. It is controlled by a movement subprogram located downstream from motor cortex. There is no doubt that cerebellar assistance is important in the execution of the postural program. It was observed in two chronically cerebellectomized cats (REGIS et al., 1976b) that the postural adjustment associated with a placing movement was deeply depressed, much more than after motor cortical ablation. The role of the cerebellar loop in the performance of the postural program is indirectly illustrated by the fact that neurons of the red nucleus, which form one of the main relays from the cerebellum to the periphery, modulate their activity during the postural adjustment (PADEL and STEINBERG, 1978). The contribution of cerebellum, red nucleus and probably also vestibular nucleus to the postural adjustment can be compared to the role of the same structures in locomotion (ORLOVSKY, 1972a, b).

If the main contribution to the diagonal postural adjustment is made by the bulbospinal level and by the cerebellum, it appears that central structures located upstream such as motor cortex play a role in these adjustments.

The motor cortical contribution to the associated postural adjustment has three aspects.

First, the corticofugal impulses which command the movement, also command the postural program associated with it. Both effects are centrally linked.

Second, there is a contribution of the cerebello-cortical pathway not only to placing movements, as shown by AMASSIAN et al. (1972) but also to the associated postural adjustment. Units in ventrolateral nucleus projecting to motor cortex and receiving cerebellar inputs from interpositus and/or dentate nucleus were among activated cells when the contralateral limbs participate in the postural reaction (SMITH et al., 1978). It is interesting to notice that the cells participating in the central control of the postural adjustment are located within the lateral half of the nucleus, that is, the part which projects to the limb cortical area and not to the part influencing axial muscles.

Third, there is no doubt that an important function of motor cortex in postural adjustments is the inhibition of the postural reflexes which are in competition with the movement and its associated postural adjustment. The bipedal diagonal stance, which is adequate for movements performed when the animal is standing with the head in the axis of the body, may compete with many other postural reflexes as soon as the animal moves the head or performs, at the same time, another motor act. Motor cortex appears, together with pyramidal tract, as a key structure which permits the performance of the adequate postural support by inhibiting those reflexes which are contrary to the movement and its associated adjustment. There are, in the literature, two interesting demonstrations of this fact. First, STEPIEN and STEPIEN (1960a) have observed that after bilateral motor cortical ablation, dogs confuse both forelimbs when performing a conditioned placing of a forelimb. Before lesion, the dog was conditioned to always use the right paw to obtain food reward. After lesion, the dog used the left or right paw depending on the position of the head. When the dog had to turn the head to the left in order to reach the food tray, the right forelimb was placed whereas the left forelimb was used when the head was turned to the right. Neck reflexes determined the choice of the placing limb. One may infer from these observations that with intact cortex, the neck reflexes which would be contrary to the performance of movement are inhibited. Another interesting example has been shown by IOFFE (1973) who observed that after motor cortical lesion or after pyramidotomy the dog cannot combine two motor performances which consist in flexion of one forelimb and eating with the head near the ground (Fig. 11), whereas a combination of forclimb flexion

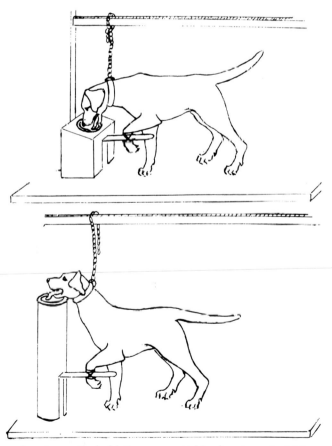

Fig. 11 Influence of motor cortical ablation on a combined motor act which consists in eating with the head down or in up right position and holding the left forepaw flexed. For further comments see text. (Modified from IOFFE, 1973)

and eating with the head in upright position is still possible.   There is a conflicting situation between the support in extension associated with the forelimb flexion movement and the support in a flexed position used for eating with the head down.   This conflict is normally resolved with intact motor cortex.

Central contribution to posture associated with complex movements

The diagonal postural pattern, which accompanies movements performed along the axis of the body is not adequate for many types of complex movements.   There is a need for dynamic changes of posture which concern not only the limb musculature but also the proximal and axial muscles.

Very little is known, at the present time, of the effective contribution of motor cortex, cerebellum and basal ganglia to the postural changes associated with complex movements. However, several theoretical and experimental considerations may be proposed which suggest the possible role of each structure in the postural changes.

Motor cortex with its topographical organization is able to influence distal, proximal, as well as axial muscles (WOOLSEY, 1958).   Distal and proximal musculature are under the control of area 4 through pyramidal and extrapyramidal pathways, whereas axial muscles are under the control of area 6 through extrapyramidal pathways (KUYPERS, 1964; ARMAND et al., 1974; PADEL et al., 1973; NIEOULLON and RISPAL-PADEL, 1976). There is thus, at the motor cortical level a tool which may be utilized for influencing the different parts of the musculature.   Besides the topographical organization, there is a more diffuse pattern of projection through the pyramidal tract along the rostrocaudal segments of the spinal cord (ASANUMA et al., 1978).   This second network of projection is not necessarily related to the command of muscular contraction which according to KOSTYUK and VASILENKO (1978) would depend on a specific path relay, but may be important in the control of networks implied in segmental and plurisegmental reflexes.   Interestingly, the shoulder and hip motor cortical areas are those which are the main sources of these more diffuse rostrocaudal projections (ARMAND et al., 1974; ARMAND and AURENTY, 1977).   That the area for proximal musculature is important for the performance of precise ballistic movements in space was illustrated by DUBROVSKY et al. (1974) who noticed that a cortical lesion within the shoulder area in the cat produces a difficulty in reaching for moving targets.

Motor cortex with its precise columnar organization may be utilized as a relay for the motor control exerted from cerebelum and basal ganglia.

That cerebellum and especially neocerebellum plays an important role in posture is strongly suggested by phylogenetic considerations.   The development of neocerebellum in primates might be explained by the increasing use of arm in space together with the progressive loss of the specific supporting function of the limb seen in quadrupeds.   The fact that no exaggeration of the tonic cervicolabyrinthine reflexes but only a neocerebellar hypotonia is observed after cerebellar ablation in primates, is explained by the decreasing contribution of paleocerebellum and the increasing contribution of the neocerebellum to posture (see MASSION, 1973).

Several sources of experimental evidence suggest that the cerebellocortical pathway is implicated not only in the organization of movement but also in the associated postural changes.   First, the dentate nucleus in the cats has a projection area upon motor cortex which corresponds mainly to areas for axial and proximal muscles (RISPAL-PADEL and LATREILLE, 1974).   These areas are of importance for the control of posture.   The same control on motor area for axial and proximal musculature is seen in monkey, where an important control on motor area for distal muscles is seen together with the appearance of the use of a prehensile hand (Sasaki, 1977).   The control of proximal and axial muscles in monkey may also be performed through the brainstem and descending pathways (Schultz et al., 1976).   Second, the cerebellocortical pathway at the unitary level is organized in such a way that a single cerebellar nuclear site influences preferentially a specific cortical site together with a very large projection onto various part of motor cortex through a diverging thalamocortical projection (Rispal-Padel et al., 1973; Asanuma et al., 1974; Asanuma and Hunsperger, 1975; Rispal-Padel and Grangetto, 1977). This type of organization would indicate that the command of precise movements might be organized by the cerebello-cortical pathway together with its accompanying postural support.   The neopostural function of the neocerebellum is also suggested by the fact that many cells in the dentate nucleus have increased activity during a sequential movement of the arm without being related to a specific part of the sequence (Robertson and Grimm, 1975).

Finally, the functions of the basal ganglia in postural adjustment associated with movement has also been put forward.   The fact that in Parkinsonian patients the postural support of movement is performed with difficulty, as for example initiation of walking, has been interpreted as indicating a specific role of these structures in postural adjustment (Martin, 1967).   Recently, evidence of postural deficit associated with caudate lesion was given by Olmstead et al. (1976).   It would thus appear that the same central structures which are important in central programming of movement are also important for central programming of associated posture.

ACKNOWLEDGEMENTS

The author is very much indebted to A. Polit who has criticized the manuscript and helped in its translation into English.

REFERENCES

Abrahams, V. C.: Cervico-lumbar reflex interactions involving a proprioceptive receiving area of the cerebral cortex.   J. Physiol. (Lond.), 209: 45–56 (1970)

Abzug, C., Maeda, M., Peterson, B. W. and Wilson, V. J.: Cervical branching of lumbar vestibulospinal axons.   J. Physiol. (Lond.) 243: 499–522 (1974)

Adkins, R. J., Cegnar, M. R. and Rafuse, D. D.: Differential effects of lesions of the anterior and posterior sigmoid gyri in cats.   Brain Res., 30: 411–414 (1971)

Alexeiev, M. A. and Naidel, A. V.: Rapports entre les éléments volontaires et posturaux d'un acte moteur chez l'homme.   Agressologie, 14-B: 9–16 (1973)

Allen, G. I. and Tsukahara, N.: Cerebro-cerebellar communication systems.   Physiol. Rev., 54: 957–1006 (1974)

Amassian, V. E. and Ross, R. J.: Developing role of sensorimotor cortex and PT neurons in contact placing in kittens.   J. Physiol. (Paris), 74: 165–184 (1978a)

Amassian, V. E. and Ross, R. J.: Electrophysiological correlates of the developing higher sensorimotor control system.   J. Physiol. (Paris), 74: 185–201 (1978b)

Amassian, V. E., Ross, R., Wertenbaker, C. and Weiner, H.: Cerebellothalamocortical interrelations in contact placing and other movements in cats.   In Frigyesi, T., Rinvik, E. and Yahr, M. D. (eds.): Corticothalamic Projections and Sensorimotor Activities. pp. 395–444, Raven Press, New York (1972)

Armand, J. and Aurenty, R.: Dual organization of motor corticospinal tract in the cat.   Neurosci. Lett., 6: 1–7 (1977)

Armand, J., Padel, Y. and Smith, A. M.: Somatotopic organization of the corticospinal tract in cat motor cortex.   Brain Res., 74: 209–227 (1974)

Asanuma, H., Fernadez, J., Scheibel, M. E. and Scheibel, A. B.: Characteristics of projections from the nucleus ventralis lateralis to the motor cortex in the cats: an anatomical and physiological study. *Exp. Brain Res.*, *20*: 315–331 (1974)

ASANUMA, H., HONGO, T., JANKOWSKA, E., MARCUS, S., SHINODA, Y. and ZARZECKI, P.: Pattern of projections of individual pyramidal tract neurons to the spinal cord of the monkey. *J. Physiol. (Paris)*, *74*: 235–236 (1978)

ASANUMA, H. and HUNSPERGER, R. W.: Functional significance of projection from the cerebellar nuclei to the motor cortex in the cat. *Brain Res.*, *98*: 73–92 (1975)

BARD, P.: Studies on the cerebral cortex. I. Localized control of placing and hoping reactions in the cat and their normal managment by small cortical remnants. *Arch. Neurol. Psychiat. Chicago*, *30*: 40–74 (1933)

BARD, P. and RIOCH, D. McK.: A study of four cats deprived of neocortex and additional portions of the forebrain. *Johns Hopkins Hosp. Bull.*, *60*: 73–147 (1937)

BELENKIY, V. E., GURFINKEL, V. S. and PALTSEV, E. I.: On elements of control of voluntary movements. *Biofizica (Rus.)*, *12*: 135–141 (1967)

BERTHOZ, A.: Rôle de la proprioception dans le contrôle de la posture et du geste. *In* HECAEN, H. et JEANNEROD, M. (eds.): *Du contrôle moteur à l'organisation du geste"*, pp. 187–225. Masson, Paris, (1978)

BROOKHART, J. M., PARMEGGIANI, W. A., PETERSEN, W. A. and STONE, S. A.: Postural stability in the dog. *Amer. J. Physiol.*, *208*: 1047–1057 (1965)

BROOKHART, J. M. and TALBOTT, R. E.: The postural response of normal dogs to sinusoidal displacement. *J. Physiol. (Lond.)*, *243*: 287–307 (1974)

BROOKS, V. B.: Roles of cerebellum and basal ganglia in initiation and control of movements. *Canad. J. Neurol. Sci.*, *2*: 265–277 (1975)

BRUTKOWSKI, S.: Functions of prefrontal cortex in animals. *Physiol. Rev.*, *45*: 721–746 (1960)

CORJAVA, N., GROFOVA, I., POMPEIANO, O. and WALBERG, F.: The lateral reticular nucleus in the cat. I. An experimental anatomical study of its spinal and supraspinal afferent connections. *Neuroscience*, *2*: 537–554 (1977)

DICHGANS, J., HELD, R., YOUNG, L. and BRANDT, T.: Moving visual scenes influence the apparent direction of gravity. *Science*, *178*: 1217–1219 (1972)

DOBRZECKA, C.: The effect of postural reflexes on the acquisition of the left foreleg-right foreleg differentiation in dogs. *Acta Neurobiol. Exp.*, *35*: 361–367 (1975)

DUBROVSKY, B., GARCIA-RILL, E. and SURKES, M. A.: Effects of discrete precruciate cortex lesions on motor behavior. *Brain Res.*, *82*: 328–333 (1974)

FORSSBERG, H., GRILLNER, S. and SJÖSTRÖM, A.: Tactile placing reactions in chronic spinal kittens. *Acta physiol. scand.*, *92*: 114–120 (1974)

GAHERY, Y. and NIEOULLON, A.: Postural and kinetic coordination following cortical stimuli which induce flexion movements in the cat's limbs. *Brain Res.*, *155*: 25–37 (1978)

GILMAN, S., LIEBERMAN, J. S. and MARCO, L. A.: Spinal mechanisms underlying the effects of unilateral ablation of areas 4 and 6 in monkeys. *Brain*, *97*: 49–64 (1974)

GILMAN, S. and MARCO, L. A.: Effects of medullary pyramidotomy in the monkey. I. Clinical and electromyographic abnormalities. *Brain*, *94*: 495–514 (1971)

GILMAN, S., MARCO, L. A. and EBEL, H. C.: Effects of medullary pyramidotomy in the monkey. II. Abnormalities of spindle afferent responses. *Brain*, *94*: 515–530 (1971)

GLASSMAN, R. B.: Discrimination of passively received kinesthetic stimuli following sensorimotor cortical ablations in cats. *Physiol. Behav.*, *7*: 239–243 (1971)

GLASSMAN, R. B.: Similar effects of infant and adult sensorimotor cortical lesions on cats' posture. *Brain Res.*, *63*: 103–110 (1973)

GRILLNER, S.: Locomotion in vertebrates: central mechanisms and reflex interaction. *Physiol. Rev.*, *55*: 247–304 (1975)

GURFINKEL, V. S., LIPSHITS, M. I. and POPOV, K. Y.: Is the stretch reflex the main mechanism in the system of regulation of the vertical posture of man? *Biophysics*, *19*: 744–748 (1974)

HAOUR, R., MASSARINO, R., MASSION, J. and SWETT, J. E.: A device used for study of postural reactions in the quadruped. *Electroencephal. clin. Neurophysiol.*, *40*: 427–431 (1976)

HICKS, S. P. and D'AMATO, C. J.: Motor-sensory and visual behavior after hemispherectomy in newborn and mature rats. *Exp. Neurol.*, *29*: 416–438 (1970)

IOFFE, M. E.: Pyramidal influences in establishment of new motor coordinations in dogs. *Physiol. Behav.*, *11*: 145–153 (1973)

IOFFE, M. E.: *Cortico-spinal Mechanisms of Instrumental Motor Reactions* (in Russian). Nauka, Moscow (1975)

IOFFE, M. E. and ANDREYEV, A. E.: Interextremities coordination in local motor conditioned reactions of dogs (in Russian), *Zh. Vyssh. nerv. Deyat. Pavlova*, *19*: 557–565 (1969)

JEANNEROD, M., KIYONO, S. and MOURET, J.: Effects des lésions frontalés bilaterales sur le comportement oculo-moteur chez le chat. *Vision Res.*, *8*: 575–583 (1968)

KONORSKI, J.: *Integrative Activity of the Brain. An Interdisciplinary Approach.* The University of Chicago Press, Chicago (1967)

KOSTYUK, P. G. and VASILENKO, D. A.: Propriospinal neurones as a relay system for transmission of cortico-spinal influences. *J. Physiol. (Paris)*, *74*: 247–250 (1978)

KUYPERS, H. G. J. M. (1964): The descending pathways to the spinal cord, their anatomy and function. In ECCLES, J. C. and SCHADÉ, J. P. (eds.): *Organization of the spinal cord, Vol. II. Progress in Brain Research.* pp. 178–202, Elsevier, Amsterdam, (1964)

LAPLANE, D., TALAIRACH, J., MEININGER, V., BANCAUD, J. and ORGOGOZO, J. M.: Clinical consequences of corticectomies involving the supplementary motor area in man. *J. Neurol. Sc.*, *34*: 301–314 (1977)

LESTIENNE, F., SOECHTING, J. and BERTHOZ, A.: Postural readjustments induced by linear motion of visual scenes. *Exp. Brain Res.*, *28*: 363–384 (1977)

LLOYD, D. P. C.: Mediation of descending long spinal reflex activity. *J. Neurophysiol.*, *5*: 435–458 (1942)

MAGNUS, R.: *Körperstellung*, Springer, Berlin (1924)

MARTIN, J. P.: *The Basal Ganglia and Posture.* Pitman, London (1967)

MASSION, J.: Intervention des voies cérébello-corticales et cortico-cérébelleuses dans l'orgaisation et la régulation du mouvement. *J. Physiol. (Paris)*, *67*: 117A–170A (1973)

NASHNER, L. M.: Adapting reflexes controlling the human posture. *Exp. Brain Res.*, *26*: 59–72 (1976)

NASHNER, L. M.: Fixed patterns of rapid postural responses among leg muscles during stance. *Exp. Brain Res.*, *30*: 13–24 (1977)

NIEOULLON, A. and GAHERY, Y.: Influence of pyramidotomy on limb flexion movements induced by cortical stimulation and on associated postural adjustment in the cat. *Brain Res.*, *155*: 39–52 (1978)

NIEOULLON, A. and RISPAL-PADEL, L.: Somatotopic localization in cat motor cortex. *Brain Res.*, *105*: 405–422 (1976)

OLMSTEAD, C. E., VILLABLANCA, J. R., MARCUS, R. J. and AVERY, D. L.: Effects of caudate nuclei or frontal cortex ablations in cats. IV. Bar pressing, maze learning, and performance. *Exp. Neurol.*, *53*: 670–693 (1976)

ORLOVSKY, G. N.: Activity of vestibulospinal neurons during locomotion. *Brain Res.*, *46*: 85–98 (1972a)

ORLOVSKY, G. N.: Activity of rubrospinal neurons during locomotion. *Brain Res.*, *46*: 99–112 (1972b)

PADEL, Y., SMITH, A. M. and ARMAND, J.: Topography of projections from the motor cortex to rubrospinal units in the cat. *Exp. Brain Res.*, *17*: 315–332 (1973)

PADEL, Y. and STEINBERG, R.: Red nucleus cell activity in awake cats in the course of placing reaction *J. Physiol. (Paris)*, *74*: 265–282 (1978)

PENFIELD, W. and WELCH, K.: The supplementary motor area of the cerebral cortex. *Arch. Neurol. Psychiat. (Chic.)*, *66*: 289–317 (1951)

RADEMAKER, G. G. J.: Das Stehen. Statische Reaktionen Gleichgewichtsreaktionen und Muskeltonus under besonderer Berücksichtigung ihres Verhaltens bei kleinhirnlosen Tieren. Springer, Berlin (1931)

REGIS, H., TROUCHE, E. and MASSION, J.: Movement and associated postural adjustment. In SHAHANI, M. (ed.): *The Motor System: Neurophysiology and Muscle Mechanisms.* pp. 349–361. Elsevier, Amsterdam, (1976a)

REGIS, H., TROUCHE, E. and MASSION, J.: Effect de l'ablation du cortex moteur ou du cervelet sur la coordination posturocinetique chez le chat. *Electroencephal. clin. Neurophysiol.*, *41*: 348–356 (1976b)

RISPAL-PADEL, L. and GRANGETTO, A.: The cerebello-thalamocortical pathway. Topographical investigation at the unitary level in the cat. *Exp. Brain Res.*, *28*: 101–123 (1977)

RISPAL-PADEL, L. and LATREILLE, J.: The organization of projections from the cerebellar nuclei to the contralateral motor cortex in the cat. *Exp. Brain Res.*, *19*: 36–60 (1974)

RISPAL-PADEL, L., MASSION, J. and GRANGETTO, A.: Relations between the ventrolateral thalamic nucleus and motor cortex and their possible role in the central organization of motor control. *Brain Res.*, *60*: 1–20 (1973)

ROBERTS, T. D. M.: *Neurophysiology of Postural Mechanisms.* Butterworths, London (1967)

ROBERTSON, L. T. and GRIMM, R. J.: Responses of primate dentate neurons to different trajectories of the limb. *Exp. Brain Res.*, *23*: 447–462 (1975)

ROSENKILDE, C. E. and LAWICKA, W.: Effects of medial and dorsal prefrontal ablations on a go left-go right time discrimination task in dogs. *Acta Neurobiol. Exp.*, *37*: 209–221 (1977)

SASAKI, K.: The cerebro-cerebellar interconnections. *Proceedings of the Internat. Union of Physiol. Sc.*, *12*: 619 (1977)

SCHULTZ, W., MONTGOMERY, E. B. and MARINO, R.: Stereotyped flexion of forelimb and hindlimb to microstimulation of dentate nucleus in cebus monkeys. *Brain Res.*, *107*: 151–155 (1976)

SHERRINGTON, Sir Charles: The *Integrative Action of the Nervous System*, 2nd ed. University Press, Cambridge (1947)

SHINODA, Y., ARNOLD, A. P. and ASANUMA, H.: Spinal branching of corticospinal axons in the cat. *Exp. Brain Res.*, *26*: 215–234 (1976)

SHINODA, Y., GHEZ, C. and ARNOLD, A.: Spinal branching of rubrospinal axons in the cat. *Exp. Brain Res.*, *30*: 203–218 (1977)

SMITH, A. M., MASSION, J., GAHERY, Y. and ROUMIEU, J.: Unitary activity of ventrolateral nucleus during a placing movement and an associated postural adjustment. *Brain Res.*, *151*: 329–346 (1978)

STEPIEN, I., STEPIEN, L. and KONORSKI, J.: The effects of bilateral lesions in the motor cortex on type II conditioned reflexes in dogs. *Acta biol. exp.*, *20*: 211–224 (1960a)

STEPIEN, I., STEPIEN, L. and KONORSKI, J.: The effects of bilateral lesions in the premotor cortex on type II conditioned reflexes in dogs. *Acta biol. exp.*, *20*: 225–242 (1960b)

TARNECKI, R.: The formation of instrumental conditioned reflexes by direct stimulation of sensorimotor cortex in cats. *Acta biol. exp.*, *22*: 35–45 (1962)

THOMAS, E.: Role of postural adjustments in conditioning of dogs with electrical stimulation of the motor cortex as the unconditioned stimulus. *J. Comp. Physiol. Psychol.*, *76*: 187–198 (1971)

VILLABLANCA, J. and MARCUS, R.: Sleep-wakefulness, EEG and behavioral studies of chronic cats without neocortex and striatum: the "diencephalic" cat. *Arch. ital. Biol.*, *110*: 348–382 (1972)

VILLABLANCA, J. R., MARCUS, R. J., OLMSTEAD, C. E. and AVERY, D. L.: Effects of caudate nuclei or frontal cortex ablations in cats: III. Recovery of limb placing reactions, including observations in hemispherectomized animals. *Exp. Neurol.*, *53*: 289–303 (1976)

WAGNER, A. R., THOMAS, E. and NORTON, T.: Conditioning with electrical stimulation of motor cortex: evidence of a possible source of motivation. *J. Comp. Physiol. Psychol.*, *64*: 191–199 (1967)

WIESENDANGER, M.: The pyramidal tract. Recent investigations on its morphology and function. *Ergebn. Physiolog.*, *61*: 73–136 (1969)

WIESENDANGER, M., SEGUIN, J. J. and KUNZLE, H.: The supplementary motor area. A control system for posture? *In* STEIN, R. B., PEARSON, K. B., SMITH, R. S. and REDFORD, J. B. (eds.): *Control of Posture and Locomotion.* pp. 331–346, Plenum Press, New York (1973)

WOOLSEY, C. N.: Organization of somatic sensory and motor areas of the cerebral cortex. *In* HARLOW, H. F. and WOOLSEY, C. N. (eds.): *Biological and Biochemical Basis of Behaviour.* pp. 63–81. University of Wisconsin Press, Madison (1958)

DISCUSSION PERIOD

CAREW: Have you tried to dissociate the postural component of the program from the reflex component, for example by loading the limb during the reflex or conversely, putting the animal under a more severe gravitational problem like tilting it, so that the postural adjustments get to be more challenging for the same small reflex movement?

MASSION: Limb loading experiments using 100 or 200 g have been performed recently by GAHÉRY and LEGALLET (1978). Under these conditions, the movement and the associated postural adjustment produced by motor cortical stimulation are still observable without marked changes for the loaded limb. In particular, the loaded limb shows the change in weight with the same latency as before and the peak change is reached after the same delay.

TEODORU: In your view, would the postural mechanisms operate in the same fashion if the supporting limbs or one of the moving limbs were deafferented?

MASSION: Of course, this would be an interesting experiment to do, but was not done in the present experimental seires.

NEAL MILLER: Did I understand you to say that if the movement was a rapid, ballistic one, you did not always get adequate postural compensation?

MASSION: The point I was discussing at the end of my topic concerned the adequacy of the primitive diagonal bipedal postural support used in locomotion and for various types of limb movement the animal may perform. I made the suggestion that this pattern would be convenient for certain movements performed in the same direction as the body axis but that it would not provide adequate support during others such as ballistic movements, projected in various directions in space. For these movements, a supplementary postural support is needed. I would suggest that neocerebellum and dentate nucleus should play an important role in the postural support required by this type of movement.

MILLER: The reason I ask this is because of some experiments on conditioning done by Earl THOMAS, a student at Yale, about 7 years ago. He found that when leg flexion was caused by stimulating the motor cortex of a dog, the dog would tend to fall over if there was no conditioned stimulus to serve as a warning signal. Whether it was the strength of stimulation, the placement of electrodes, or something else, the dog didn't make an adequate postural adjustment as a part of the pattern of response to the stimulation of the brain.

MASSION: The observation you mention is interesting. A comparable description of the effect of cortical stimulation was made by TARNECKI (1962), who also noticed that during a movement produced by stimulation of area 4, there was a tendency to fall. These observations are different from those made in my laboratory. Possibly, it might be a matter of stimulus intensity. We used chronically implanted intracortical electrodes which rest iet the stimulated area much more than surface electrodes. Another difference might be in the experimental procedure. The stimulation was always applied first with near threshold intensities before using higher intensities. We never tried an intense stimulation in a "naive" cat. It is not excluded that the link between the cortically induced movement and its associated postural support is built up by learning during the first near threshold stimulations applied to the cortex.

AMASSIAN: I wounder if the reaction which you so elegantly studied could be called proprioceptive correction because this does survive very extensive removal of sensorimotor cortex, somewhat more complete even than you've shown. There is one interesting difference. The cat's forepaw rests on its digits. When the wrist is bent, complete correction may not occur at the digits, but does occur at the wrist. Now, by contrast, we found that a red nuclear lesion had much more serious effects on proprioceptive correction, and your account of the effect of cerebellectomy in abolishing the form of placing you studied made me wonder if this reaction is mediated by nucleus interpositus driving the red nucleus. (Reference: AMASSIAN, V. E., ROSS, R., WERTENBAKER, C., and WEINER, H.: Cerebello-thalamo-cortical interrelations in contact placing and other movements in cats. *In* FRIGYESI, T., RINVIK, E. and YAHR M. D. (eds.), *Corticothalamic Projections and Sensorimotor Activities.* pp. 396–444, Raven Press, New York. 1972).

MASSION: There is no doubt that the red nucleus plays an important role in the reaction, both during the prelift off phase, during achievement of postural support, and during the late displacement phase, as recently shown by PADEL and STEINBERG (1978). Were you suggesting a proprioceptive origin of the reaction elicited in our animals?

AMASSIAN: Yes. Rather than, for example, the tactile placing reaction. Incidentally, your technique would provide a way of finding out of the gain of the proprioceptive correction is reduced by cerebral cortical lesions.

MASSION: The first time the animal receives the stimulation from the moving plate, he has a kind of startle reaction. After a few trials, the placing reaction occurs with its associated postural changes. In this case, the postural reaction starts before any marked change in limb position takes place and the reaction is initiated on the basis of tactile stimulation. By contrast, after motor-cortical ablation, there is a marked increase in the latency of the changes in weight, and one may propose as an explanation that the tactile cues are no longer effective and that proprioceptive cues are now the curcial ones. Thus, under normal conditions, the animal uses mainly tactile cues, whereas after cortical ablation, proprioceptive cues are required.

PETERSON: To what extent do you think the deficits following cortical lesions might be due to removal of a tonic facilitation of a reflex executed by a lower center, rather than to the removal of a reflex pathway including a cortical loop?

MASSION: I think that this is something which has been extensively studied, in particular by Dr. AMASSIAN, and he will probably discuss the matter in his presentation.

CORTICAL AND SUBCORTICAL INTEGRATION (2)

Chairman: Harry GRUNDFEST

THE CORTICO-SPINAL PATHWAY OF PRIMATES

Charles G. PHILLIPS

Department of Anatomy, University of Oxford
Oxford, England

A significant corticospinal pathway is the prerogative of those mammals which use their forelimbs as well as, or instead of, their muzzles for the functions of tactile exploration, prehension and manipulation of objects. The pathway is fairly well developed in cats, but is much more prominent in primates, and bulks largest in man. Other contributors to this Symposium have written of its cortical origin and of the inputs which excite or suppress the discharges of its corticospinal neurons. From the starting-point of this essay the view will be wholly caudalward. The corticospinal tract of primates will be arbitrarily wrenched from the complex networks of which it forms an integral part, and treated simply as a common path which leads from the forebrain and cerebellum to the spinal segments. A collaborative attempt to view it in its proper perspective has been made elsewhere (PHILLIPS and PORTER, 1977).

The Symposium in New York was held in honour of two men who have made major advances in our knowledge of this pathway, in the devising and application of powerful techniques and in fertile reasoning as well as in new discovery. LORENTE DE NÓ (1938) first perceived the radially-orientated circuitry of the neocortex which discharges its output through the large pyramidal neurons. In the sensorimotor cortex there are important populations of pyramidal neurons which send their long axons to the brainstem and spinal cord. The first unravelling of their distribution in the spinal segments was David LLOYD's (1941).

By the nineteen-thirties the tremendous impetus which had been given to the subject in the 1870's had largely spent itself. The discoveries of FRITSCH and HITZIG and FERRIER, though hailed at the time as a breakthrough in cerebral physiology, had amounted mainly to an electroanatomical demonstration of the existence of a localized area of motor outflow from the cerebral cortex (FRANÇOIS-FRANCK, 1887). It is noteworthy that they came before the practical possibility of accurate microscopical mapping of pathways by the tracing of Wallerian degeneration resulting from ablation of their cells of origin. True, WALLER had enunciated the principle twenty years earlier. 'It is really remarkable that WALLER, who was essentially a physiologist, and who lived at a time when histological technique was so defective that one was unable to make precise structural observations, was able to formulate... the true solution of the problem, orienting himself without difficulty in a puzzling field in which even distinguished modern scientists have lost their way' (RAMÓN Y CAJAL, 1928). So anterograde degeneration resulting from lesions of the excitable cortex could only be followed by FERRIER and YEO (1884) in monkeys, and by SHERRINGTON (1885) in dogs, by soaking the brainstem and cord in ammonium bichromate for a few weeks, or by staining with carmine. In one monkey, after 19 months' survival, the nerve fibres had almost entirely disappeared from the pyramid, 'their place being taken by connective tissue staining deeply with carmine'. The Marchi method for degenerating myelin was introduced in 1884. According to RAMÓN Y CAJAL (1909) it caught on slowly.   GUDDEN and VULPIAN made lesions of the excitable sigmoid gyri in dogs, and CHARCOT and DEJERINE examined the brains and cords of patients with cortical disease, and traced the course of degeneration of the thickest myelinated axons through the internal capsule, brainstem and spinal cord (DEJERINE, 1901).   But the method, though excellent for tracing the course of this relatively compact tract, could not reveal the existence of its more numerous unmyelinated axons, nor could it follow the unmyelinated terminals of the myelinated axons into the spinal grey matter.   In man, COLLIER and BUZZARD (1903) could follow degenerating fibres into the grey matter in only 2 out of 16 cases of hemiplegia, and then not into the ventral horns.   In chimpanzee, LEYTON and SHERRINGTON (1917) detected some Marchi degeneration in the ventral horn of the 7th and 8th cervical segments following excision of the contralateral cortical area 'yielding primary movements of thumb, index finger, wrist and elbow'.   They obtained more convincing results, however, by the 'Schafer combination of the Marchi and Kulschitzky methods; the minute blue-black ring surrounding the pale axis cylinder, which many of the very small fibres in the grey matter give by that method, when seen in cross-section, is altered to a minute blob containing no axis cylinder.   In other words, the fine collaterals are degenerated, and their sheaths, with that element of it which the haematoxylin stain after the mordant tinges deeply, is broken up, and the axis cylinder also; and this kind of minute degeneration is scattered widely and liberally through the ventral horn'.

Microanatomical methods were not to give a decisive confirmation for another forty years, until the Nauta method made it possible to stain degenerating axons as distinct from degenerating myelin sheaths (KUYPERS, 1960).   Silver staining of degenerating *boutons terminaux*, though capricious, can be seen in retrospect to have achieved a limited degree of success (HOFF and HOFF, 1934).   Meanwhile, the initiative was regained by electro-anatomy.   COOPER and DENNY-BROWN (1928) stimulated the cortex at different frequencies and made electromyographic and myographic records of the responses of muscles of the monkey's forelimb.   After a 'summation period' lasting a few seconds the motoneurones began to discharge in response to each stimulating pulse.   The 'true latent period', measured from the pulse to the corresponding primary wave in the EMG, was about 14 msec, but could be reduced to 9 msec by a 'light dose of strychnine'.   Of this time, 2.5 msec was due to peripheral conduction time, measured from a shock to the motor nerve to the onset of the EMG.   There was in those days no way of measuring the conduction time from cortex to spinal segment, and the value of the synaptic delay was unknown.   But the ability of the primary EMG waves to follow stimulus frequencies up to 180 Hz, taken together with LEYTON and SHERRINGTON's description of pyramidal collaterals ramifying among the anterior horn cells, led COOPER and DENNY-BROWN to the conclusion that there is 'a very simple synaptic relation between the pyramidal tract and the anterior horn cell'.   'A direct synaptic relation seems most likely'.   As important as the evidence of excitation was the abundant evidence of inhibition, seen sometimes as the earliest response to a train of stimuli: the slight tonic contraction of a muscle would relax and the background discharge of its motoneurones would be silenced.   When two antagonist muscles were examined simultaneously, there was usually reciprocal innervation, but sometimes co-contraction.   The central actions were not confused by reflex effects from the contracting and relaxing muscles, for the dorsal roots were cut in control experiments.   It has always been a supreme merit of electroanatomy that it reveals inhibitory as well as excitatory connexions.   But in the 1920's it could only do this by suppressing the discharge of already-firing motoneurones, or by preventing their firing by a testing excitatory stimulus.

Such was the state of knowledge at the time of publication of LLOYD's seminal paper, 'The Spinal Mechanism of the Pyramidal System in Cats' (1941).   The technical innovations and discoveries made by the people working at what was then called the Rocke-feller Institute have passed into our common heritage, and need now be recalled only briefly. LORENTE DE NÓ with motoneurones in the brain stem, and RENSHAW with those in the spinal cord, had obtained measurements of synaptic delay of less than one millisecond—essential information which COOPER and DENNY-BROWN had lacked. This had enabled LLOYD to make the crucial distinction between a fixed synaptic delay and variable nuclear delays. The discovery of the segmental monosynaptic reflex by RENSHAW had provided a test with which to measure the general level of excitability of motoneurone pools, allowing one to plot the time courses of excitation and inhibition which had been generated by prior conditioning inputs. LLOYD was soon to discover that the monosynaptic reflex originated from muscle receptors, so that the motoneurone pools could be tested by mono-synaptic Group Ia inputs from specific muscles. The pioneering use of microelectrodes permitted the recording and timing of conditioning and testing volleys in tracts of the central nervous system, and of the activities of interneurones synaptically excited and inhibited during the variable nuclear delays. Though this essay is about the corticospinal projection of primates, so much progress has depended, and will continue to depend, on the application of techniques and concepts derived from work on the cat that no excuse is needed for staying with that animal a little longer, though stopping well short of the most modern developments which LUNDBERG has reported to this Symposium.

LLOYD's (1941) corticospinal work was done too soon to make use of the Group Ia inputs from specific muscles for testing the actions of pyramidal volleys on the spinal mechanism. As was appropriate at the pioneering stage, the conditioning and testing inputs were of blunderbuss type, just as they had been in the experiments of the SHERRINGTON school in which large mixed nerve trunks had often been used for conditioning and testing volleys. The massive conditioning volleys were sent down the lateral corticospinal tract (LCST) from a stimulus site located rostral to a brainstem section which spared only the pyramids, and the testing volleys entered by the mixed population of large-calibre afferents in a dorsal root. The motoneurones discharging reflexly were recorded from the ventral root of the same segment, and were therefore not sorted out into those belonging to different muscle groups. A single corticospinal volley had no effect on the excitability of these mixed populations of motoneurones. LLOYD pointed out that the absence of such effect excludes any significant monosynaptic connection from the LCST. At least three volleys (at about 400 Hz) were needed to evoke detectable facilitation. Measured from the time of arrival of the earliest LCST impulses in the segment, the specific latency of the response to the third volley was about 2 msec. The increasing bombardment of the motoneurones was revealed by the curve of facilitation of the segmental monosynaptic reflex which reached its maximum in about 10 msec. Four, five or six LCST volleys acted on the motoneurones with a shorter specific latency for each successive volley. To evoke subliminal depolari-zation of motoneurones, the LCST volleys must actually *discharge* some interneurones. The shortening nuclear delays would therefore have signalled the discharges of interneurones lying nearer to the motoneurones along the chains which link them to the LCST. In other experiments the discharges of interneurones were recorded with microelectrodes. To fire any interneurones in the dorsal horn, at least three LCST volleys were required. Some interneurons in the intermediate region were 'driven' by volleys at 300 Hz, which would strongly suggest monosynaptic coupling to LCST axons. The background discharges of some other neurones were suppressed by LCST volleys. The overall picture is of response building up in the dorsal and intermediate region and then spreading ventrally to the motoneurones.

It is right to acclaim this paper as the conceptual and methodological starting point of all subsequent electroanatomical work on the spinal mechanism of the corticospinal projection, in monkeys as well as in cats. It was another 15 years before intracellular recording began to be used as a tool for teasing out complex integrative networks, as distinct from investigating the biophysical properties of neurones. Intracellular recording has never displaced monosynaptic testing for assessing excitability changes in whole pools of motoneurones. The mapping of the distribution of corticospinal excitation and inhibition to the motoneurone pools of the main muscle-groups of the fore- and hindlimbs of cats and primates was accomplished by this method (PRESTON, SHENDE and UEMURA, 1967). Extracellular recording has continued to be invaluable in recording the activities of interneurones. Interneurones remain more difficult than motoneurones for intracellular recording, but intracellular recording from motoneurones of identified muscles gives essential indirect information about the excitatory and inhibitory synaptic actions of pools of interneurones which converge upon them. Some of these belong to 'proprioceptive' networks: the Ia inhibitory interneurones, and the inhibitory and excitatory interneurones which are interposed in the Ib line from the Golgi tendon organs. Less is known about the specific interneuronal connexions of Group II muscle afferents and joint afferents. Other interneurones are exteroceptive, shared between cutaneous inputs and the LCST. The γ motoneurones have also been added to the picture. The actions of the LCST on these segmental networks in the lumbosacral cord of the cat were reviewed by LUNDBERG (1964). The exciting new work of the Gothenburg school on the networks which control the cats forelimb have been reported to this Symposium by LUNDBERG. The cat's hind-limbs are used to project its muzzle and forelimbs on to its prey, but it is the forelimbs which constitute the more direct menace to birds and mice.

In 1941 there had been no reason to think of the cat's pyramidal tract as anything other than a fairly simple and direct projection to purely motor targets. In Weigert material its cross-sectional appearance seemed as self-contained as that of a nerve-trunk. KUYPERS' (1958) pictures of longitudinal sections of the brainstem, stained by the Nauta method after cortical ablations, revealed for the first time the wealth of its collateral branching. ENDO, ARAKI and YAGI (1973) followed much of this branching electro-anatomically. And SHINODA, ARNOLD and ASANUMA (1976) have proved electroanatomi-cally that 30 per cent of the cat's CST neurones supply branches to the lumbar as well as to the cervical enlargement of the spinal cord. ASANUMA, SHINODA and ZARZECKI (1976) find similar branching in monkeys. We do not yet know to what combinations of how many targets a single CST neurone may project. But we do know that not all the targets are 'motor'. Apart from collaterals to basal ganglia, red nucleus, etc., there are presynaptic and postsynaptic connexions which would transmit corollary discharges to neurones of ascending systems, both somaesthetic and spinocerebellar. The relative preponderance of the different actions of these multiple collateral branchings, every one of which would be invaded by every impulse discharged by the CST neurone as required by the all-or-none law, could be varied only by changes in background excitation and inhibition imposed on the different target neurones by other inputs, peripheral or central. Without such independent controls, the different actions of the multiple anatomical linkages of the pyramidal axons would be indissoluble. One can imagine that some of the branchings of CST axons would be appropriate to certain patterns of movement but not to others, and that the post-synaptic actions of different collaterals would have to be selectively suppressed or enhanced during the course of complex movements. The branching of Group Ia axons to give monosynaptic excitation both to α motoneurones and to Ia-inhibitory interneurones, the latter being switchable by other inputs according to the need for reciprocal innervation or co-contraction (see below), furnishes a possible model.

In what follows we shall look at the results of some experiments on the spinal mechanism of the CST in primates, and finally at a few experiments on normal people and on patients with lesions of the brain, chosen because the continuing influence of LLOYD's work may be felt in them.

Very much less work has been done on primates than on cats. A *priori* it would seem probable that the elemental segmental networks are essentially similar in all limbed vertebrates, so that, after a few confirmatory tests in another species, one could justifiably proceed on the assumption of similarity with the cat unless and until some anomalous result turned up. An immediately obvious difference is the slower conduction velocity of Group I axons in monkeys and man: the higher velocities in cat may be peculiar to that species. Fortunately, however, there is a clear difference in electrical threshold between the Group I and the α motor axons in primates, in spite of the smaller difference in conduction velocity, so that selective electrical stimulation is possible.

But in investigations of descending control of the segments from the much bigger and more 'encephalized' brain, differences from the cat are only to be expected. These are most likely to be found in the distribution and actions of the much bigger CST. Other important descending pathways, which we are here choosing to ignore, would presumably continue to supply postural and righting signals from the vestibular and visual systems to the motoneurones of proximal and axial muscles, and to retain control of the prehensile use of the hands in climbing, even in monkeys in which pyramidotomy has permanently abolished the relatively independent movements of the fingers in tactile exploration and in the taking hold of objects (LAWRENCE and KUYPERS, 1968; LAWRENCE and HOPKINS, 1976) and in which the normal reactions of the hands to tactile stimulation have been permanently lost (DENNY-BROWN, 1966).

The monosynaptic cortico-motoneuronal component of the CST is an important taxonomic feature of primates (PHILLIPS, 1971). It gives to the forebrain and cerebellum, acting through the motor cortex, a preferential excitatory access to the α motoneurones which control the hand, and to a lesser extent the foot. Also present in primates (JANKOWSKA, PADEL and TANAKA, 1976), and absent from cats (HULTBORN, ILLERT and SANTINI, 1976b), is a monosynaptic connexion between the CST and the Ia-inhibitory interneurones which supply reciprocal inhibition to the α motoneurones of antagonist muscles. In the distribution of polysynaptic corticospinal excitation and inhibition to homologous muscle groups there is another important difference between cats and primates: PRESTON et al. (1967) found excitation of elbow flexors in cat, but inhibition in baboon. This difference they related to 'the transition from quadruped to biped posture'. They timed and quantified these polysynaptic actions of the CST by monosynaptic testing of the excitability of the motoneurone pools—in other words, by LLOYD's method.

Electroanatomical proof of monosynaptic excitation of α motoneurones by the CST was given first by timing of the earliest motoneurone discharge into a ventral root in relation to the time of arrival of the CST volley in the spinal segment (BERNHARD, BOHM and PETERSÉN, 1953); next, by monosynaptic testing (BERNHARD et al., 1953; PRESTON and WHITLOCK, 1960); and finally by intracellular recording from α motoneurones (PRESTON and WHITLOCK, 1961; LANDGREN, PHILLIPS and PORTER, 1962). Intracellular measurements showing its preferential distribution to the α motoneurones of distal forelimb muscles were published by PHILLIPS and PORTER (1964) and CLOUGH, KERNELL and PHILLIPS (1968). The enhancement by repetitive volleys of monosynaptic transmission by CST synapses was reported by LANDGREN et al. (1962) and PHILLIPS and PORTER (1964) and has since been analyzed in detail by PORTER (1970) and MUIR and PORTER (1973). The disynaptic inhibition from the CST was found, in monosynaptic testing, to be extremely sensitive to small doses of barbiturate (PRESTON and WHITLOCK, 1960), and the yield of intracellularly-recorded IPSPs was small (PRESTON and WHITLOCK, 1961). To reveal the common EPSP-IPSP sequence evoked by a pyramidal volley, it is often necessary to depolarize the motoneurone by passing current through the microelectrode: the IPSPs may otherwise be missed JANKOWSKA, PADEL and TANAKA, 1976).

Strong evidence that the disynaptic inhibition of α motoneurones is due to monosynaptic excitation of Ia inhibitory interneurones by the CST comes from the experiments of JANKOWSKA and TANAKA (1974) and JANKOWSKA, PADEL and TANAKA (1976). The first step was to impale an α motoneurone and identify it antidromically. The next was to send in a Group Ia volley from an antagonist muscle group and also a CST volley, timed to arrive simultaneously in the same segment (Fig. 1). The strength of each volley was adjusted to produce a minimal IPSP in the motoneurone. Together they evoked a larger IPSP. This would have been due to spatial facilitation in a common pool of inhibitory interneurones, resulting in a larger number projecting their inhibitory discharges on to the motoneurone. Another test strengthened the identification of these inhibitory inter-neurones with the Ia-inhibitory interneurones: in the cat, the Ia interneurones are the only interneurones which receive the characteristic combination of (1) excitation from the Ia in-put from muscles antagonistic to the motoneurones they inhibit, with (2) inhibition from Renshaw cells belonging to the antagonists (R, Fig. 1). Assuming this to be the arrangement in monkeys, the equal effectiveness of an antidromic ventral root volley in suppress-ing the Ia IPSP and the CST-IPSP in the test motoneurone supports the identification the inhibitory interneurones as Ia-inhibitory interneurones. It is essential that the test motoneurone should itself receive no recurrent (Renshaw) inhibition from the antidromic ventral root volley to complicate the issue. Conveniently for this experiment, not all motoneurones in a pool are inhibited by Renshaw cells, as indicated by the dotted lines in Figure 1.

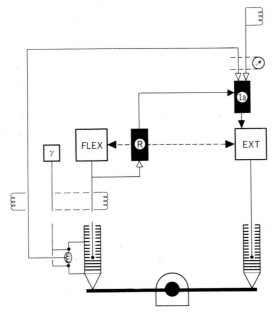

Fig. 1 Convergence of Group Ia and CST volleys on a pool of Ia-inhibitory interneurones in monkeys. Identification of Ia-inhibitory interneurones by action of Renshaw cells upon them (see text). Open arrowheads: excitation; Filled arrowhead; inhibition, in this and subsequent figures.

Figure 2 summarizes the elemental electroanatomical data. The only datum additional to those already presented is the mutual inhibitory interaction between the antagonistic pools of Ia-inhibitory interneurones, newly discovered in the cat by HULTBORN, ILLERT and SANTINI (1976a). No connexions are shown for the Group Ib and Group II inputs. The diagram has functional implications which are now being widely invoked in discussions of motor control. If the brain co-activates the α and γ motoneurones, e.g. of flexors in Figure 2, in initiating a movement (Granit's '$\alpha\gamma$ linkage') the spindle primaries (and secondaries) could continue to discharge throughout the movement instead of being silenced by the shortening of the prime mover muscles, and could provide servoassistance if the moving part encountered an external load which had not been predicted by the motor programme (MATTHEWS, 1972). HONGO, JANKOWSKA and LUNDBERG (1969) have proposed, further, that the operation of $\alpha\gamma$ linkage extends to reciprocal inhibition. The

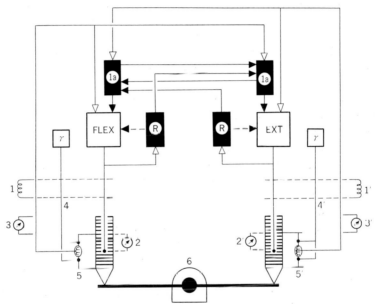

Fig. 2 Elemental components of segmental control networks which are available to exteroceptive reflexes and to commands descending from the brain. Their existence is well established in cat, confirmed at points so far tested in primates, and assumed provisionally for man. Diagram shows pools of α and γ motoneurones of flexor and extensor muscles and their associated pools of Renshaw cells and Ia-inhibitory interneurones. The monosynaptic Group Ia excitatory input from primary endings of muscle spindles is shown. The disynaptic excitatory input carried by Group II axons from secondary endings (LUNDBERG, MALMGREN and SCHOMBURG, 1975, 1977) and the di- and trisynaptic inhibitory inputs from Golgi tendon organs carried by Group Ib axons are omitted. The mechanical linkage is to indicate that muscles cannot shorten without lengthening their antagonists.

In human studies the system can be probed at the following points, either at rest or during reflex or voluntary movement:

1,1': Electrical stimulation of muscle nerves. It is possible, in healthy volunteers, to record the resulting afferent volleys by needle electrodes in the vicinity of the dorsal roots (MAGLADERY, PORTER, PARK and TEASDALL, 1951; INOUYE and BUCHTHAL, 1977).

2,2': Recording of reflex volleys (H-reflexes) and unitary and integrated EMGs.

3,3': Recording from single Group Ia axons in muscle nerves in healthy volunteers (HAGBARTH and VALLBO, 1969).

4,4': Blockage of fusimotor axons by injection of local anaesthetics or alcohol.

5,5': Selective excitation of primary endings of muscle spindles by percutaneous vibration of tendons.

6: Mechanical recording of isometric force, isotonic acceleration and deceleration, etc.

fusimotor-sustained discharge would not only help to drive the α motoneurones of the prime mover but would also drive the Ia-inhibitory interneurones to its antagonist, as shown in Figure 2.   Those Ia-inhibitory interneurones can also be driven by the brain. The functionally related fusimotor neurones, α motoneurones and Ia-inhibitory interneurones could thus be driven as a quasi-unitary effector apparatus by the CST.

All this can be readily applied to the case of muscles which act across a single hinge joint and are always in an uncomplicated antagonistic relationship to one another when the joint is moving.   But if the muscles are to be able to co-contract in fixation of the joint, there must be some way of switching off the reciprocal interconnexions.   In the cat, Renshaw cells can inhibit Ia interneurones, and are under supraspinal control; antagonistic Ia-inhibitory interneurones can mutually inhibit one another; and intracellular records from Ia-inhibitory interneurones have revealed that activation of the CST usually evokes a mixture of (polysynaptic) excitation and inhibition (HULTBORN et al., 1976b).   If the inhibitory CST connexions can be activated separately during motor performance, possibly in association with cortical excitation of Renshaw cells of the class which inhibits Ia-inhibitory interneurones but does not inhibit α motoneurones, there would seem to be ample provision for co-contraction of antagonists.   Greater complication must arise in the case of groups of muscles acting across more than one joint, and where joints have more than one degree of freedom.   Examples are to be found in plenty in the classic monographs of DUCHENNE (1867) and BEEVOR (1904).   BERNSTEIN (1967) remarks: 'The concept of antagonism may be applied unconditionally only to cases of muscles operating on joints with a single axis and, further, to those which cross only this one joint.   The number of muscles of this type is extremely small......   All other muscles may be only functionally antagonistic in a single situation and in quite different relationships in other situations'. Supraspinal and reflex control of the Ia-inhibitory apparatus must be powerful and flexible enough to cope with the continuously-varying relationships between different muscle groups in the course of a complex flowing sequence of movement.   In finger movements, in which the antagonistic action of gravity is unimportant, there is usually some degree of co-contraction—the moderating action of DUCHENNE (LONG and BROWN, 1964).

The cat's Ia-inhibitory interneurones are foci of convergence from several central and peripheral sources (LUNDBERG, 1975), and might therefore be expected to be able to provide a wide range of control, extending from absolute reciprocal innervation at one end of the scale to uninhibited co-contraction at the other.   An observation of MARSDEN, ROTHWELL and TRAUB (1978) is interesting in relation to the possible action of inputs to Ia-inhibitory interneurones from the skin.   The effect of cutaneous anaesthesia on voluntary flexion of the distal joint of the human thumb was to add some co-contraction of the antagonist, extensor pollicis longus.   Since, in the cat, low-threshold cutaneous afferents excite the Ia-inhibitory interneurones (FEDINA and HULTBORN, 1972), the effect of cutaneous anaesthesia might be to disfacilitate these interneurones and thus to reduce the level of reciprocal inhibition.

If the distribution of monosynaptic excitation to α motoneurones and to Ia-inhibitory interneurones is by branching of the same Ia axons, we have here, as remarked above, a possible model for the dissociation of the post-synaptic actions of collateral branches of pyramidal axons, despite their all-or-none invasion by every impulse.

The diagram of Figure 2 may be provisionally assumed to be valid for man; the connexions of the CST to fusimotor neurones (GRIGG and PRESTON, 1971; CLOUGH, PHILLIPS and SHERIDAN, 1971), α motoneurones and Ia-inhibitory interneurones may be assumed to be at least as well developed in man as in monkeys, and to be best developed in relation to the hand.   The diagram, with its functional implications, is already being found useful in the planning and interpretation of studies of normal people and of patients with brain lesions. The points at which the networks are being probed are indicated in Figure 2 and its legend. An idea of the large and growing volume of human work now coming forward can be gained from two recent series of books (DESMEDT, 1973, 1977). Here there is space only to cite a few illustrative examples. The first must be the demonstration in normal people that $\alpha\gamma$ coactivation is a fact (VALLBO, 1970, 1973). During voluntary flexion of a finger, whether isotonic or isometric, the discharge of the α motoneurones of the prime mover is accompanied by discharge of its muscle spindles. Since the spindles of the shortening muscle would otherwise be silenced, this is proof of parallel excitation of fusimotor neurones. And since the necessary connexions exist in monkeys, it seems probable that this coactivation of α and γ motoneurones can be effected by the CST in man.

We need to be able to test the responsiveness of the networks of Figure 2 to the input from the primary endings of the muscle spindles, that is, to one part of the input which is aroused by fusimotor activation. Unfortunately the length-measuring secondary endigs, which supply the other part, cannot be stimulated in isolation, but the dynamically-sensitive primaries can be selectively stimulated by percutaneous vibration of tendons, the very valuable method which HAGBARTH and EKLUND (1966) and DE GAIL, LANCE and NEILSON (1966) have introduced into human neurophysiology. Vibration evokes a 'tonic vibration reflex' in the muscle whose tendon is vibrated, with reduction of the EMG of an antagonist. If the muscle is already engaged in voluntary activity, for example, the biceps in holding the elbow at a right-angle against gravity, the reflex begins promptly, but it does not end abruptly when the vibration is withdrawn: 'the forearm usually sinks down slowly to its original position'. If however the muscle is relaxed initially, the response may be long delayed: 'when the foot passively hangs in plantar flexion, the first signs of activity in tibialis anterior may appear more than 30 sec after vibration is applied to the tendon of this muscle' (HAGBARTH and EKLUND, 1966). Clearly therefore the input from the spindle primaries has no overpowering effect when delivered in isolation in resting man. This contrasts with the prompt onset and equally prompt cessation of the tonic vibration reflex of the soleus muscle in the decerebrate cat (MATTHEWS, 1966). The slow onset of excitation of agonists and inhibition of antagonists may depend on complex and widespread effects; it is unlikely that it depends solely on the monosynaptic driving of the α motoneurones and the relevantly-coupled Ia-inhibitory interneurones by the Group Ia input. The efficacy of this input must depend on the prevailing settings of background facilitation of these neurones, which no doubt, and especially in the case of voluntary use of the fingers, would be determined in part by the known connexions of the CST.

Reciprocal Ia inhibition is in abeyance in resting man. In the experiments of TANAKA (1974) the Group Ia input was provided by a brief burst of three electrically-evoked volleys in Group Ia axons (instead of by vibration). This conditioning input was sent in along the lateral popliteal nerve which carries the Group Ia axons from dorsiflexors of the ankle, and reciprocal inhibition of the motoneurone pool of the antagonist plantar flexor, triceps surae, was tested monosynaptically by a Group Ia afferent volley in the medial popliteal nerve.* When the subject was relaxed the conditioning burst evoked no H-reflex in the dorsiflexors, and had no inhibitory effect on the testing H-reflex in the plantar flexor. Thus, under these conditions, either the Ia-inhibitory interneurones, as well as the dorsiflexor motoneurones, were without essential background facilitation, or they were under active tonic inhibition. During sustained voluntary dorsiflexion of the ankle, however,

---

* The familiar electrically-evoked monosynaptic reflex of the calf muscles was discovered by Paul HOFFMANN (cf. JUNG, 1969), who speculated in the 1920's that it might be monosynaptic; it was named H-reflex by MAGLADERY and McDOUGAL (1950) in his honour.

the conditioning burst evoked an H-reflex in the dorsiflexors and reduced the H-reflex in the plantar flexor to about 70 per cent of its control amplitude. This effect could well be due to the CST. In electroanatomical experiments on anaesthetized baboons, HONGO, LUNDBERG, PHILLIPS and THOMPSON were impressed by the remarkable lack of reciprocal Ia IPSPs in lumbosacral motoneurones in response to Group Ia volleys in muscle nerves of the hindlimb, as compared with their common occurrence in cats under similar experimental conditions.

If the networks of Figure 2 are so unresponsive at rest, something must happen to turn them on in preparation for voluntary movement. As is well known, there is abundant evidence of increased and very widespread cerebral activity during the reaction time of brief and circumscribed movements made in response to visual or auditory signals, or during up to 500 msec preceding the onset of self-paced movements, both in monkeys and men (PHILLIPS and PORTER, 1977, for references). There is also widespread spinal activity preceding movement. PAILLARD (1955) drew attention to the astonishing disproportion between the narrow localization of a motor act and the very widespread facilitation of motoneurones which can be detected in advance of it. Thus COQUERY and COULMANCE (1971) found that when a subject suddenly clenches his *fist*, the motoneurones of *soleus* show an increase in reflex excitability which begins 50 to 100 msec before the EMG of the finger flexors. There is also evidence that the Ia-inhibitory apparatus is brought into a state of readiness about 80 msec before the onset of an abrupt dorsiflexion of the ankle made in response to a visual signal with a reaction time (RT) of 100 to 250 msec (SIMOYAMA and TANAKA, 1974). Paired conditioning and testing stimuli were given to the lateral and medial popliteal nerves, as in TANAKA's experiment (1974) on the facilitatory effect of voluntary dorsiflexion of the ankle on reciprocal Ia inhibition of triceps surae. The interval between the last of the three conditioning pulses and the testing pulse was fixed at 1.5 to 2.0 msec, the optimum interval for reciprocal Ia inhibition. This whole brief conditioning-testing complex was then injected at various times during the RT to the visual signal and after the abrupt onset of the EMG of the dorsiflexors of the ankle. An H-reflex appeared in the ankle dorsiflexors, associated with reciprocal inhibition of the H-reflex of triceps surae, from 80 msec before the onset of dorsiflexion until more than 100 msec after the onset.

In the direct activation of α motoneurones in human voluntary movement, the monosynaptic cortico-motoneuronal component of the CST presumably plays an important role. Often, however, the first detectable action is inhibition of the antagonist (HUFSCHMIDT and HUFSCHMIDT, 1954; HALLETT, SHAHANI and YOUNG, 1975; MARSDEN, MERTON, MORTON, HALLETT, ADAM and RUSHTON, 1977). This suggests that the earliest excitatory action is on the Ia-inhibitory interneurone. The next event is a centrally-programmed, rapid stereotyped sequence of agonist-antagonist excitation which was originally discovered by WACHHOLDER and ALTENBURGER (HALLETT et al., 1975; MARSDEN et al., 1977). The duration of this burst is apparently incapable of modification: the force required can be adjusted only by changes in the amplitude of the burst (MARSDEN et al., 1977). Our voluntary movements have a strong tendency to begin in this ballistic manner, and it is quite difficult to produce a perfectly smooth ramp movement.

For the execution of learned patterns of skilled movement, the forebrain and cerebellum must have available to them the possibility of synthesizing new combinations of motor output from the spinal segments (LEYTON and SHERRINGTON, 1917). The great development of the CST in primates, and the appearance of its monosynaptic corticomotoneuronal component, suggests that this pathway may have conferred evolutionary advantage in this regard. The degree to which the human motor apparatus can allow selective voluntary addressing of α motoneurones is therefore interesting, and has been made clear in experiments by KATO and TANJI (1972). They found that people who were provided with visual or auditory feedback of the potentials of single motor units, mostly in intrinsic muscles of the thumb and extensor digitorum communis (those muscles whose motoneurones receive the largest corticomotoneuronal EPSPs in baboons) could select single units, with a high degree of accuracy, from among those motor units that were recruited in gentle voluntary contractions, but could not single out any that were recruited only at higher force thresholds (cf HENNEMAN, SOMJEN and CARPENTER, 1965).

The foregoing techniques and concepts are all applicable to the analysis of disorders of posture and of voluntary, pre-programmed and reflex movements in neurological patients, who can cooperate in the clinical and instrumental examinations and can produce, on request, performances which could be produced by monkeys, if at all, only after prolonged and careful training. Such analytical work on the effects on the spinal segments of interruption of descending pathways holds great promise. The time will come when blanket expressions like 'spinal shock, 'diaschisis' and 'release' will be outmoded and will be replaced by precise statements about the disfacilitation and disinhibition of specific pools of interneurones, resulting in identifiable alterations of transmission in segmental networks which should not only explain the patients' disabilities but also help in the planning of treatment.

The preponderance of extensor reflexes in the legs of patients with lesions of descending pathways is obvious clinically, but a lesser degree of exaggeration of flexor reflexes is also present. In normal people there is no H-reflex in the dorsiflexors of the ankle, but in patients with lesions of lower brainstem and spinal cord a good H-reflex can be elicited in these muscles by a single Group I volley (stimulus below M threshold) in the lateral popliteal nerve (TEASDALL, PARK, LANGUTH and MAGLADERY, 1952). MIZUNO, TANAKA and YANAGISAWA (1971) found that such a volley caused no reciprocal inhibition of an H-reflex in the calf muscles when conditioning and testing volleys were delivered at the interval which is optimal for disynaptic inhibition. But in 4 out of 6 patients with bilateral athetosis, who showed minimal rigidity and no involuntary movements at rest, but in whom 'disturbance of reciprocal innervation was observed during coordinate movements,' the paired volleys revealed inhibition of the H-reflex in triceps surae. The level of background facilitation of the Ia-inhibitory interneurones which are interposed between the Group Ia afferents from the dorsiflexors and the α motoneurones of the plantar flexor was therefore abnormally high in these patients.

YANAGISAWA, TANAKA and ITO (1976) have examined the state of the reciprocal Ia-inhibitory networks which interlink the dorsiflexors and plantar flexors of the ankle in eleven patients with spastic hemiplegia. All had H-reflexes in triceps surae, but only 5 had H-reflexes in pretibial muscles: these were the only patients in whom these muscles retained any voluntary power. In two cases only was there any reciprocal Ia inhibition of triceps surae motoneurones. (In three there was facilitation, possibly by the Group Ib input: cf. LAPORTE and LLOYD, 1952). But in those patients who showed pre-tibial H-reflexes at rest, those reflexes were powerfully inhibited by Group I volleys from triceps surae. The balance was thus heavily tipped against the dorsiflexors, which are 'doubly crippled by reduced descending impulses and strong reciprocal inhibition by the Ia impulses from the spindles of the extensor muscles.' Figure 3 is an abstraction from Figure 2 which shows only those segmental interconnexions discussed by YANAGISAWA et al. in interpreting their findings. On the extensor side they invoke excessive fusimotor activity as the basic effect of the cerebral lesions. One might add that since some γ motoneurones in primates receive inhibition from the CST (GRIGG and PRESTON, 1971; CLOUGH et al.,

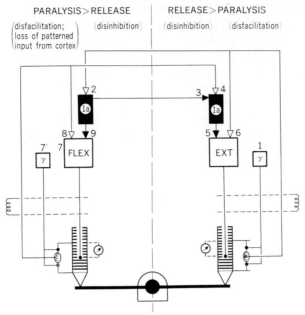

Fig. 3 Abstraction from Fig. 2 of networks invoked by YANAGISAWA et al. (1976) to explain unbalanced reciprocal innervation at ankle joint in hemiplegia (See text).

	Extensors	*Effects of alcohol blockade of extensor fusimotor axons*
Abnormalities		
1.	Pathological fusimotor hyperactivity	Transmission blocked
2.	Excessive excitation	Reduced
3.	Excessive inhibition	Reduced
4.	Disfacilitation (due to 7′)	—
5.	Disinhibition	Removed
6.	Excessive excitation	Reduced

Effects of abnormalities on—
Voluntary power:

Weakness mitigated by excessive reflex support (spasticity)	Weakness increased / Spasticity reduced

H-reflex:
Present in all cases
Uninhibitable by Ia input from flexors in most cases — Becomes inhibitable in some cases.

Dorsiflexors

Abnormalities
7, 7′. Pathological reduction of αγ driving — —
8. Disfacilitation — —
9. Excessive inhibition (due to 1, 2) — Reduced

Effects of abnormalities on—
Voluntary power:
Weakness aggravated by diminished reflex support — Subjective and objective improvement of power.

H-reflex:
Absent in severe paralysis —
Present when some power preserved —
Powerfully inhibited by Ia input from extensors —

1971), disinhibition of fusimotor neurones by the lesion could be a contributory factor. The excessive fusimotor activity would drive the α motoneurones of the extensors and reciprocally inhibit those of the flexors. The efficacy of the Ia-inhibitory interneurones which might otherwise restrain the extensors would be reduced by two factors; first, by the relative lack of fusimotor-driven excitation from the spindle afferents of the flexors, as a result of the central lesion; and secondly, by inhibition from the Ia-inhibitory interneurones of the antagonistic pool. On the flexor side, disfacilitation of α and γ motoneurones preponderates over the disinhibition which is revealed in some cases by the presence of an H-reflex in the flexors.

YANAGISAWA et al. have interpreted the consequential changes in reflexes and voluntary control, and of the beneficial effects of blocking the extensor fusimotor axons by injecting alcohol into the motor points of the muscles, in the ways summarized in the legend to Figure 3. Though these authors hold to the belief that the monosynaptic Group Ia control of α motoneurones and of their associated Ia-inhibitory interneurones welds these pools into a tightly coupled functional unit, their observations show that the coupling can be dissociated under abnormally-balanced descending control from the brain. In monkeys, JANKOWSKA et al. (1976) did not report any preponderance of cortical excitation to Ia-inhibitory interneurones to ankle dorsiflexors or extensors.

LLOYD's classic paper on the Spinal Mechanism of the Pyramidal System in Cats opened a rich vein of electroanatomical research which is still showing no signs of exhaustion. We still lack, however, methods for investigating the actions of the very thin axons which form the major bulk of the corticospinal pathway. Perhaps this vein too will be opened by present or future workers at the Rockefeller University.

REFERENCES

ASANUMA, A., SHINODA, Y. and ZARZECKI, P.: Branching of cortico-spinal fibres in the monkey. *Neurosci. Abst.*, *2*: 537 (1976)

BEEVOR, C. E.: *The Croonian Lectures on Muscular Movements and their Representation in the Central Nervous System.* Adlard, London (1904)

BERNHARD, C. G., BOHM, E. and PETERSÉN, I.: Investigations on the organization of the cortico-spinal system in monkeys. (*Macaca mulatta*). *Acta physiol. scand.*, *29*: Suppl. 106, 79–105 (1953)

BERNSTEIN, N.: *The Coordination and Regulation of Movements.* Pergamon Press, Oxford (1967)

CLOUGH, J. F. M., KERNELL, D. and PHILLIPS, C. G.: The distribution of monosynaptic excitation from the pyramidal tract and from primary spindle afferents to motoneurones of the baboon's hand and forearm. *J. Physiol.*, *198*: 145–166 (1968)

CLOUGH, J. F. M., PHILLIPS, C. G. and SHERIDAN, J. D.: The short-latency projection from the baboon's motor cortex to fusimotor neurones of the forearm and hand. *J. Physiol.*, *216*: 257–279 (1971)

COLLIER, J. and BUZZARD, E. F.: The degenerations resulting from lesions of posterior nerve roots and from transverse lesions of the spinal cord in man. A study of twenty cases. *Brain*, *26*: 559–591 (1903)

COOPER, S. and DENNY-BROWN, D. E.: Responses to stimulation of the motor area of the cerebral cortex. *Proc. Royal Soc. B*, *102*: 222–236 (1928)

COQUERY, J.-M. and COULMANCE, M.: Variations d'amplitude des réflexes monosynaptiques avant un mouvement volontaire. *Physiology and Behaviour*, *6*: 65–69 (1971)

DE GAIL, P., LANCE, J. W. and NEILSON, P. D.: Differential effects on tonic and phasic reflex mechanisms produced by vibration of muscles in man. *J. Neurol. Neurosurg. Psych.*, *29*: 1–11 (1966)

DEJERINE, J.: *Anatomie des Centres Nerveux*, vol. 2, pp. 82–90. Rueff, Paris (1901)

DENNY-BROWN, D.: *The Cerebral Control of Movement.* Liverpool University Press, Liverpool (1966)

DESMEDT, J. E. (ed.): *New Developments in Electromyography and Clinical Neurophysiology* in 3 vols. Karger, Basel (1973)

DESMEDT, J. E. (ed.): *Progress in Clinical Neurophysiology*. Vols. 4, 5, 8, 9. Karger, Basel (1977)

DUCHENNE DE BOULOGNE, G. B.: *Physiologie des Mouvements*. Bailliére, Paris (1867)

ENDO, K., ARAKI, T. and YAGI, N.: The distribution and pattern of axon branching of pyramidal tract cells. *Brain Res.*, *57*: 484–491 (1973)

FEDINA, L. and HULTBORN, H.: Facilitation from ipsilateral primary afferents of interneuronal transmission in the Ia inhibitory pathway to motoneurones. *Acta physiol. scand.*, *86*: 59–81 (1972)

FERRIER, D. and YEO, G. F.: A record of experiments on the effects of lesion of different regions of the cerebral hemispheres. *Philosophical Transactions of the Royal Society*, Part II, 479–564 (1884)

FRANÇOIS-FRANCK, C. E.: *Leçons sur les Fonctions Motrices du Cerveau*. Doin, Paris (1887)

GRIGG, P. and PRESTON, J. B.: Baboon flexor and extensor fusimotor neurons and their modulation by motor cortex. *J. Neurophysiol.*, *34*: 428–436 (1971)

HAGBARTH, K.-E. and EKLUND, G.: Motor effects of vibratory muscle stimuli in man. *In* GRANIT, R. (ed.): *Muscular Afferents and Motor Control*, pp. 177–186, Almqvist and Wiksell, Stockholm (1966)

HAGBARTH, K.-E. and VALLBO, Å. B.: Single unit recordings from muscle nerves in human subjects. *Acta physiol. scand.*, *76*: 321–334 (1969)

HALLETT, M., SHAHANI, B. T. and YOUNG, R. R.: E. M. G. analysis of stereotyped voluntary movements in man. *J. Neurol. Neurosurg. Psych.*, *38*: 1154–1162 (1975)

HENNEMAN, E., SOMJEN, G. and CARPENTER, D. O.: Functional significance of cell size in spinal motoneurones. *J. Neurophysiol.*, *28*: 560–580 (1965)

HOFF, E. C. and HOFF, H. E.: Spinal terminations of the projection fibres from the motor cortex of primates. *Brain*, *57*: 454–474 (1934)

HONGO, T., JANKOWSKA, E. and LUNDBERG, A.: The rubrospinal tract II. Facilitation of interneuronal transmission in reflex paths to motoneurones. *Exp. Brain Res.*, *7*: 365–391 (1969)

HUFSCHMIDT, H.-J, and HUFSCHMIDT, T.: Antagonist inhibition as the earliest sign of a sensory-motor reaction. *Nature*, *174*: 607 (1954)

HULTBORN, H., ILLERT, M. and SANTINI, M.: Convergence of interneurones mediating the reciprocal Ia inhibition of motoneurones. I. Disynaptic Ia inhibition of Ia inhibitory interneurones. *Acta physiol. scand.*, *96*: 193–201 (1976a)

HULTBORN, H., ILLERT, M. and SANTINI, M.: Convergence of interneurones mediating the reciprocal Ia inhibition of motoneurones. III. Effects from supraspinal pathways. *Acta physiol. scand.*, *96*: 368–391 (1976b)

INOUYE, Y. and BUCHTHAL, F.: Segmental sensory innervation determined by potentials recorded from cervical spinal nerves. *Brain*, *100*: 731–748 (1977)

JANKOWSKA, E. and TANAKA, R.: Neuronal mechanism of the disynaptic inhibition evoked in primate spinal motoneurones from the corticospinal tract. *Brain Res.*, *75*: 163–166 (1974)

JANKOWSKA, E., PADEL, Y. and TANAKA, R.: Disynaptic inhibition of spinal motoneurones from the motor cortex in the monkey. *J. Physiol.*, *258*: 467–487 (1976)

JUNG, R.: Paul Hoffmann 1884–1962. *Ergebnisse der Physiologie, 61*: 1–17 (1969)

KATO, M. and TANJI, J.: Conscious control of motor units of human finger muscles. *In* SOMJEN, G. G. (ed.): *Neurophysiology Studied in Man*. Excerpta Medica, Amsterdam (1972)

KUYPERS, H. G. J. M.: An anatomical analysis of cortico-bulbar connexions to the pons and lower brain stem in the cat. *J. Anat.*, *92*: 198–218 (1958)

KUYPERS, H. G. J. M.: Central cortical projections to motor and somatosensory cell groups. (An experimental study in the Rhesus monkey). *Brain*, *83*: 161–184 (1960)

LANDGREN, S., PHILLIPS, C. G. and PORTER, R.: Minimal synaptic actions of pyramidal impulses on some alpha motoneurones of the baboon's hand and forearm. *J. Physiol.*, *161*: 91–111 (1962)

LAPORTE, Y. and LLOYD, D. P. C.: Nature and significance of the reflex connections established by large afferent fibers of muscular origin. *Am. J. Physiol.*, *169*: 609–621 (1952)

LAWRENCE, D. G. and HOPKINS, D. A.: The development of motor control in the rhesus monkey: evidence concerning the role of corticomotoneuronal connections. *Brain*, *99*: 235–254 (1976)

LAWRENCE, G. G. and KUYPERS, H. G. J. M.: The functional organization of the motor system in the monkey. I. The effects of bilateral pyramidal lesions. *Brain*, *91*: 1–14 (1968)

LEYTON, A. S. F. and SHERRINGTON, C. S.: Observations on the excitable cortex of the chimpanzee, orang-utan and gorilla. *Quart. J. Exp. Physiol.*, *11*: 135–222 (1917)

LLOYD, D. P. C.: The spinal mechanism of the pyramidal system in cats. *J. Neurophysiol.*, *4*: 525–546 (1941)

LONG, C. and BROWN, M. E.: Electromyographic kinesiology of the hand: muscles moving the long finger. *J. Bone Joint Surg.*, *46-A*: 1683–1706 (1964)

LORENTE DE NÓ, R.: Cerebral cortex: architecture, intracortical connexions, motor projections. *In* FULTON, J. F.: *Physiology of the Nervous System.* Oxford University Press, London (1938)

LUNDBERG, A.: Supraspinal control of transmission in reflex paths to motoneurones and primary afferents. *In*: *Progress in Brain Research*, Vol. 12, pp. 197–221. Elsevier, Amsterdam, London, New York (1964)

LUNDBERG, A.: Control of spinal mechanisms from the brain. *In* TOWER, D. B. (editor-in-chief): *The Nervous System.* Vol. 1: *The Basic Neurosciences.* Raven Press, New York (1975)

LUNDBERG, A., MALMGREN, K. and SCHOMBURG, E. D.: Characteristics of the excitatory pathway from group II muscle afferents to alpha motoneurones. *Brain Res.*, *88*: 538–542 (1975)

LUNDBERG, A., MALMGREN, K. and SCHOMBURG, E. D.: Comments on reflex actions evoked by electrical stimulation of group II muscle afferents. *Brain Res.*, *122*: 551–555 (1977)

MAGLADERY, J. W. and McDOUGAL, J. B., Jr.: Electrophysiological studies of nerve and reflex activity in normal man. I. Identification of certain reflexes in the electromyogram and the conduction velocity of peripheral nerve fibres. *Bull. Johns Hopkins Hosp.*, *86*: 265–290 (1950)

MAGLADERY, J. W., PORTER, W. E., PARK, A. M. and TEASDALL, R. D.: Electrophysiological studies of nerve and reflex activity in normal man. IV. The two-neurone reflex and identification of certain action potentials from spinal roots and cord. *Bull. Johns Hopkins Hosp.*, *88*: 499–519 (1951)

MARSDEN, C. D., MERTON, P. A., MORTON, H. B., HALLETT, M., ADAM, J. and RUSHTON, D. N.: Disorders of movement in cerebellar disease in man. *In* ROSE, F. C. (ed.): *Physiological Aspects of Clinical Neurology.* pp. 179–199. Blackwell, Oxford (1977)

MARSDEN, C. D., ROTHWELL, J. C. and TRAUB, M. M.: Changes in perceived heaviness in man after thumb anaesthesia are associated with corresponding changes in the degree of muscle activation. *In*: *Proceedings of the Physiological Society, March* 1978, p. 82 (1978)

MATTHEWS, P. B. C.: The reflex excitation of the soleus muscle of the decerebrate cat caused by vibration applied to its tendon. *J. Physiol.*, *184*: 450–472 (1966)

MATTHEWS, P. B. C.: *Mammalian Muscle Receptors and their Central Actions.* Arnold, London (1972)

MIZUNO, Y., TANAKA, R. and YANAGISAWA, N.: Reciprocal Group I inhibition on triceps surae motoneurons in man. *J. Neurophysiol.*, *34*: 1010–1017 (1971)

MUIR, R. B. and PORTER, R.: The effect of a preceding stimulus on temporal facilitation at cortico-motoneuronal synapses. *J. Physiol.*, *228*: 749–763 (1973)

PAILLARD, J.: *Réflexes et Regulations d'Origine Proprioceptive chez l'Homme.* Librairie Arnette, Paris (1955)

PHILLIPS, C. G.: Evolution of the corticospinal tract in primates with special reference to the hand. *In*: *Proceedings of the Third International Congress of Primatology, Zurich, 1970, 2*: 2–23. Karger, Basel (1971)

PHILLIPS, C. G. and PORTER, R.: The pyramidal projection to motoneurones of some muscle groups of the baboon's forelimb. *In* ECCLES, J. C. and SCHADE, J. P. (eds.): *Progress in Brain Research: Physiology of Spinal Neurones*, vol. 12, pp. 222–242. Elsevier, Amsterdam (1964)

PHILLIPS, C. G. and PORTER, R.: *Corticospinal Neurones. Their role in movement.* Academic Press, London (1977)

PORTER, R.: Early facilitation at corticomotoneuronal synapses. *J. Physiol.*, *207*: 733–745 (1970)

PRESTON, J. B., SHENDE, M. C. and UEMURA, K.: The motor cortex-pyramidal system: patterns of facilitation and inhibition on motoneurons innervating limb musculature of cat and baboon and their possible adaptive significance. *In* YAHR, M. D. and PURPURA, D. P. (eds.): *Neurophysiological Basis of Normal and Abnormal Motor Activities.* pp. 61–72, Raven Press, New York (1967)

PRESTON, J. B. and WHITLOCK, D. G.: Precentral facilitation and inhibition of spinal motoneurons. *J. Neurophysiol.*, *23*: 154–170 (1960)

PRESTON, J. B. and WHITLOCK, D. G.: Intracellular potentials recorded from motoneurons following precentral gyrus stimulation in primate. *J. Neurophysiol.*, *24*: 91–100 (1961)

RAMÓN Y CAJAL, S.: *Histologie du Système Nerveux de l'Homme et des Vertébrés.* Vol. 1. Maloine, Paris (1909)

RAMÓN Y CAJAL, S.:   *Degeneration and Regeneration of the Nervous System*, translated and edited by R. M. MAY, Vol. 1.   Oxford University Press, Oxford (1928)

SHERRINGTON, C. S.:   On secondary and tertiary degenerations in the spinal cord of the dog. *J. Physiol.*, *6*: 177–191 (1885)

SHINODA, Y., ARNOLD, A. P. and ASANUMA, H.:   Spinal branching of corticospinal axons in the cat. *Exp. Brain Res.*, *26*: 215–234 (1976)

SIMOYAMA, M. and TANAKA, R.:   Reciprocal Ia inhibition at the onset of voluntary movements in man.   *Brain Res.*, *82*: 334–337 (1974)

TANAKA, R.:   Reciprocal Ia inhibition during voluntary movements in man.   *Exp. Brain Res.*, *21*: 529–540 (1974)

TEASDALL, R. D., PARK, A. M., LANGUTH, H. W. and MAGLADERY, J. W.:   Electrophysiological studies of reflex activity in patients with lesions of the nervous system.   II.   Disclosure of normally suppressed monosynaptic reflex discharge of spinal motoneurones by lesions of lower brainstem and spinal cord.   *Bull. Johns Hopkins Hosp.*, *91*: 245–256 (1952)

VALLBO, Å. B.:   Slowly adapting muscle receptors in man.   *Acta physiol. scand.*, 78: 315–333 (1970)

VALLBO, Å. B.:   Muscle spindle afferent discharge from resting and contracting muscles in normal human subjects.   *In* DESMEDT, J. E. (ed.):   *New Developments in Electromyography and Clinical Neurophysiology.*, vol. 3. pp. 251–262.   Karger, Basel (1973)

YANAGISAWA, N., TANAKA, R. and ITO, Z.:   Reciprocal Ia inhibition in spastic hemiplegia of man. *Brain*, *99*: 555–574 (1976)

THE USE OF CONTACT PLACING IN ANALYTICAL AND SYNTHETIC STUDIES OF THE HIGHER SENSORIMOTOR CONTROL SYSTEM*

Vahé E. Amassian

Department of Physiology, SUNY-Downstate Medical Center
New York, NY

INTRODUCTION

The continuing survival and evolution of a central nervous system is generally held to reflect the success with which the organism exhibits adaptive behaviors and controls the internal environment within narrow limits. The Symposium title includes "Integration", which is apt in relation to such crucial functions of the central nervous system, although reminding us only of the name of the problem and not providing the solution. From the Oxford English Dictionary (1933) we learn that "Integration" is "a making up or composition of a whole by adding together or combining the separate parts or elements;...". Especially when considering the mammalian nervous system, two questions arise; first, the nature of the whole—be it the social unit, the individual organism, individual areas of the brain, etc. The term is now used transitively, integration at one level serving as a building stone at the next functional or structural level. Secondly, it is implied that a prerequisite of the integration is the identification of the constituent elements, that is, analysis appears to precede synthesis. However, a powerful test of whether an element is a necessary component of an overall system is to attempt to synthesize the overall system without the putative component. That is, *analysis* and *synthesis* are not necessarily sequential operations, but are interwoven, admittedly to a varying extent, in any significant enquiry of the nervous system.

Although Sherrington's contributions (1906) as the Master Analyst of the reflexes are the familiar starting point for those beginning the study of the nervous system, he attached no less significance to the synthetic principles governing the relationships between reflexes. The notion of a priority structure, now so mundane in computer system functioning, converted what would otherwise be a chaotic jumble of reflexes into an orderly sequence of the simplest kinds of behavior.

At first sight studying the neural basis of a particular behavior and using the behavior as an aid in studying how portions of the nervous system function separately and together would seem to be convergent activities. However they can be antithetical; for example, suppose it were found that the behavior could be accounted for by a reduced fragment of the CNS, such as the spinal cord, with its peripheral connections. The possibility of eventually explaining the behavior would thereby be improved. By contrast, the possibility of understanding how the higher level sensorimotor (SM) control components interrelate would be diminished.

Exploiting a behavior in synthesis and analysis of higher level neural networks requires that the behavior be clearly separable from other behaviors, the stimuli eliciting the

* This research was supported by USPHS, NIH grants NS 10987 and 11219.

behavior and the context of the behavior be clearly definable, the behavior be readily measurable, be reproducible—yet not be so consistent as to deny the possibility of seeking correlations between neural and behavioral variables.

Concerning *developmental* aspects, the behavior ideally would be present soon after birth, subsequently maturing and perfecting at a well defined age.

Finally, if present, *plasticity* of the behavior introduces the possibility not only of studying the neural correlates of plasticity but of dissociating neural and behavioral events (FETZ and FINOCCHIO, 1972) and distinguishing thereby circumstantial and cause-effect relationships.

The tactile placing reaction or contact placing (CP) is an example of a behavior in the adult mammal, which has long been known to depend on the cerebral cortex (RADEMAKER, 1931) and more particular on the SM cortex (BARD, 1933, 1938). Using sterotaxic lesions or local cooling, our laboratory defined two major thalamocortical projection systems, the VP→SM cortex and the Cerebello→VL-VA→motor cortex, as normally required for the full placing reaction. Recording from individual neurons during CP disclosed that while the VP projection system could contribute dynamically to the earliest muscle activity in CP, the VL-VA system could contribute dynamically only to *later* components of lifting-withdrawal, the first phase of CP (AMASSIAN et al., 1972a, b).

Thus, CP is subserved by many of the elements of the higher SM control system. Furthermore, the involvement of both the VP and the VL-VA thalamocortical projection systems in this behavior is mirrored by the participation of both systems in the load compensation reflex (cf. EVARTS, 1973; TATTON et al., 1975; CONRAD et al., 1974), that is, the study of the circuitry subserving CP has generality for other types of motor response. The *gain* of the circuitry subserving CP is usually adequate over a wide range of object heights to secure placing of the paw on top of the object contacted. (Gains of stretch and "triggered" components in load compensation are discussed by CRAGO et al., 1976.)

Similarly, CP fulfills many of the criteria listed above for a behavior suitable for use in synthetic and analytical operations (AMASSIAN et al., 1972a, b). The advantages are also manifest in developmental studies (AMASSIAN and ROSS, 1978a, b), because CP is present from birth onwards, becoming perfected by the seventh postnatal week (AMASSIAN and RUDELL, 1978). CP also exhibits plasticity (WERTENBAKER et al., 1973) with at least some of the circuitry subserving the plasticity separable from that subserving CP (AMASSIAN et al., 1974).

A "naturally" occurring behavior such as CP necessarily entails an acceleration of the inertial mass of the limb following the brief initial isometric contraction of the muscles, terminated ultimately by deceleration to stand still of the limb. Given overt movements over considerable distances, the possibility arises (and is readily confirmed) that the trajectory of the limb can vary in successive trials, despite the attainment of a similar goal. Such variability and the difficulties implicit in measuring the many parameters of multidimensional movement contrast with those encountered when, for example, a primate is taught to perform a stereotyped, quasi-isometric task with a selected muscle (EVARTS, 1968). However, it has long been known that activity in distant muscles, for example, axial muscles, may change prior to an intended movement by one muscle; that is, the apparent advantage of a restricted output in *learnt* movements is relative and not absolute. More significantly, it may be argued that the major function of the higher SM control system is to generate movements resulting in the attainment of goals rather than to generate isometric forces.

The focus of this report is a re-examination of the evidence that CP in the adult cat is subserved by at least two types of dynamic transcortical loop; by contrast, in the kitten

CP is subserved at first by a subcortical circuit, the subsequent involvement of the cerebral cortex, specifically PT neurons, initially occurring through tonic rather than dynamic activity.   The Results section deals with: (1) The experimental strategy; (2) a description of the movements and muscle activities in the behavior-CP; (3) the differentiation of CP from stepping.   The role in CP by the adult cat of (4) the VP thalamocortical projection system, (5) the cerebello-VL and VA projection system, (6) the cerebello-rubral outflow.   In the young kitten, (7) the initial role of the subcortical circuitry and (8) the emerging role of the SM cortex and PT neurons; (9) the transition from juvenile to adult circuitry subserving CP.

METHODS

General

The techniques used in the adult cat or kitten for lesion making, cooling brain structures, stimulation of brain structure, recording from individual central neurons and from muscles during CP, recording the parameters of CP (other than trajectory of the paw) and for eliciting plasticity of CP are described in the appropriate references cited above, together with the histological controls.   The techniques used in data processing and analysis with a computer are described in AMASSIAN, et al. (1972a).

Recording movement of the forepaw

A technique has been developed (references in RUDELL, 1979) for tracking the position of the forepaw as a function of time (AMASSIAN and RUDELL, 1978).   Briefly, a 6.25 mm diameter paper spot, which is coated with a green fluorescing pigment, is glued to the side of the terminal phalanx either of digit V (right forepaw) or digit II (left forepaw). The spot is illuminated with UV light, permitting data to be collected from animals with white fur and in the presence of dim ambient light.   The light in the video field passes through a green filter into a Sony AVC-3210 camera, where it falls on a photosensitive surface which is scanned at a rate of 60 Hz with rasters, each composed of $262^{1}/_{2}$ lines.   The spot is detected by the change in voltage output from the camera when the scanning electron beam crosses the illuminated area in the field.   This change in voltage triggers a one-shot, which triggers a sample-and-hold of the horizontal sawtooth.   After A/D conversion of this analog voltage and a (digital) count of the number of horizontal sweeps elapsing since the start of the raster, the time delays and hence the positions of the sites of increased illumination are calculated by a PDP 11/45 computer.   The spot covers a variable number of horizontal lines, the mean being taken as the center of the spot.   The system is statically calibrated by moving a spot through known distances in X and Y axes.

The technique suffers from a number of limitations.   Temporal resolution is limited to 1/60 sec, and is worse if the spot is not detected during fast hypermetric movements, especially when twisting of the paw causes a smaller area of spot to be presented to the camera.   Undetected spots are linearly interpolated between those detected, introducing a probable error in the trajectory and an underestimate of its length.   Persistence of the trace also tends to lead to an underestimate of the distance travelled.   The lag between true and computed positions of the spot is usually about 50 msec, as timed by electrical contact of a moving conductor with the placer.   In addition, the small movements occurring in the 3rd dimension are not measured.   However, despite such limitations, the technique has proved valuable in measuring CP movements.

RESULTS

Strategy

The types of procedure used in examining the hypothesis of a dynamic transcortical loop include:

1) Determining the effect on CP of changing the activity of the nucleus by a) making permanent lesions, b) cooling the nucleus and c) applying electrical pulses or polarizing currents. Essentially, procedures a) and b) help determine the relevance of the nucleus to some aspect of CP, without distinguishing tonic from dynamic modes of functioning. The temporal resolving power is never less than many seconds with the faster of these two procedures—cooling. By contrast, modifying the activity of the nucleus by electrical currents permits a resolving power of the order of milliseconds.

2) Comparing the timing of CP, activities of muscles, and of individual neurons located in central stations shown to be relevant to CP by procedure (1). The outcome of such comparison is either to *reject* or to *fail* to *reject* the *hypothesis* of *dynamic participation* when the neural activities follow, or precede with appropriate timing the behavioral events, respectively. At best, the hypothesis of dynamic participation is circumstantially supported but it is not proved by an analysis of time relations alone.

3) Comparing changes in CP and in individual neuronal activites during; a) spontaneous variations, b) different behavioral states, for example, in the awake versus drowsy or sleeping cat, c) lack of support and support of the tested limb and d) type II conditioning, using water as an adversive agent. Such procedures test the contingency relations between central neural events and the behavior, constituting a more powerful test of functional relationships when the dynamic transcortical loop hypothesis cannot be rejected by procedure (2).

Patterns of movement and muscle activities in CP

CP is present in some kittens to gentle stimulation of the dorsal or medial aspects of the unsupported forepaw on the day of birth (Fig. 1). CP to stimulation of the lateral and posterior aspects is present before the end of the first week. Because CP very rarely exhibits water conditioning before the 7th postnatal week, it seems likely that the neural circuitry required for CP starts functioning through genetic specification rather than depending on learning.

At first, the withdrawal phase of CP has a very long latency usually taking over 1 sec,

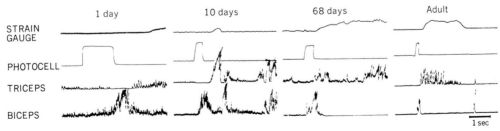

Fig. 1 CP and associated EMG activity as a function of age. Contact of the dorsum of the forepaw with the front of the apparatus occludes a light beam falling on a photocell, causing an upward deflection of the trace. Subsequent lifting-withdrawal of the forepaw restores photocell output. Landing of the forepaw on top of apparatus cause an upward deflection on the strain gauge output. The EMGs are integrated with a 10 msec decay time constant. (from Fig. 1, AMASSIAN and Ross, 1978b)

but by the middle of the first week it has markedly accelerated. However, the extra-ordinary economy of CP movements characteristically present in the normal adult is absent in young kittens until about the 7th postnatal week (AMASSIAN and RUDELL, 1978). In younger kittens, following dorsal contact, the forepaw swings high above the corner of the placing apparatus in the initial lifting-withdrawal phase of CP, subsequently placing far inward from the corner in the second, directed-landing phase. Not only are the movements hypermetric, but the trajectory of the paw is close to 45° to the horizontal, thus differing from the more mature trajectory, which is initially more vertical and subsequently more horizontal before descending (Fig. 2, cf. left forepaw at 39 and 44 days). Given that flexion occurring at the shoulder, the elbow, or at the wrist would cause the tip of the paw to move in an arc, the near rectilinear component of the trajectory present after CP movements are perfected in the 7th week implies a *highly coordinated rotation occurring* at a *minimum* of *two* joints.

Electromyographic recordings have disclosed that the prime movers in the lifting-withdrawal phase of CP to dorsal stimulation of the paw include the biceps and the long flexors of the digits. Significantly, *any activity in the extensor digitorus longus prior to dorsal contact is inhibited during this initial phase of CP.* Because the dorsal cutaneous surface is in the line of action of the extensor digitorum longus, it is evident that the initial response in dorsal CP is the opposite of that expected from the action of the motor cortical input-output columns described by ASANUMA et al. 1968 (although consistent with that described by SAKATA and MIYAMOTO, 1968). Indeed, were the extensor digitorum longus not inhibited, contraction of the biceps in the dependent forelimb would cause the paw to move in an arc, attempting to push the contacted object forward instead of ascending its vertical surface.

At first, the latency of biceps activation is quite prolonged, ranging from 0.4–1.3 sec. By the middle of the first week, the latency of biceps activation had fallen markedly to 0.15 0.6 sec. However, even as late as the 6th–7th week, biceps activation had a latency of 50–60 msec, that is, the adult latency range of 20–40 msec had still not been achieved. Figure 1 shows at 68 days (10th week), clearly distinguishable *initial* and *later* phases of biceps activation, a pattern also detectable in the adult CP.

In the adult cat, when the initial and second phases of biceps activation were distin-guishable, only the latencies of second phases and of initial phases with a latency of more than 50 msec were related to the latency of withdrawal, implying a *dual* process of biceps *activation* in which the later process is especially important in CP withdrawal (Fig. 5 in AMASSIAN et al., 1972a).

CP is initiated by stimulation of cutaneous mechanoreceptors and, in the limiting case, by hair stimulation alone. Sensory control *during* CP can also be demonstrated when the forepaw touches the placing apparatus many cms below the top corner (long travel). In clearing the top edge, the forepaw is lifted an increased distance as compared with that occurring when contact occurs high up near the top corner (short travel) and biceps output is correspondingly increased (Fig. 7 in AMASSIAN et al., 1972a). Such travel related increase in biceps output is present even during the first postnatal week (Fig. 3), at 3–6 days commencing 160–120 msec after the forepaw *would have cleared the top corner* of the placing apparatus had the contact occurred close to the top. Maturation occurs by 45 days (7th week), the delay for the increased biceps output decreasing to 40 msec, similar to that (50 msec) in the adult cat.

In the adult cat, the extensor digitorum longus is activated when the forepaw clears the top corner of the placing apparatus, triceps activation usually occurring later. The activation of the extensors cannot be a long latency response to "positive feedback" motor

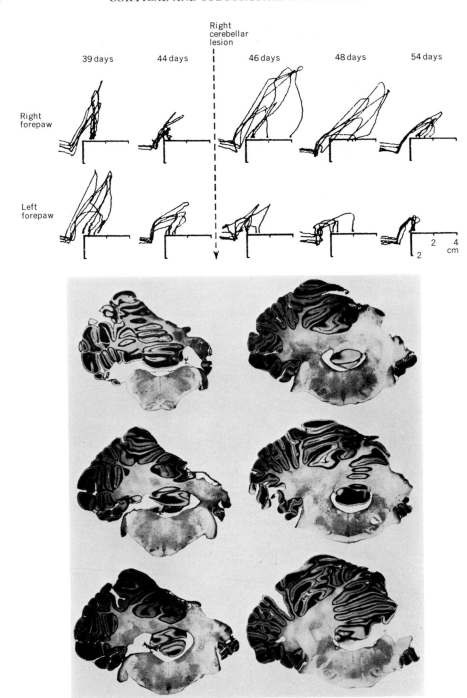

Fig. 2 CP trajectories in the 6th and 7th weeks and after a cerebellar cortical lesion. *Above*: from left to right, each record shows 5 superimposed, computed trajectories of a forepaw being passively moved to contact the front of the apparatus and subsequently actively placing. Positions of front and top of apparatus indicated by calibrated lines. Tip of paw projects anteriorally and ventrally to the fluorescent spot. After series at 44 days, a large lesion was made in right intermediate and lateral zone cerebellar cortex with minor damage to posterior vermis; the roof N. were spared. (from Fig. 1, AMASSIAN and RUDELL, 1978)

Below: representative photomicrographs through lesion. Sections stained with cresyl violet.

cortical input-output columns activated by the initial contact, because the extensor activation is *postponed* during a long travel.

The delay for extensor activation after the forepaw has cleared the top corner of the placer is remarkably prolonged in the first postnatal week. At 3–6 days, the delay during short travel CP was 280–100 msec, falling to 20 msec in the 7th week.

Significantly, timed from the same reference point- the forepaw clearing the top edge, the delay for extensor activation was greatly *reduced* during long as compared with *short* travel during the first postnatal week. Such finding implies differing neural bases for extensor activation after long as compared with short travels.

The context of CP includes the lack of support of the paw tested. In an alert cat, transient stimulation of hairs alone elicits activation of biceps and indeed may elicit an attempted place. By contrast, such stimulation of hairs in the *supported* forepaw failed to elicit biceps activation (Fig. 4 in AMASSIAN et al., 1972a).

Differentiation of CP and stepping

Spontaneously occurring stepping movement of the unsupported limb are quite common in kittens (FORSSBERG et al., 1974). The question arises whether forepaw CP is simply a step triggered by cutaneous contact or whether it is a different type of behavior. Even during the first postnatal week, CP and steps can be distinguished by their differing EMG patterns. Figure 4 compares 5 summed short travel CPs with 5 spontaneously occurring steps (The comparison is made with short rather than with long travel CPs to minimize the effect of cutaneous stimulation other than the initial contact). Using an increase in biceps activity as the '0' reference for alignment of the responses by the computer, the steps clearly differ from CPs in the *larger amplitude* of *biceps* activity and the *earlier activation* of the *extensors*. These differences are useful in distinguishing triggered steps from true CPs, for example, in 2 day kittens where both types of response are interspersed.

The role of the VP thalamocortical projection system in CP by adult cats

a) Synaptic basis and connectivities. The types of afferent input and their synaptic connectivities with PT neurons are of special interest because CP is either abolished or impaired by pyramidotomy in the adult cat (LIDELL and PHILLIPS, 1944; CHAMBERS and LIU, 1957; LAURSEN and WIESENDANGER, 1966). To such evidence from lesions may be added the similar effect on lateral CP of cooling the bulbar pyramid, manifested as early as the second postnatal week (AMASSIAN and ROSS, 1978a). Nevertheless, it must be emphasized that the PT system is not the only higher level motor output likely to be important in CP (see section on role of Red N. below).

The VP projections to large PT neurons are obligatorily polysynaptic, while those from VL-VA are monosynaptic and polysynaptic (AMASSIAN and WEINER, 1966). The *added* minimum delay (at least 1.2 msec) for discharge by PT neurons following a VP stimulus is within the range of *monosynaptic* delays for discharge by PT and uninvaded motor cortical neurons (0.75–1.34 msec in Figs. 3 and 4, ROSENTHAL et al., 1967). Thus, the earliest PT response to VP stimulation is disynaptically mediated. Later, the rising phase of the PT response to VP stimulation periodically increments as though mediated by excitatory cortical interneuronal chains, whose existence was postulated long ago by LORENTE DE NÓ (1938).

The interneuronal relays between VP and large PT neurons are located at several sites. Thus, extirpation of SI cortex behind the dimple or along the coronal sulcus *reduces* the *peak* components, but *spares* the *earliest* component of the bulbar PT response to VP stimulation, and all components of the response to VL-VA stimulation (AMASSIAN, 1967). Simi-

6 DAYS

SHORT TRAVEL CP

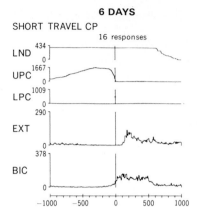

LONG TRAVEL CP

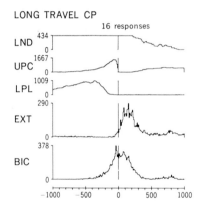

SUPERIMPOSED 2X GAIN

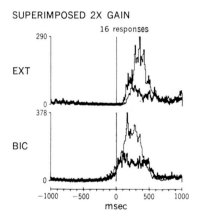

Fig. 3 Relationship in a 6 day kitten of EMG activities in CP to the distance traversed to the top corner of the placer. From above downwards, 16 summed pre- and postcontact histograms are shown of the landing indicator (LND), the output from the upper photocells (UPC), the output from a lower photocell (LPC), integrated EMGs from extensor digitorum longus (EXT) and biceps (BIC). LND indicates small currents generated by dissimilar metal potentials when kitten completes circuit on landing. Short and long travel placing, produced by contact near, and 5 cm below, top corner respectively, with the trials interspersed. The restoration of the upper photocell output (that is, when the forepaw clears the top corner) is used as the 'O' reference prior to summing the responses. Bottom histograms obtained by superimposing start of biceps response during long travel (thin trace) on that during short travel (heavy trace). The ability to superimpose the initial portions of the responses implies kitten had no warning as to type of travel. Other details in text.

larly cooling (Fig. 5), or starting a spreading depression in post dimple SI (AMASSIAN, 1967) reduces the peak components before any reduction of the *initial* disynaptic component of the bulbar PT response occurs. Extirpating SII also reduces the bulbar PT response to VP stimulation, the peak component usually being more affected than the initial, disynaptic component.

Such findings imply that the excitatory interneuron responsible for the *initial* activation of large PT neurons by VP is located closeby, that is, it is a "short" interneuron supplied

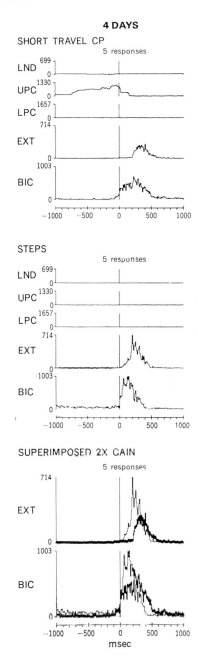

Fig. 4 Comparison in a 4 day kitten of EMG activities in CP and stepping. Abbreviations as in Fig. 3. The start of biceps activity is used as the 'O' reference in summing the responses. Bottom histograms obtained by superimposing start of CP (heavy trace) and step (thin trace). Other details in text.

by VP thalamocortical projections terminating near large PT neurons (cf. STRICK, 1975). By contrast, interneurons mediating the *later* components have long projection axons.

The sensory modalities projecting to individual PT neurons and their columnar organization in the adult cat have been amply described by WELT et al. (1967) and ASANUMA et al. (1968). We found that both sustained, high frequency driving during, for example, rubbing forelimb skin and short latency (10–20 msec) responses of large individual PT neurons to contact with the contralateral forepaw were lost after destruction of VP

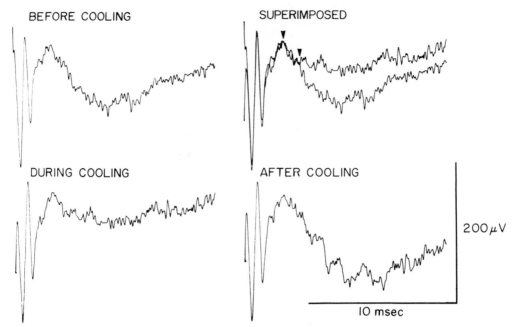

Fig. 5 Effect of cooling SI on ipsilateral bulbar pyramidal responses to VP stimulation. Each record shows summed, 10 sequential responses to stimulation at 1 per 4 sec. Positivity of PT electrode indicated by downward deflection. Cooling probe covered most of exposed SI, with anterior edge 3 mm behind the cruciate sulcus. Thermistor on pia close to cooling probe recorded temperatures initially of 34°C (before cooling record), 8–14°C (during cooling record) and 27°C (after cooling record). Series for record 'during cooling' started approximately $5\frac{3}{4}$ min after ethanol-dry CO_2 mixture in probe; record 'after cooling' started $3\frac{3}{4}$ min after cooling discontinued. Arrow heads in superimposed record indicate disynaptic PT component. Prior initially positive, triphasic response is volume recording of antidromic response in underlying medial lemniscus. (AMASSIAN and WEINER, 1966; AMASSIAN, 1967)

(AMASSIAN et al., 1972a). Long latency (60–150 msec) changes could still be evoked in PT neurons by contralateral contact, a finding consistent with the sparing of less direct afferent inputs to PT neurons, for example, those relaying through VL-VA.

The pathway for short latency responses of large PT neurons following contact with skin, especially hairs, might either be relayed by VP to the 'short' motor cortical interneuron or through projections from SI coronal or postdimple cortex or SII (see above). The ability to drive PT neurons from the periphery persists after locally cooling SI, suggesting the importance of the short interneuron relay (THOMPSON et al., 1970). However, the evidence does not exclude coronal cortex or SII as other possible sites of the relay, or the possibility that the SI relay might adequately replace the short interneuron if the latter could be eliminated.

b) Motor correlates of the VP projection system. The loss of contralateral CP following massive lesions or cooling in VP has been described elsewhere (AMASSIAN et al., 1972a). Lesions that are incomplete ventrally, tend to spare CP to stimulation of the digits but abolish CP to stimulation of proximal parts of the limb.

The early phase (20–40 msec latency) of biceps activation in forelimb CP is also lost following VP destruction. Any biceps responses recorded are quite delayed (for example, 68–234 msec) and are unaccompanied by inhibition of the extensor digitorum longus. (Fig. 6, bottom right).

Given the evidence that the VP projection system is normally required for adult CP

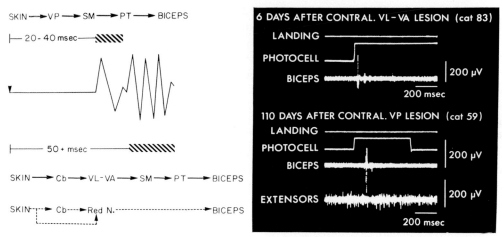

Fig. 6 Proposed modes of activation of prime movers in adult CP and effects thereon of VL-VA and VP lesions. At left, diagrammatic representation of initial contributions by VP and cerebello-VL & VA projection systems to early and later activations of prime movers, for example, biceps (Note that later contribution by VP system is not precluded). Delay for contribution by cerebello-rubral outflow is believed closer to that for VL & VA than for VP circuit (Details in appropriate sections and discussion).

At right, examples of early and late biceps responses, respectively, to contact stimulation after VL-VA (top) and VP lesions (bottom). CP negative after both lesions.

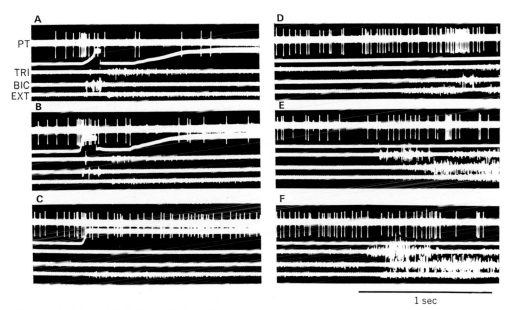

Fig. 7 Activity of individual bulbar PT axon during CP and ongoing movements of contralateral forepaw. From above downwards each record shows PT unit discharges, output from photocell which if forepaw withdraws is replaced by output from strain gauge to signal landing, contralateral triceps, biceps and extensor digitorum longus EMGs. A, B and C show effect of contact stimulation. D, E and F show different types of ongoing movement.

and for short latency, dynamic driving of large PT neurons, the question arises as to whether the VP→large PT neuron link accounts for some aspect of CP.   Certainly, individual PT neurons with cutaneous fields that are stimulated when the contralateral forepaw contacts the placer are powerfully driven at short latency.   Figure 7, (A) and (B) show such examples of discharge by the PT neuron preceding any EMG changes or CP.   The contact in (C) resulted in a lesser discharge by the PT neuron without activation of biceps or later of triceps, or inhibition of the extensor digitorum longus or CP.   The discharge of the PT neuron was not linked to biceps activation in other types of ongoing movement (E and F), but was apparently linked in (D).

Figure 13 in AMASSIAN et al. (1972a) displays the pre- and postcontact histograms of a local hairfield PT neuron which similarly discharged prior to any changes in EMG activity or CP of the stimulated contralateral forepaw.

Nevertheless, the VP→large PT neuron link is an insufficient cortical output for CP. Thus destruction of VL-VA temporarily abolishes CP, but not the *early* activation of biceps; high frequency driving of a PT neuron by ongoing cutaneous stimulation is also spared even during sleep (Fig. 8).

Does the VP→PT link account for at least the early activation of biceps in CP?   Timing the delays around the putative loop yielded latencies of 8–12 msec for the population VP

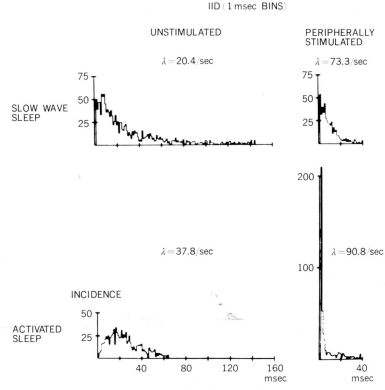

Fig. 8 Effect of physiological stimulation during sleep on discharge by an individual bulbar PT axon recorded after ipsilateral VL-VA destruction. Interspike interval distributions shown of discharge during slow wave (above) and activated sleep (below) without peripheral stimulation (left) and during tapping of contralateral forelimb (right). Regardless of the type of sleep, the mean rate and relative incidence of very brief intervals is markedly increased by peripheral stimulation.

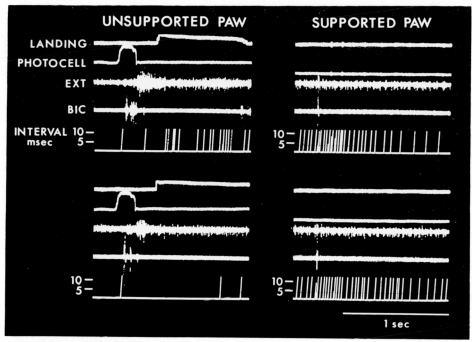

Fig. 9 Effect of supporting the paw on responses to peripheral stimulation by an individual bulbar PT axon and by forelimb muscles. At left, from above downwards, outputs from landing indicator, photocell indicating contact, contralateral extensor digitorum longus and biceps EMGs, and 12 msec ramp which is interrupted and restarted by each discharge of the PT axon. Two examples of CP shown. At right, two examples of supported paw being gently tapped, yielding briefer intervals between discharges, but less EMG response.

response and 12–16 msec for the initial discharge by the individual PT neuron, respectively and 8 msec for the earliest biceps response to an electrical stimulus to motor cortex (Fig. 17 (A) in AMASSIAN et al., 1972a). These delays are consistent with biceps activation occurring as early as 20–24 msec after contact, provided that spatiotemporal summation of PT discharges on the lower motor centers occurs during CP equivalent to that engendered by an electrical stimulus to motor cortex.

The motor effects of repetitive discharge by cutaneous field PT neurons appears to be powerfully controlled by a gate, perhaps located at the level of the spinal interneuron (ILLERT et al., 1974). Thus, single PT neurons can be driven at high frequency (over 200/sec) by mechanical stimulation of the *supported* or held forepaw, but produce little or no movement; by contrast, stimulation only of the *unsupported* paw leads to CP (Fig. 9). Presumably, lifting the forepaw off a support "opens the gate", increasing thereby the motor consequences of the PT discharge.

The role of the cerebello-VL & VA projection system in CP by adult cats
   a) Synaptic basis and connectivities. The VL-VA projection system activates large PT neurons both monosynaptically and polysynaptically (AMASSIAN and WEINER, 1966). YOSHIDA et al. (1966) demonstrated an overall disynaptic circuit from cerebellar outflow to large PT neurons.

The behavioral state strongly inflences the efficacy of the polysynaptic input, which is depressed in the awake cat, but is prominent during slow wave sleep (WEINER and

AMASSIAN, 1970). Thus, VL-VA drives large PT and probably other corticofugal neurons monosynaptically during the behavioral state when CP can best be elicited.

Even a 'maximal' VL-VA stimulus caused *monosynaptic* discharge by only a small fraction (10–15%) of the pool of large PT neurons. Potentiation up to 80% occurs following tetanic stimulation, but was much less than that observed by LLOYD (1949) at the moto-neuron. The inability to discharge a higher fraction of large PT neurons, even after a tetanus, may result from a number of factors. We suggested that VL-VA projections were sparsely distributed in the PT population. Recent studies on such projections while not settling this issue, showed by morphological and physiological methods that projections from a given focus in VL were remarkably wide spread (MASSION et al., 1972; STRICK, 1973; ASANUMA et al., 1974). Another factor may be the large core resistance of the spiny process synapse which limits the flow of outward current from central portions of the neuron (RALL and RENZEL, 1971). Possibly, the evolution of such synaptic processes allows a *consistency* in synaptic activation associated with high quantal transmitter release to be combined with a *subthreshold* effect on discharge appropriate for an integrating output neuron from the SM cortex.

The cerebellar roof nuclear inputs to VL-VA and the red N. have been extensively studied and were reviewed by EVARTS and THACH (1969) and recently by ALLEN and TSUKAHARA (1974).

b) Motor correlates of the cerebello-VL & VA projection system.

Cerebellum. The temporary loss of ipsilateral CP following massive lesions or cooling of N. interpositus and dentatus has been described elsewhere (AMASSIAN et al., 1972a, b). When CP had returned following such lesions, or during mild cooling, CP had an increased latency and was markedly hypermetric in both vertical and horizontal axes.

Inhibition of CP by aversive conditioning with water occurred after massive unilateral lesions of N. interpositus alone, or with N. dentatus, or of N. fastigius (AMASSIAN et al., 1974). Evidently, the cerebellum does have an important role in the coordination of movements in adult CP, but is dispensable in the *occurrence* of CP and of *plasticity* of this type of behavior.

The effect of lesions or cooling of the cerebellar roof N. on biceps activity in CP is variable. Although early biceps activation was spared when later components were reduced by cooling sufficiently to abolish CP (Fig. 23 in AMASSIAN et al., 1972a), biceps activation was markedly delayed early in recovery (3 days) after a N. interpositus-dentate lesion (Fig. 10, left). CP was fast and the biceps was activated early by 14 days (Fig. 10, right). Similarly, anodically polarizing these roof N. resulted in loss of CP and even the initial component of biceps activation (Fig. 24 in AMASSIAN et al., 1972a).

The latency of response by individual cerebellar roof N. neurons during CP is of crucial importance in interpreting the alterations in biceps activation described above. Most N. interpositus neurons projecting to VL which responded during CP were initially activated and subsequently were depressed. Only exceptionally did activation occur prior to the 20–30 msec period after contact (AMASSIAN et al., 1972a). Thus, a dynamic pathway through N. interpositus could not account for the earliest biceps activity recorded in CP, but clearly occurs early enough to contribute dynamically later during lifting-withdrawal. It is of interest that the increase in interpositus neuronal firing was better correlated with the promptness of withdrawal than with the amount of early biceps activation. Thus, the loss of even the earliest biceps activation when N. interpositus-dentate activities are reduced probably depends on the removal of tonic (precontact) facilitation of the dynamic circuit driving biceps. The latencies of discharge by N.

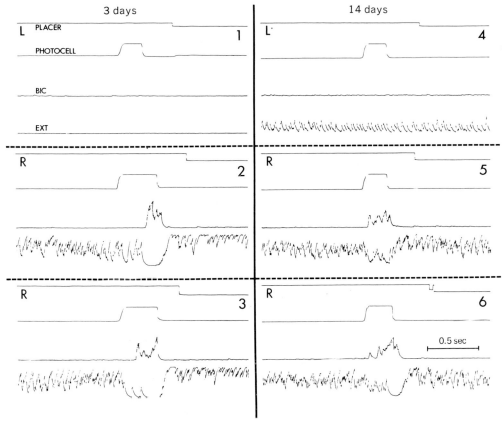

Fig. 10 Effect of lesion of N. interpositus and dentatus on CP and on responses by ipsilateral forelimb muscles. From above downwards, each record shows output of landing keys, photocell indicating contact, biceps and extensor digitorum longus integrated EMGs. The larger the deflection on the keys output, the greater was the horizontal distance reached by the paw on landing (AMASSIAN et al., 1972a). Side (L) contralateral to lesion shows normal CPs at 3 days (1) and 14 days (4) after lesion. Side (R) ipsilateral to lesion shows at 3 days (2, 3), hypermetric CP, slowed withdrawal and delayed biceps activation. At 14 days (5, 6), CP still hypermetric, but withdrawal not delayed and biceps activation occurred early. Right interpositus N. mainly destroyed; anteriorly some medial cells and posteriorly some ventral cells spared. Small ventral portion of dentate N. spared throughout rostrocaudal extent.

interpositus neurons recorded by ECCLES et al. (1975) to tapping the forelimb in acute preparations, peaked at 19 msec and thus were usually shorter than those we recorded during CP. However, our conclusions are based largely on the estimated *interval* between neuronal and muscle activities, so that any absolute errors in latency measurements in the behaving cat should be minimized.

VL-VA. The prolonged loss of contralateral CP following massive lesions of VL-VA and the temporary loss of CP following cooling of these nuclei have been described elsewhere (AMASSIAN et al., 1972a). The loss of CP following destruction of VL-VA is rather specific, proprioceptive correction recovering long before CP, and CP to stimulation of dorsal or medial aspects of the forepaw long before the response to lateral stimulation, which may still be depressed one month postoperatively. Elsewhere, we have suggested that lateral CP is a more recently evolved and complex movement than dorsal CP, a *synergy* of flexors and extensors of the ulnar carpals being required for lateral deviation of the forepaw at the wrist (AMASSIAN and ROSS, 1978a).

During recovery from a massive VL-VA lesion, the response to contact is at first a prominent 'jerk', which often becomes repetitive before an occasional delayed placing is achieved. More strikingly, antero-ventral lesions in VL-VA, sparing much of the motor cortical response to stimulation of the cerebellar outflow, are followed within a few days by the return of CP with a pronounced 'jerky' quality. However, inhibition of contra-lateral CP during water conditioning (WERTENBAKER et al., 1973) is absent, as shown in Figure 1 of AMASSIAN et al. (1974). Such lack of conditioning does not depend on the loss of the aversive quality of the water, because the passively immersed paw is rapidly withdrawn from water. We proposed that both the 'jerky' quality of CP and the lack of water conditioning reflected the loss of an inhibitory function of the VA-VL complex, distinct from the function of processing the cerebellar outflow.

The early phase of biceps activation not only persists after a VL-VA lesion but over-shadows in amplitude any later components (Fig. 6, top right). Presumably, the pro-minent early phase of biceps activity accounts for the jerk, the failure to place being explained by an insufficient total output by the flexors (especially biceps) and of forward protrusion of the forelimb.

A single electrical stimulus delivered to VL-VA either when contact of the forepaw occurs or soon after, delays or prevents CP and alters the pattern of biceps activation (Fig. 11). The sustained, later phase of biceps activation normally following the initial phase (top left record) is replaced by a periodic discharge with reduced reciprocal innerva-

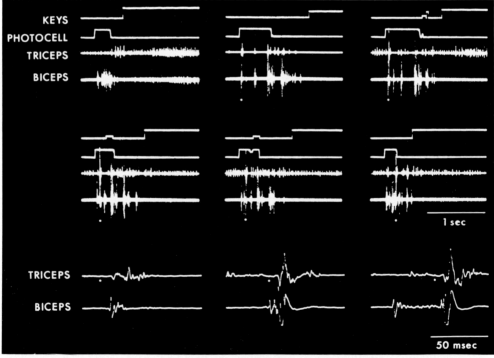

Fig. 11 Effect of single electrical stimulus to anterior VA on contralateral CP and muscle responses. Same cat as in Fig. 10; VA stimulated contralateral to the N interpositus-dentate lesion. Top and middle records show from above downwards, output of landing keys, photocell indicating contact, triceps and biceps EMGs. Top left shows placing to contact above. Subsequent records from series in which VA stimulus (indicated by dot) delivered 15, 38, 55, 105 and 180 msec after contact. Bottom records, at faster sweep speed, show increasing EMG responses to stimulus when delay increased from 15 to 38 to 55 msec.

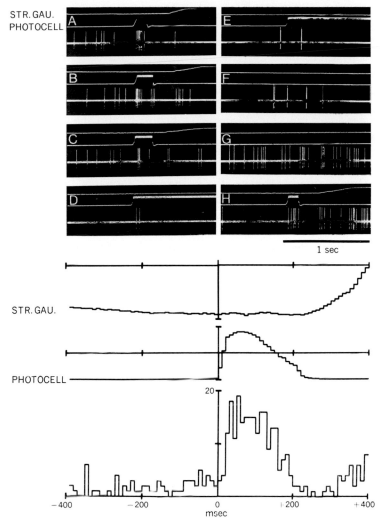

Fig. 12 Early responses by an individual VA neuron during contralateral CP and effect of drowsiness. Above, each record in series A to H shows strain gauge output indicating landing, photocell output indicating contact, and discharges by VA neuron. Contact in A, B and C followed by high frequency response and placing. CP failed and responses reduced in D and absent in E. Spindling pattern of high frequency discharge (F) desynchronized by massaging paw (G). Neuronal response and placing to contact restored (H).

Below, pre- and postcontact histograms of neuronal discharges and transducer outputs. 35 CPs summed. (from Fig. 2, AMASSIAN et al., 1972b)

tion of triceps, unless the stimulus is presented a long delay after contact (180 msec in middle right record). CP depression could also be elicited by a VL-VA stimulus, which when presented alone caused no movement. Backfiring of N. interpositus and dentate fibers projecting to VL-VA was probably not responsible for the CP depression because in the experiment illustrated these nuclei had largely been destroyed by an antecedent lesion. Furthermore, direct activation of PT fibers was not required for the CP depression, which was lessened when the stimulating electrodes were lowered deep to the thalamus, producing large direct activation of PT fibers. Presumably, the CP depression results from a disruption either of the VL-VA or the SM cortical activity which drives the later component of biceps and other muscles required for effective lifting-withdrawal in CP.

The earliest discharge by individual VL-VA neurons following contralateral contact stimulation occurred significantly later than that by cutaneous type PT neurons. An early response commencing in the 20–30 msec bin of the pre- and postcontact histogram is shown in Figure 12, A, B and C. An additional response by the neuron occurred long after the top corner of the placing apparatus had been cleared, that is, after *activity of the antagonists had commenced* (also Fig. 13 below). Figure 12 also shows the reduction (C) or the loss (D) of the response by the VA neuron and the loss of CP when the cat became drowsy. In the drowsy behavioral state the irregularly occurring, isolated resting discharges were replaced by grouped high frequency "spindling" type discharges (cf. A-C with E-F). After massaging a paw, the pattern of discharge became desynchronized (G), both the response of the neuron and placing returning to contact stimulation (H).

The use of water conditioning permits a further test of the contingency relationship between VL-VA neuronal activity and CP. The pre- and postcontact histograms in Figure 13, show discharges by the VL neuron commencing soon after the preconditioning contact and continuing until landing. During water conditioning, the behavioral responses to contact could be classified either as 'placing' or 'no placing'. The VL neuron gave slightly delayed and no responses, respectively, during these behavioral responses. Both the early responses by the neuron and CP were restored after disinhibition by passively resting the forepaw on a solid surface.

When the resting discharge by a VL-VA neuron was *inhibited* by contact in the control period, inhibition of CP during water conditioning resulted in a loss of the inhibition of the discharge. Thus water conditioning does not simply reduce excitability of VL-VA neurons, but reduces the changes, be they excitatory or inhibitory, following contact stimulation.

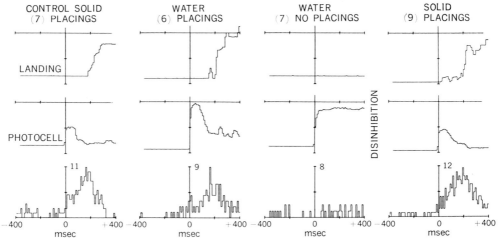

Fig. 13 Effect of water conditioning on forepaw CP and responses by contralateral individual VL neuron. From left to right pre- and postcontact histograms of transducer outputs and discharges by neuron before conditioning, during water conditioning when outcome was either 'placing' or 'no placing' and after disinhibition by resting the forepaw on a solid surface for many seconds (conditioning apparatus described in WERTENBAKER et al., 1973 and AMASSIAN et al., 1974). Neuron was fired at 1.8 msec by stimulation of contralateral cerebellar outflow. From left to right, mean rates of discharge were 4.7/trial, 2.7/trial, 1.6/trial and 2.3/trial respectively, for the 400 msec period preceding contact.

The precontact mean rate of discharge often changed as a result of water conditioning, particularly when the rate before control successful contacts was compared with that preceding inhibited placings. Less commonly, after disinhibition the changed precontact mean rate of discharge reverted to the control rate.

The role of the cerebello-rubral outflow in CP by adult cats

The depression of contralateral CP following destruction of the red N. rivals in severity that following extirpation of the SM cortex. Because destruction of N. interpositus and dentatus cause only a transient depression of CP, the effect of red N. destruction is not attributable to the concomittant loss of the nearby cerebellar input to the higher SM control system, but implies an important role in adult CP of the red N. (AMASSIAN et al., 1972a).

The role of the rubral outflow in adult CP must likely depends on cerebellar roof N. input to this nucleus. Thus, cooling N. interpositus (with dentatus) in a cat in which CP had recovered following a lesion disconnecting VL-VA from the cerebellar outflow, resulted in the reversible loss of CP (Fig. 32, ibid).

We have not yet recorded pre- and postcontact histograms of activities of individual rubral neurons during CP. PADEL and STEINBERG (1978) demonstrated early firing of rubral neurons during a modified (perhaps proprioceptive) placing reaction, but the time resolution available does not permit a direct comparison with our data on muscle activities in CP. In acute preparations, ECCLES et al. (1975) found latencies of response by individual rubral and interpositus neurons to stimulation of peripheral nerves were usually similar. If the argument is accepted that N. interpositus neurons fire too late to contribute dynamically to the *earliest* biceps activity but may contribute to later activity during lifting-withdrawal (see above), then the rubral outflow could be expected to make a similar contribution. These authors also discuss an input to red N. bypassing the cerebellum.

Subcortical circuitry subserving CP in the young kitten

By contrast with the adult cat, unilateral removal of SM cortex, the nearby mesial surface and varying amounts of SII prior to the 4th postnatal week is followed by recovery of CP to stimulation of each of the 4 forepaw fields (refs in AMASSIAN and Ross, 1978a). When the operated kitten ages to 5–9 weeks, CP becomes secondarily depressed, but may be restored by administration of d-amphetamine. An extirpation made *initially* after the 5th postnatal week is followed by a severe deficit in CP.

The 'stand alone' capacity of the subcortical circuit to manage forelimb CP in the young kitten requires supraspinal structures (AMASSIAN et al., 1977). Thus, transecting the spinal cord at C1-C2, with the kitten artificially respirated, abolishes all forepaw CP, even when withdrawal reflexes are present. Full CP could not be elicited after decerebration below the low pontine level. Unilateral, high frequency lesions made in midbrain decerebrate kittens were followed by ipsilateral loss of CP when the vestibular N. complex was destroyed (Fig. 1, ibid). Whether the vestibular N. function dynamically or tonically in CP has not yet been determined.

Analysis of the circuitry subserving hindlimb CP is complicated by the release of stepping following either a high cervical or a low thoracic transection. We have been unable to confirm the claim that the circuitry for *full* hindlimb CP is present in the spinal kitten (FORSSBERG et al., 1974). Responses to stimulation of dorsal (and medial) aspects of the hindpaw can be elicited an hour after spinal transection, but lateral CP is virtually absent and posterior CP absent during observation periods up to 34 days (In very rare trials where CP appeared to have occurred to lateral stimulation, lateral carriage of the hindpaw was minimal).   Given the omnipresent stepping, it seems unwise to interpret the responses to dorsal and medial stimulation as true CPs rather than triggered steps.   The failure to elicit posterior CP in the spinal kitten may be especially significant because the patterns of activity in tibialis anterior and gastrocnemius are quite different in stepping and posterior CP (Amassian, 1975).   It may also be noted that the phase dependent reflex reversal present in spinal kittens (Forssberg et al., 1975) is not apparent in CP by the intact kitten, the forepaw undergoing lifting-withdrawal whether initially contacted in the extended or the flexed position.

Emerging role of SM cortex and PT neurons in young kittens

During the 2nd and 3rd postnatal weeks, extirpation of SM cortex under a volatile anesthetic is followed by a *transient* asymmetry between lateral CP by the two forepaws, contralateral CP exhibiting the greater depression.   The implication that SM cortex might have a role in CP prior to the loss of the stand alone capacity of the subcortical circuitry was directly tested using the cooling technique.   Starting at the 2nd week, cooling the SM cortex, internal capsule or bulbar PT selectively depressed contralateral placing to lateral contact.   Cooling the SM cortex was tested during the first postnatal week, but was usually inffective.

The role in lateral CP of SM cortical neurons, in particular PT neurons, did not depend on dynamic inputs relayed by the VP and VL-VA thalamocortical projection systems. Thus cooling VP and VL-VA sufficiently to block the SI and MI responses to stimulating contralateral periphery and cerebellar outflows, respectively, did not abolish contralateral lateral CP.   The conclusion—that starting at the second week PT neurons subserve lateral CP by tonic activity is supported by the finding of a marked increase in resting discharge by PT neurons in the second as compared with the first postnatal week (This brief account is based on Amassian and Ross, 1978a, b).

The relative unimportance of thalamic inputs in mediating CP by the 4 week old kitten is underscored by the lack of increase in the pre-existing hypermetria following a combined lesion of intermediate and lateral cerebellar cortex and N. interpositus and dentatus (Amassian and Rudell, 1978).   Furthermore, individual VL-VA neurons recorded in a kitten as young as 3 weeks showed only small increases or decreases in discharge rate during CP as compared with the responses in 7 week or older kittens (following section).

The transition from juvenile to adult circuitry subserving CP

Lesions or cooling of intermediate and lateral zones of cerebellar cortex from the 7th postnatal week onwards (that is, after CP movements have become perfected) resulted in markedly hypermetric CP (Fig. 2).   The average speed of lifting either increased or was unchanged, but, significantly, the *latency* of *lifting was not increased.*   By contrast, cooling N. interpositus abolished or delayed CP (Amassian and Rudell, 1978; Amassian et al., 1978).   We proposed that N interpositus drives the prime movers of CP (for example, biceps), hypermetria being prevented by an inhibitory output from cerebellar cortex unless reduced by a lesion or by cooling.

Significantly, VL-VA cooling during the 6th to 10th week, or permanent lesions in VL-VA made during the 7th to 9th week resulted in deficits in contralateral CP approaching those seen in the adult cat (Amassian and Ross, 1978a).   Furthermore, recordings from individual VL-VA neurons from the 7th week onward revealed either marked increases or decreases in activity occurring during CP.   Figure 14, left shows pre- and postcontact histograms of a VL neuron recorded at 43 days.   This neuron commenced responding in the 240–260 msec bin after contacts that resulted in successful placings.

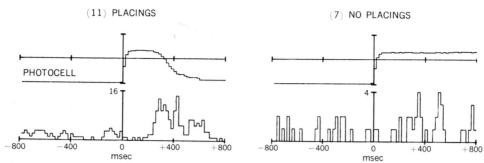

Fig. 14   Activity of individual VL neuron in 43 day old kitten during placing by contralateral forepaw.   Pre- and postcontact histograms of photocell output (above) and neuronal discharge (below) when outcome of contact was 'placing' (left) or 'no placing' (right).   Neuron responded usually at 2.1–2.5 msec to stimulation of contralateral cerebellar outflow.   Technique used in recording from individual neurons in kittens during CP similar to that in AMASSIAN et al. (1972a).   Differences in precontact rate of discharge discussed in text.

Because biceps activation started much earlier (60–80 msec), this VL neuron could only have contributed to later components in lifting—withdrawal.   Unsuccessful placings (right) were unaccompanied by such increases over the precontact rate of discharge. The mean rates of discharge were 6.1 spikes/trial and 3.6 spikes/trial during the 0.8 sec periods preceding contacts followed by 'placing' and 'no placing', respectively.   Therefore, the *precontact rate of discharge can serve as a predictor of the outcome of the contact stimulus.*

Thus, by the 7th postnatal week, the cerebellar outflow is functionally part of the higher SM system controlling CP and a major cerebellar target, VL-VA has acquired many of the properties of the adult nuclear complex in CP.

DISCUSSION

The use of a variety of experimental procedures has led to the conclusion that adult CP is subserved by multiple circuits in the higher SM control system.   Dynamic (transcortical) loops in the VP and cerebello- VL & VA thalamocortical projection systems most likely start contributing to the initial and later components, respectively, of liftingwithdrawal in the first phase of CP (Fig. 6, left).   The cerebello-rubral outflow is also implicated in CP, but probably contributes after the earliest component of the response. Given the bilateral afferent input to the red N. (ECCLES et al., 1975), the rubral projection system is a possible contributor to crossplacing seen after VL-VA lesions (AMASSIAN et al., 1972a) and a possible alternative to the VP system in accounting for recovery of CP following such lesions.

The VP and the VL-VA projection systems are not simply parallel systems, differing only in the shorter transit time of the VP→PT link.   Thus, the VP projection system permits the driving of PT neurons at high frequency by cutaneous stimulation under a variety of conditions (for example, supported limb or during sleep) in which motor responses are small or absent.   Such findings do not contradict the existence of motor cortical input-output columns (ASANUMA et al., 1968), but emphasize the importance of other conditions, perhaps the state of a 'spinal' gate, in determining whether the PT activity is expressed in movement.   Although muscle activities in dorsal CP of the forepaw are the reverse of those expected from the action of the input-output columns (but see SAKATA and MIYAMOTO, 1968), reversal of such action depending on whether the forepaw was 'not supported' versus 'supported', perhaps analogous to reflex reversal during stepping (FORSSBERG et al., 1975), would permit a role of the input-output columns in CP. Cross-correlation between PT neuronal and muscle activities (FETZ and CHENEY, 1978) in CP may help to resolve this issue, but because the link in the cat is disynaptic (ILLERT et al., 1974) rather than monosynaptic, the technique may be less successful in cat than in monkey.

The VL-VA projection system is markedly altered during behavioral conditions, including type II conditioning, which depress CP. Individual VL-VA neurons exhibit reduced responses to contact when CP is depressed, but it is unclear whether VL-VA is the decision node or merely reflects changes occurring in its inputs.

The VP and VL-VA projection systems do not merely differ functionally, they activate overlapping, but not identical populations of individual PT neurons. In a sample of 54 bulbar PT axons, 65 per cent were fired by stimulating VL-VA, 72 per cent by VP stimulation and 37 per cent by stimulation of either system (AMASSIAN and WEINER, 1968). The problem of whether PT neurons exclusively driven by VL-VA or VP have differing motor actions is unresolved, but again might be elucidated by crosscorrelation techniques.

Certain similarities in the circuitry subserving load compensation in monkeys and CP were previously discussed (Introduction). The increased output in biceps occurring when the forepaw unexpectedly is required to lift through an increased distance is similarly delayed by at least 40 msec from the onset of added sensory signals generated by the continued ascent of the forepaw up the contacted surface. Such delays for load related biceps output are sufficient for a transcortical loop. By contrast, the delay for activation of the extensors of the digits when the forepaw has cleared the top corner after a long ascent is very brief in adult cats, or even in kittens a few days to 7 weeks in age. The change in muscle activities occurring during CP when the top corner is cleared most likely depends on a low level, possibly spinal loop.

In the kitten, the circuitry subserving CP is at first entirely subcortical, but starting with the second week a (dispensable) participation by PT neurons was detected, which as late as the 4th week occurs through tonic activity. We have argued else where (AMASSIAN and Ross, 1978b) that the need for orderly development of the higher SM control system may conflict with the need to develop a useful behavior-CP. Given the long delays in poorly myelinated or unmyelinated pathways for afferent transmission to SM cortex and efferent transmission to forelimb muscles, the development of a fast dynamic circuit at the subcortical level permits an acceleration of CP to occur even during the first postnatal week. The subcortical circuit requires the vestibular N. complex for full CP, the spinal kitten exhibiting no forelimb CP and, equivocally, part of the full hindlimb response (section on subcortical circuitry above).

Electrophysiological analysis reveals that conduction in afferent and efferent connections of SM cortex becomes accelerated before the subcortical circuit has begun losing its 'stand alone' capacity to manage CP in the 5th week. By the 7th week, the cerebellum, VL-VA and SM cortex perform important functional roles in CP through afferent and efferent connections with transit times that, as in the adult cat, are only a small fraction of the latency of the first phase of the behavior, lifting-withdrawal (AMASSIAN and Ross, 1978b).

The development of the circuitry for adult CP seems to imply both an unduly complex basis for a 'simple postural reflex' and that multiple, dynamic transcortical loops have important advantages over the prior subcortical circuitry. However, the trajectory of the forepaw after CP has become perfected by the 7th week is not at all simple, the near vertical initial movement resulting from a *simultaneously* coordinated angular rotation occurring at *two* or *more* joints in the forelimb (section on movement and muscle activities above). Consider the simplest case of angular rotation at shoulder and elbow with a unity ratio of length of upper arm to length of extremity below the elbow and with the limb initially straight and at 90° to the trunk; then a given vertical movement of the paw is specified by unique angular rotations occurring at the elbow (flexion) and the shoulder (posterior flexion) with a constant ratio (2 : 1) between these rotations during the vertical movements. The problem in preserving the ratio between angular rotations at two joints is greatly increased if movements at a third or more joints occur, as seems likely because the flexor mass of the digits is also a prime mover in CP. The number of combinations of angular rotations at three forelimb joints satisfying the condition of a given vertical displacement of the forepaw is vastly increased over the above, two joint solution. Thus, by the 7th week, in addition to truncating the *length* of the trajectory by inhibiting N. interpositus output to the prime movers (AMASSIAN et al., 1978), a subtle role of cerebellar cortex in CP is to elicit the simultaneous angular rotations at several joints of the forelimb producing given vertical and horizontal movements of the paw.

While the utility in mature CP of the cerebellar contribution through VL-VA to the SM cortical control system is apparent, that of the VP projection system is less obvious. However, CP can only occur swiftly if the inertial mass of the unsupported limb is first rapidly accelerated by the prime movers which may be activated at short latency, if imprecisely, by the VP→large PT neuronal link. We have also commented on the possible informational role of such PT neurons, which through collaterals signal to widely separate regions of the CNS the incidence and location of a cutaneous contact (AMASSIAN et al., 1972a).

Our previous experiments disclosed that CP abolished either by lesions of SM cortex or during cooling of N. interpositus with dentatus could be partially restored by tonic 100/sec stimulation of the red N. (ibid). Figure 15 shows that after an SM cortical lesion, contact failed to elicit placing (2) except during 100/sec rubral stimulation (3). When the contact occurred far below the top corner of the placing apparatus (1), as in CP by the

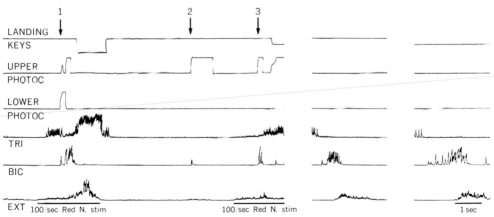

Fig. 15 Return of contralateral dorsal CP during 100/sec red N. stimulation after a previous SM cortical lesion. At left, from above downwards, output from keys indicating landing, from upper photocell indicating contact near top corner, from lower photocell indicating contact 8 cm below top corner, integrated EMGs from triceps, biceps, and extensors of digits and carpi ulnaris. 1 and 3 show successful CP during 100/sec bipolar stimulation of red N. with 50 μ sec rectangular pulses at 4.0–4.2 mA. 80 days prior to this recording, SM cortex unilateraly extirpated except for part of coronal cortex anteriorly. For comparison, two spontaneous movements shown at right.

intact cat the output from biceps was increased and activation of the triceps and the extensors delayed until the forepaw had cleared the top corner. Do such observations contradict the hypothesis of dynamic transcortical loops in adult CP? Tonic rubral stimulation never restores the fine movements exhibited by mature CP, that is, there is no evidence that the subtler aspect of cerebellar influence can be duplicated. Furthermore, tonic activity and certainly that engendered by 100/sec rubral stimulation is probably very inefficient in terms of the total number of nerve impulses expended in securing an occasional behavior. A temporarily 'opened door' for the SM cortical output systems, cued by the lack of support for the forepaw, and triggered by cutaneous contact, may economize in the impulses required to produce CP.

SUMMARY

The neural circuitry subserving contact placing of the forelimb in the adult cat and kitten is reexamined, with particular emphasis on the possible roles of dynamic, SM cortical loops. Dynamic participation of the VP and the cerebello-VL & VA thalamo-cortical projection systems in adult CP is reaffirmed and the contribution of the cerebello-rubral outflow is discussed. The functions of the VP and cerebello-VL & VA projection systems are compared and the closer relationship of the latter to the behavior is emphasized.

The circuitry subserving CP in the young kitten at first does not include SM cortex, but does require brainstem structures such as the vestibular N. Subsequently, when conduction in afferent and efferent systems of the SM cortex is still slowed, PT neurons participate in CP through tonic activities. By the 7th postnatal week, the influence of the cerebellum in securing a mature trajectory of the forepaw during CP is manifest. Maturation of the afferent and efferent SM cortical systems has also continued, providing the substrate for dynamic SM cortical control of CP in the adult.

ACKNOWLEDGEMENTS

I am indebted to my past collaborators, Richard Ross, Herbert WEINER and Christian WERTEN-BAKER for their major contributions to the work reported here. The TV-computer technique for tracking movements was designed by Alan RUDELL to whom my further thanks are owed.

REFERENCES

ALLEN, G. I. and TSUKAHARA, N.: Cerebrocerebellar communication systems. *Physiol. Rev.*, *54*: 957–1006 (1974)

AMASSIAN, V. E.: Discussion. *In* YAHR, M. D. and PURPURA, D. P. (eds.): *Neurophysiological Basis of Normal and Abnormal Motor Activities.* pp. 288–292, Raven Press, New York, (1967)

AMASSIAN, V. E.: Backward placing in intact kittens and adult cats. *J. Physiol.*, *London, 252*: 26–27 P (1975)

AMASSIAN, V. E., EBERLE, L. and RUDELL, A.: Mode of cerebellar functioning in contact placing in kittens. *J. Physiol.*, *London, 284*: 179–180 P (1978)

AMASSIAN, V. E., REISINE, H. and WERTENBAKER, C.: Neural pathways subserving plasticity of contact placing. *J. Physiol.*, *London, 242*: 67–69 P (1976)

AMASSIAN, V. E. and ROSS, R.: Developing role of sensorimotor cortex and PT neurons in contact placing in kittens. *J. Physiol.*, *Paris, 74*: 165–184 (1978a)

AMASSIAN, V. E., ROSS, R.: Electrophysiological correlates of the developing higher sensorimotor control system. *J. Physiol.*, *Paris, 74*: 185–201 (1978b)

AMASSIAN, V. E., ROSS, R., WERTENBAKER, C. and WEINER, H.: Cerebellothalamocortical inter-relations in contact placing and other movements in cats. *In* FRIGYESI, T., RINVIK, E. and YAHR,

M. D. (eds.): *Corticothalamic Projections and Sensorimotor Activities*. pp. 395–444, Raven Press, New York (1972a)

AMASSIAN, V. E., ROSS, R. and ZIPSER, B.: A role of the vestibular nuclei in contact placing by kittens. *J. Physiol. London, 266*: 97–98 P (1977)

AMASSIAN, V. E. and RUDELL, A.: When does the cerebellum become important in coordinating contact placing movements? *J. Physiol., London, 276*: 35–36 P (1978)

AMASSIAN, V. E. and WEINER, H.: Monosynaptic and polysynaptic activation of pyramidal tract neurons by thalamic stimulation. *In* PURPURA, D. P. and YAHR, M. D. (eds.): *The Thalamus*. pp. 255–282, Columbia Univ. Press, New York (1966)

AMASSIAN, V. E. and WEINER, H.: Unpublished observations (1968)

AMASSIAN, V. E., WEINER, H. and ROSENBLUM, M.: Neural systems subserving the tactile placing reaction: a model for the study of higher level control of movement. *Brain Res., 40*: 171–178 (1972b)

ASANUMA, H., FERNANDEZ, J., SCHEIBEL, M. E. and SCHEIBEL, A. B.: Characteristics of projections from nucleus ventralis lateralis to the motor cortex in cats: an anatomical and physiological study. *Expl. Brain Res., 20*: 315–330 (1974)

ASANUMA, H., STONEY, S. D., Jr. and ABZUG, C.: Relationship between afferent input and motor outflow in cat motorsensory cortex. *J. Neurophysiol., 31*: 670–681 (1968)

BARD, P.: Localized control of placing and hopping reactions in the cat and their normal management by small cortical remnants. *Arch. Neurol. & Psychiat., 30*: 40 74 (1933)

BARD, P.: Studies on the cortical representation of somatic sensibility. *Harvey Lect., 33*: 143–169 (1938)

CHAMBERS, W. W. and LIU, C. N.: Cortico-spinal tract of the cat: Attempt to correlate the pattern of degeneration with deficits in reflex activity following neocortical lesions. *J. comp. Neurol., 108*: 23–56 (1957)

CONRAD, B., MATSUNAMI, K., MEYER-LOHMANN, J., WIESENDANGER, M. and BROOKS, V. B.: Cortical load compensation during voluntary elbow movements. *Brain Res., 71*: 507–514 (1974)

GRAGO, P. E., HOUK, J. C. and HASAN, Z.: Regulatory actions of human stretch reflex. *J. Neuro physiol., 39*: 925–935 (1976)

ECCLES, J. C., SCHEID, P. and TÁBOVÍKOVÁ, H.: Responses of red nucleus neurons to antidromic and synaptic activation. *J. Neurophysiol., 38*: 947–964 (1975)

EVARTS, E. V.: Relation of pyramidal tract activity to force exerted during voluntary movement. *J. Neurophysiol., 31*: 14–27 (1968)

EVARTS, E. V.: Motor cortex reflexes associated with learned movement. *Science, 179*: 501–503 (1973)

EVARTS, E. V. and THACH, W. T.: Motor mechanisms of the CNS: cerebrocerebellar interrelations. *Ann. Rev. Physiol., 31*: 451–498 (1969)

FETZ, E. E. and FINOCCHIO, D. V.: Operant conditioning of isolated activity in specific muscles and precentral cells. *Brain Res., 40*: 19 23 (1972)

FETZ, E. E. and CHENEY, P. D.: Muscle fields of primate corticomotoneuronal cells. *J. Physiol. Paris., 74*: 239–245 (1978)

FORSSBERG, H., GRILLNER, S. and SJOSTROM, A.: Tactile placing reactions in chronic spinal kittens. *Acta physiol. scand., 92*: 114–120 (1974)

FORSSBERG, H., GRILLNER, S. and ROSSIGNOL, S.: Phase dependent reflex reversal during walking in chronic spinal cats. *Brain Res., 85*: 103–107 (1975)

ILLERT, M., LUNDBERG, A. and TANAKA, R.: Disynaptic cortiospinal effects in forelimb motoneurones in the cat. *Brain Res., 75*: 312–315 (1974)

LAURSEN, A. M. and WIESENDANGER, M.: Motor deficits after transection of bulbar pyramid in the cat. *Acta physiol. scand., 68*: 118–126 (1966)

LIDDELL, E. G. T. and PHILLIPS, C. G.: Pyramidal section in the cat. *Brain, 67*: 1–9 (1944)

LLOYD, D. P. C.: Post-tetanic potentiation of response in monosynaptic reflex pathways of the spinal cord. *J. Gen. Physiol., 33*: 147–170 (1949)

LORENTE DE NÓ, R.: The cerebral cortex architecture, intracortical connections and motor projections. *In* FULTON, J. F. (ed.): *The Physiology of the Nervous System*. pp. 291–325, Oxford Univ. Press, New York, (1938)

MASSION, J. and RISPAL-PADEL, L.:   Differential control of motor cortex and sensory areas on ventro-lateral nucleus of the thalamus.   *In* FRIGYESI, T., RINVIK, E. and YAHR, M. D. (eds.):   *Cortico-thalamic Projections and Sensorimotor Activities.*   pp. 357–374, Raven Press, New York (1972)

OXFORD ENGLISH DICTIONARY, In: Vol. 5. University Press, Oxford (1933)

PADEL, Y. and STEINBERG, R.:   Red nucleus cell activity in awake cats during of a placing reaction.   *J. Physiol. Paris, 74*: 265–282 (1978)

RADEMAKER, G. G. J.:   *Das Stehen,* Springer, Berlin (1931)

RALL, R. and RENZEL, J.:   Dendritic spine function and synaptic attenuation calculations.   *Soc. Neurosc. Abstr.,* 1: 64 (1971)

ROSENTHAL, J., WALLER, H. J. and AMASSIAN, V. E.:   An analysis of the activation of motor cortical neurons by surface stimulation.   *J. Neurophysiol. 30*: 844–858 (1967)

RUDELL, A.:   The television camera used to measure movement.   *Behav. Res. Methods Instrm.* (1979 in press)

SAKATA, H. and MIYAMOTO, J.:   Topographic relationship between the receptive fields of neurons in the motor cortex and the movements elicited by focal stimulation in freely moving cats.   *Jap. J. Physiol., 18*: 489–507 (1968)

SHERRINGTON, C. S.:   *The Integrative Action of the Nervous System.*   Scribner Press, New York (1906)

STRICK, P. L.:   Light microscopic analysis of the cortical projection of the thalamic ventrolateral nucleus in the cat.   *Brain Res., 55*: 1–24 (1973)

STRICK, P. L.:   Multiple sources of thalamic input to the primate motor cortex.   *Brain Res., 88*: 372–377 (1975)

TATTON, W. G., FORNER, S. D., GERSTEIN, G. L., CHAMBERS, W. W. and LIU, C. N.:   The effect of postcentral cortical lesions on motor responses to sudden upper limb displacements in monkeys.   *Brain Res., 96*: 108–113 (1975)

THOMPSON, W. D., STONEY, S. D. and ASANUMA, H.:   Characteristics of projections from primary sensory cortex to motosensory cortex in cats.   *Brain Res., 22*: 15–27 (1970)

WEINER, H. and AMASSIAN, V. E.:   Monosynaptic and disynaptic discharge of pyramidal tract neurons during sleep and wakefulness.   *In* BERTINI, M. (ed.):   *Psicofisiologia Del Sonno E Del Sogno,* pp. 40–47, Vita e Pensiero, Milan (1970)

WELT, C., ASCHOFF, J. C., KAMEDA, K. and BROOKS, V. B.:   Intracortical organization of cat's motorsensory neurons.   *In* YAHR, M. D. and PURPURA, D. P. (eds.):   *Neurophysiological Basis of Normal and Abnormal Motor Acticities.*   pp. 255–293, Raven Press, New York, (1967)

WERTENBAKER, C., ROSS, R. and AMASSIAN, V. E.:   Modification of contact placing by aversive conditioning.   *Brain, Behav. Evol., 8*: 304–320 (1973)

YOSHIDA, M., YAJIMA, K. and UNO, M.:   Different activation of the two types of the pyramidal tract neurons through the cerebello-thalamo-cortical pathway.   *Experientia, 22*: 331–332 (1966)

CONTRIBUTIONS OF CENTRAL PROGRAMS TO RAPID LIMB MOVEMENT IN THE CAT

Claude GHEZ

The Rockefeller University
New York, NY
and
Division of Neurobioogy and Behavior, College of Physicians and Surgeons
Columbia University, New York, NY

INTRODUCTION

Sherrington considered that integration in the nervous system represented "interaction for a purpose" (Granit, 1977). In the case of voluntary responses directed towards a target, these interactions allow the translation of information about stimulus topography into an appropriate pattern of contraction of particular muscles. To be appropriate, however, the magnitude of the underlying neural output must be accurately scaled to particular stimulus variables. Voluntary responses are neither limited by "local sign" nor by the receptor surface transducing the stimulus. Their direction and magnitude is dependent only on the purpose to be achieved. Because of the large array of potential stimulus-response relations, the operation of presetting mechanisms has generally been postulated to reduce the time required for the selection of a particular response (Welford, 1976). Evidence exists that such presetting mechanisms may, in fact, determine the direction of intended responses to kinesthetic perturbations (Evarts and Tanji, 1976). Since quick and accurate responses may be fully completed within less than a single reaction time from their onset, it is also generally recognized that critical parameters of the entire response must be determined by "central programs". There is little information however, concerning the output variables controlled by such central programs or about the control policy governing the generation of responses of different magnitudes. An analysis of these problems is complicated by the fact that, once a motor output is initiated, interactions between the ongoing central commands and afferent activity resulting from the response itself may occur at multiple sites in the nervous system. The function of presetting mechanisms, the response parameters specified by central programs and the constraints imposed by reflex interactions are all critical to an understanding of the physiology of sensory-motor integration in voluntary movement. To obtain a general framework within which these problems could be approached, we have studied tracking performance in the cat. The tracking task we have developed requires rapid and precise movement of the limb or, alternatively, a change in force applied to a lever in accord with sensory information provided by a display. First, we will consider the isometric adjustments in force exerted against a stationary lever. Such isometric conditions provide a simpler circumstance to analyze the commands which control motor responses, since the effects of limb inertia and the viscoelastic properties of limb and muscle may, to a first approximation, be neglected. In addition, variations in active tension and reflex interactions resulting from changes in muscle length are also minimized. Then, from a consideration of the configuration and latency of these responses, we will suggest a function for presetting mechanisms in governing the input-output relations which characterize these responses. From a parametric analysis of output variables, a general control policy will be proposed which governs rapid force adjustments of different magnitudes (GHEZ and VICARIO, 1978c). Finally, from preliminary data, we will show the applicability of this model to the control of limb position and point out certain constraints which appear to be imposed by segmental mechanisms.

METHODS

The experimental procedure is more fully described elsewhere (GHEZ and VICARIO, 1978b). Figure 1 illustrates its major features. The animal was restrained snugly in a sleeve, its head and left humerus rigidly fixed to an external frame. The animal's forearm was strapped in a splint attached to the lever of a torque motor controlled manipulandum. Transducers indicated its angular position, velocity and the force applied to the lever.

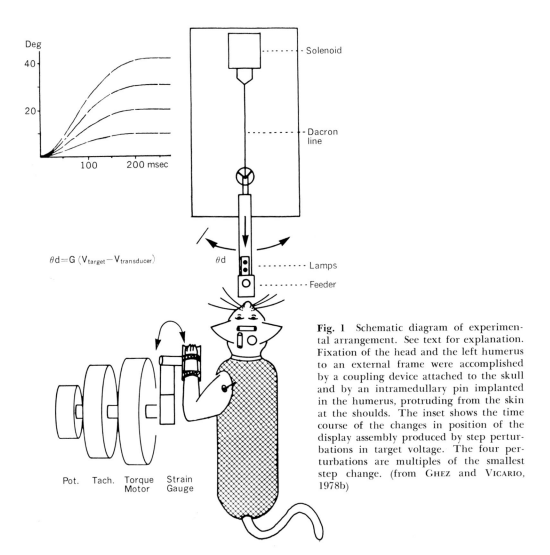

Fig. 1 Schematic diagram of experimental arrangement. See text for explanation. Fixation of the head and the left humerus to an external frame were accomplished by a coupling device attached to the skull and by an intramedullary pin implanted in the humerus, protruding from the skin at the shoulds. The inset shows the time course of the changes in position of the display assembly produced by step perturbations in target voltage. The four perturbations are multiples of the smallest step change. (from GHEZ and VICARIO, 1978b)

A display assembly in front of the animal consisted of a retractable feeder operated by a solenoid, and a pair of lamps. This assembly could move from side to side by means of another, servo operated, torque motor. The angular position of the assembly, θd, was a function of an error signal representing the voltage difference between the output of one of the transducers in the manipulandum and a 'target' level. Position or force adjustments could be elicited in the same animal by either clamping or releasing a lock on the manipulandum and changing the feedback conditions governing the display. Accordingly, if the transducer voltage was derived from the output of the strain gauge, the display assembly moved from side to side with fluctuations in the force exerted by the animal. If the potentiometer voltage was used, the display reflected changes in the lever position. In addition, the display assembly moved whenever the target voltage was stepped in one direction or another.

The animals were trained to adjust the force they applied to the lever, or its angular position, so as to align the display assembly with their midsagittal axis, in order to obtain a food reward. This was delivered by releasing the feeder which then came close to their mouths. Rapid changes in the position of the lever or the force exerted upon it were elicited by stepping the target voltage level at random times when the animal was steadily aligning the display. This perturbation moved the display assembly and required a corrective adjustment in force or position on the part of the animal. The food reward was given after a second period of stable alignment following target reacquisition.

The amount of displacement of the display system corresponding to a perturbation in target level or to a change in transducer voltage was under experimental control. The magnitude of display motion requiring a given response could be varied over an eight fold range by changing the gain, G, of the error signal controlling the display, as indicated, in Figure 1. Because of inertia and friction in the display device, approximately 200 msec were required for it to fully respond to a step perturbation. Responses of the display to step inputs of increasing size are illustrated as a function of time in Figure 1 (inset, upper left). The peaks of both the first and the second derivatives of its motion were approximately linear functions of the target perturbation. Thus, although the response of the display was slow, the full display trajectory was predictable from the early values of the derivatives of its motion. The changes in display position and its derivatives could be detected by the animal in either of two ways: by the deflection of its vibrissae as the display moved away from the midline, and by vision.

The behavior required of the animal in this experimental arrangement can be considered as an input-output transformation: the direction and magnitude of arbitrary stimulus variables must be converted by the animal into a response of a given direction and magnitude. Alterations in the gain or polarity of the signals controlling the display require the animal, in its turn, to change the gain and polarity of any internal transfer function it may have established.

RESULTS AND DISCUSSION

Isometric control of force

The distinctive features of rapid isometric adjustments in force are seen for two superimposed trials in Figure 2. About 60 msec after the perturbation in target level, a burst of activity in the agonist EMG occurs, associated with the rising phase of the first derivative of force, dF/dt. The force registered by the strain gauge increases to a maximum (with some overshoot) and is ultimately realigned with the new target level. Since the change in angular position of the display (which provides the actual stimulus for the animal) is

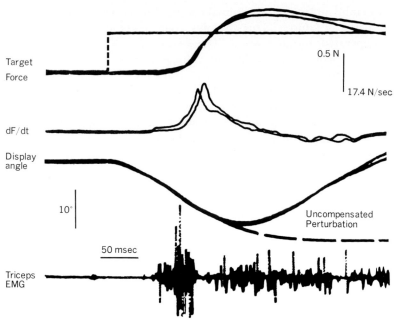

Target Force

0.5 N

17.4 N/sec

dF/dt

Display angle

10°

Uncompensated Perturbation

50 msec

Triceps EMG

Fig. 2 Isometric responses to two equal step perturbations in target level. See text for explanation. (from GHEZ and VICARIO, 1978c)

controlled by a force error, its initial deflection is produced by the step in target voltage while the terminal portion of the trace (returning the display towards its initial position) results from the change in force generated by the animal.   The dashed line indicates the trajectory of the display to the same perturbation when the animal was prevented from exerting force on the lever.   In this and in virtually all cases, both the burst of agonist activity and the peak dF/dt occur before the display has fully responded to the perturbation. Moreover, the sluggishness of the display is such that these early response events are over before the corresponding change in force exerted by the animal can modify its trajectory.

1) Response scaling.   When the perturbation in target level was randomly varied from trial to trial, the peak force, the peak dF/dt and the integrated value of the agonist EMG remained scaled to the final force required (GHEZ and VICARIO, 1978c).   Thus, derivatives of display motion must provide the animal with sufficient information to both initiate a response and scale its magnitude.   To use this early information appropriately, the animal must draw on its previous experience with the device to extrapolate the full extent of the display trajectory from the early sensory information.

The animal's reliance on experience and the role of learning can be demonstrated by unexpectedly changing the gain (G) of the display while the cat is holding the initial alignment and awaiting the perturbation.   Figure 3 illustrates the results of experiments where the gain of the display was either increased or decreased by a factor of two.   The perturbation in target level was maintained unchanged.   The animal was thus required to generate the same response, but the magnitude of the sensory input was different.   In Figure 3A the gain was increased by a factor of two and the first responses following the change in gain were approximately twice the size of control responses made earlier.   Over several trials the magnitude of this initial force response decreased progressively.   A decrease in gain (Fig. 3B) produced the converse effect.   The initial responses are approximately one half of those obtained during the control period.   These observations indicate

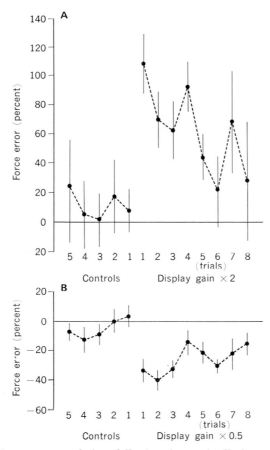

Fig. 3 Rescaling of input-output relations following changes in display gain. The display gain was either increased (**A**) or decreased (**B**) by a factor of two. The change was made during the initial alignment prior to the perturbation. The numbers on the abscissa represent the trial number before (controls) and after the change in display gain. The points and bars show the average of the error in peak force in four runs and the standard error of the mean. (from GHEZ and VICARIO, 1978c)

that the metrics of the transformation relating input and output magnitudes must be set prior to the stimulus itself.

2) Response latency. The extremely short latency of the responses supports the hypothesis of a preset transfer function. In the cases illustrated in Figure 2, the time from the perturbation to the burst of agonist EMG was about 60 msec. There, the animal relied on information provided by the deflection of vibrissae following the sudden movement of the display. When the animals relied on visual information alone, their response latencies were increased by about 20 msec over those with vibrissae alone (GHEZ and VICARIO, 1978b). This difference corresponds approximately to the retinal transfer time determined in Y cells (SHAPLEY and KAPLAN, personal communication), which provide velocity information to the central nervous system (IKEDA and WRIGHT, 1972).

The response latency using either modality was dependent on two separate factors: the display motion produced by the perturbation, and the peak rate of force change generated by the animal. With perturbations of increasing size, both factors contribute to a progressive decrease in latency towards an asymptote. To dissociate the two factors,

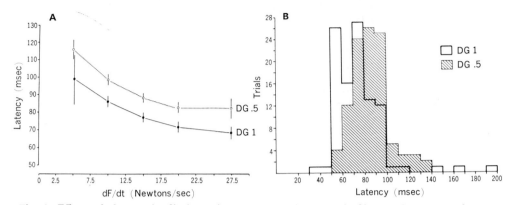

Fig. 4 Effects of changes in display gain on response latency. *A*: Changes in response latency as a function of dF/dt. Perturbations were of constant amplitude and required the same response magnitude, but the display gain was varied between two different values (DG 1, filled circles; DG 0.5, open circles). The points show the mean values and standard errors of the latencies of responses occurring in the intervals on the abscissa. Mean latencies are plotted above the mid-point of the range of the dF/dt. *B*: Latency histograms of responses elicited under the two display gain conditions. (from GHEZ and VICARIO, 1978b)

responses elicited by perturbations displayed at different gains were compared (GHEZ and VICARIO, 1978b). The results of such an experiment are illustrated in Figure 4. In A, the mean latencies of the first change in dF/dt are plotted as a function of the peak value of this parameter under two conditions of display gain. There is a gradual decrease in latency with increasing dF/dt, and the latencies of the responses elicited at the higher display gain (where the actual neural input may be assumed to be greater), are shorter at all values of dF/dt. This uniform shift suggests that two independent processes underlie the changes in latency. The histograms in Figure 4B show the latencies of response pairs matched for peak dF/dt; the two are statistically different (Mann-Whitney U test). The dependence of latency on input and output mangitudes is undoubtedly the result of spatial and temporal summation occurring in both afferent and efferent pathways. Neurons responding to movement of a visual target as well as those responding to cutaneous stimuli have shorter latencies and more brisk responses with increasing stimulus velocities. Similarly, increasing rates of force change are produced by an increase in the rate of recruitment of motoneurons (TANJI and KATO, 1973). When the predictability of the time of onset of the perturbation and the predictability of either the magnitude or direction of the required response were varied systematically, no effect on the response latency was found.

On the basis of their short latency, these tracking responses must be mediated by relatively simple pathways in which only a small number of serial relays are likely to be interposed between afferent and efferent stations. Decision processes underlying the selection of response topography and metrics are not likely to take place during the reaction time interval itself. Rather these processes are likely to be determined by gating and biasing mechanisms operating prior to the stimulus. Since, on the one hand, the force adjustments were scaled from their onset to demands set by the initial sensory events, and since rescaling of the motor responses required 10–20 trials when the properties of the display were altered, it is likely that these presetting mechanisms operate to adjust the gain of a preset or "resident" transfer function.

3) "Pulse-step" control. To determine how different output parameters are controlled, it is necessary to consider the configuration of the responses themselves in greater detail. The cardinal features of isometric force adjustments of different magnitudes

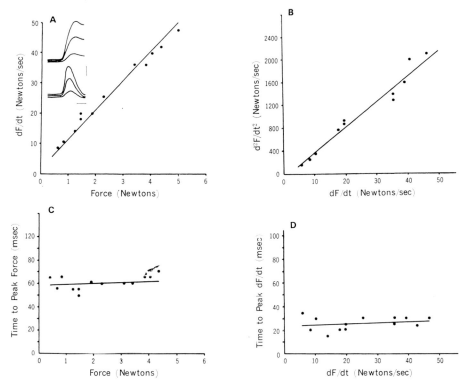

Fig. 5 Relations between output parameters under isometric conditions. *A*. Relation between peak force and peak dF/dt. The inset shows sample records of force and dF/dt for movements of different sizes. Horizontal calibration: 60 msec. Vertical calibration: 0.5 N, 12.5 N/sec. *B*: Relation between dF/dt and peak d²F/dt². *C*: Relation between peak force and the time between the first change in dF/dt and the peak force. *D*: Relation between peak dF/dt and time from onset to peak. (modified from GHEZ and VICARIO, 1978c)

are shown in Figure 5 which is representative of cases where the peak dF/dt increases mototonically to its peak and then decreases smoothly. Examples are illustrated in the inset in the upper left hand corner which shows the force above and dF/dt below. Increases in peak force were accompanied by increases in the peak of its first derivative and two parameters were linearly related, as shown in A. Similarly, a linear relationship bound the peak dF/dt and the peak of the second derivative of force (d²F/dt²) (B). By contrast, the time from onset to peak value of either force (C) or its first derivative (D) did not vary with increasing magnitudes of these parameters. Thus higher peak forces and dF/dt's were achieved without increases in time.

The linearity of the relationship between the initial force change and the peak value of its first derivative suggests that the underlying response pattern is stereotyped in its general configuration and that adjustments of different magnitudes may be related to one another by different scaling factors. To interpret the time course of the changes in dF/dt it is necessary to recall that skeletal muscles have profound low-pass characteristics. As shown by PARTRIDGE (1964), the muscle tension produced by a frequency modulated neural input decreases markedly with increasing frequency of modulation and dramatic time lags are introduced by muscle properties. As a result, for the time to peak force and the time from onset to peak dF/dt to remain essentially constant as is characteristically the case, it is necessary that the initial phase of the adjustment be governed by the transient recruitment of additional motor units and that they initially fire at higher frequency than

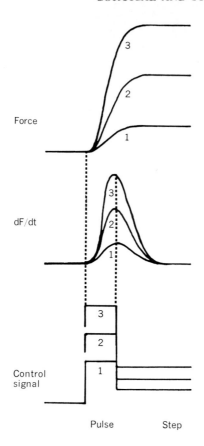

Force

dF/dt

Control
signal

Pulse   Step

Fig. 6 Pulse-step model of rapid force adjustments. See text for explanation.

during the application of the terminal steady state force.   In a first approximation the
motor outputs observed here may thus be described by a pulse-step model in which the
dynamic phase of the adjustment is controlled by the height or amplitude of an initial
pulsatile output.   This is illustrated schematically in Figure 6.   The duration of the
proposed initial control pulse approximates that of the rising phase of dF/dt and remains
essentially constant.   Its amplitude governs the rate of increase of dF/dt and thereby the
peak force as well.   The terminal steady state force can be assumed to be governed by a
step increase in neural output.   The suggestion that these force adjustments are determined
by an initial pulsatile output, modulated in amplitude rather than in duration, is supported
by our finding that the rising phase of dF/dt is accompanied by a burst of EMG activity
in the agonist muscle (as seen in Fig. 2) whose integrated value is proportional to the peak
dF/dt but whose duration does not vary with this parameter (GHEZ and VICARIO, 1978c).
Similar observations have recently been made in the human by FREUND and BÜDINGEN
(1978).
    Pulse-step models have also been proposed to account for the control of eye position
during ocular saccades (ROBINSON, 1964, 1970; BAHILL et al., 1975).   In that system
however, the magnitude of a saccade is governed primarily by the duration rather than
the amplitude (or spike frequency) of an initial burst of activity of oculomotor neurons
(ROBINSON, 1970).   In the present context the pulse-step model must be understood as the
final result of phasic and tonic descending commands controlling the force output and
its derivatives.   Thus, in limb muscles, this final output must also reflect the particular
constraints imposed by regulatory properties of motoneurons (BURKE and RUDOMIN, 1977)

and feedback actions following the activation of peripheral receptors once the motor output is initiated.

These observations suggested the possibility that in rapid voluntary muscle contraction, descending commands may specifically control the derivatives of force. In parallel with these behavioral investigations, we have studied the relationship of the activity of single neurons in the red nuclei of these cats during isometric tracking (GHEZ and VICARIO, 1978a). These neurons were sampled in areas where microstimulation produced localized contraction of forelimb muscles and often responded to peripheral stimuli applied to the forelimb. The activity of cells was modulated when the animals exerted isometric force in either flexion or extension, and this change in activity occurred prior to the contraction of the agonist muscles. The vast majority of neurons in the red nucleus exhibited a pattern of discharge which paralleled the first derivative of force with a phase lead. Over a large range the magnitude of the peak dF/dt was a linear function of the preceding peak firing of these units. Neurons showing more tonic characteristics were rarely observed in the red nucleus. By contrast, from published accounts it would seem that output neurons of the motor cortex of monkeys do show a predominant tonic pattern of activity correlating with the steady state force (SMITH et al., 1975; FETZ, personal communication), and as shown recently by HEPP-REYMOND and WYSS (1978), individual units may have a threshold force level at which their activity is recruited. Although such data suggest that different neural structures may be responsible for the phasic and tonic control of output parameters, it is necessary to reserve final judgement on this matter since differences in species and in task conditions could also have contributed to the different properties observed.

From the present parametric studies of the force output and its derivatives we conclude that the initial sensory input, derived here from parameters of display motion, ultimately control the amplitude of both an initial pulsatile event and a terminal steady state output according to a preset transfer function. To implement this control policy, the subject must have prior information not only about the full target trajectory, as described earlier, but also of the peak force likely to result from the brief initial burst of neural output. Moreover, while the time to peak force and the time to peak dF/dt remained stable within any given day, two to three fold differences in these times occurred from day to day. This suggests that the duration of the initial pulsatile command is regulated by a higher order strategy rather than by the initial sensory events.

Control of rapid limb displacement

Recently, we have focussed our attention on the kinematics of limb displacements to determine whether a pulse-step control policy, similar to that noted under isometric conditions, also determined rapid movements of the limb and whether the input-output transformations underlying tracking performance could be considered to reflect the presetting of a relation between stimulus variables and the forces required to displace the limb. Given the wide variation in loads which may be encountered in the course of limb movements, an alternative hypothesis might have suggested that central programs preset a particular angular displacement in relation to the target variables. In this case length servo mechanisms would compensate for variations in load.

To examine these problems, the display was made to reflect an error in position of the lever. Under these conditions perturbations in target level, which shifted the display, elicited rapid adjustments of the angular position of the lever by the cats. The extent and direction of the initial lever displacement was invariably correlated with the amplitude and direction of randomly varied perturbations and response latencies (measured again to the first change in dF/dt) were similar to those observed under isometric conditions,

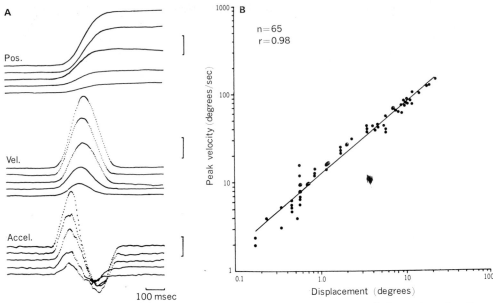

Fig. 7 Relations between parameters of movement. *A*: Displacement, velocity and accelerations of responses to perturbations of five different sizes. The traces are the average of eight trials for each perturbation. Calibrations: position 12°, velocity 67°/sec, acceleration 1000°/sec². *B*: Relationship between displacement and peak velocity for 65 separate movements (different experiment from Fig. 7A).

The peak velocity achieved during these adjustments was characteristically a quasi linear function of the displacement over an extensive range, as can be seen in Figure 7B. These increasing velocities were accomplished by corresponding increases in the peak acceleration (Fig. 7A). While the duration of movement often increased somewhat as the movement became larger, the time from onset to peak acceleration and velocity did not.

The peak velocity is, of course, determined by the magnitude and duration of the acceleration resulting from the sudden change in the contraction of agonist and antagonist muscles. It was not surprising therefore, that EMG recordings of agonist muscles showed a conspicuous burst of activity of approximately constant duration. As also noted by many investigators (MERTON, 1951; ANGEL et al., 1965; LESTIENNE, 1974; SOECHTING et al., 1976), a silent period interrupted the agonist activity just before the peak acceleration. After the silent period, EMG activity resumed at a level dependent upon the opposing forces.

If, for a moment, we neglect the factors controlling deceleration and the silent period in agonist muscles, these observations suggest that rapid limb displacements are also governed by an initial pulsatile output, modulated in amplitude and of approximately constant duration, and a terminal step-like output which determines the final position of the limb. The amplitude of this pulsatile output, which controls the peak angular acceleration, also determines the peak velocity and displacement corresponding to the change in intended position. This phasic initial output is needed to overcome the inertia of the limb and the viscoelastic properties of muscles and joints as well as the low-pass properties of muscles. A terminal step is also necessary, since gravitational and elastic forces acting on the limb vary with its angular position. Even when the mass of the forearm is considered against a constant gravitational field (and no antagonist activity is present), the central nervous system must provide additional input to the agonist in the

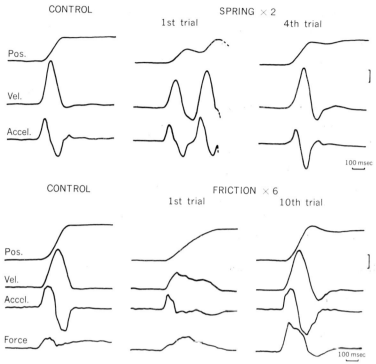

Fig. 8 Movement parameters following unexpected changes in opposing forces. See text for explanation. Calibrations: upper traces: position 6°, velocity 33°/sec, acceleration 500°/sec²; lower traces: position 12°, velocity 47°/sec, acceleration 250°/sec², force 1 Newton.

terminal position to compensate for its loss of tension due to shortening and the increased tension of the antagonist which is stretched.

To investigate the possibility that the initial pulsatile component and the later tonic events can be controlled independently, we have determined, in preliminary studies, the changes in the time course and extent of movement when lever displacement was unexpectedly opposed by loads of different configurations. These loads were generated by changing the feedback conditions controlling the torque of the manipulandum. Figure 8 illustrates the changes in response variables following an unexpected increase in opposing forces. The upper left hand traces (control) show the displacement, velocity and acceleration when the animal adjusted the lever position against a light spring load. Just prior to the perturbation eliciting the response shown in the center (first trial) the spring constant was doubled without changing the force required for the initial alignment. The increase in terminal steady state force required for alignment was 25 g. The response to the first perturbation at the new spring constant (first trial) fell short of the intended position and a second movement was made after a brief interval. Again, however, the tonic forces generated were inadequate to maintain postural stability. Nevertheless, after a few trials the animal learned the new conditions and produced movements which were similar to controls in their displacement, velocity and acceleration.

The lower frames show the alterations in movement trajectory when, again unexpectedly, the frictional force opposing movement was increased by a factor of six. The first response in the new condition differs from that seen when the spring constant was increased: while the final position following the load change was similar to the control, the peak

velocity was markedly lower.   Nevertheless, again following an adaptation period, the
animal readjusted its output so that the peak velocity and acceleration approximated
those of the controls.   The bottom traces document that this adaptation was achieved by
a marked increase (here about 200 g) in the forces generated during the initial phase of
movement.

    These observations show that when the task requires the control of limb position (rather
than force), the input-output transformations also relate derivatives of display motion to
an intended force output.   This is evident from the fact that the increase in spring constant
opposing both phasic and tonic components of the force output resulted in an undershoot
of the final limb position.   Such undershoots were still seen when only 10 g opposed the
final position.   While the frictional load, which is a function of angular velocity, prevented
the initial phasic events from resulting in a normal velocity of movement, it did not interfere
with the achievement of a correct final position.   Thus, as in the case of the head movements studied by BIZZI et al. (1976), a normal final position is achieved as a result of the
terminal muscle tension in agonist and antagonist muscles.   The different modes of compensation, which occur when the animal has learned the particular nature of the load to
be expected, indicate that the phasic and tonic components of the motor program may
be separately adjusted.   Just as a change in display gain required the animal to rescale the
transfer function relating a given sensory input to the amplitudes of an initial pulsatile
output and a terminal step, a change in the anticipated load results in a comparable reset-
ting.   When loads oppose primarily the dynamic phase of movement, the initial pulsatile
output is reset.   When the load opposes both the dynamic and static phases, both the early
and late components of the output are readjusted.   Finally, while load-compensating
position servos may be brought into action as a result of differences between actual and
intended muscle shortening, they appear to have limited impact on the trajectory of the
limb.   These observations strongly suggest that rapid limb movements are primarily
governed by central programs specifying the force output as a function, not only of input
variables, but also of the magnitude and configuration of anticipated loads.

    In the previous comments the mechanisms underlying deceleration of the limb were
disregarded.   However, although our data on this matter are incomplete, some consideration of this problem is in order.   Indeed, once the acceleration of the limb crosses
zero, the momentum will tend to passively propel the limb to a new position which depends
on the balance of active and passive forces.   It has long been known that concomitant
with the increased EMG activity in agonist muscles, the antagonists become silent.   In
addition, a burst of EMG activity in antagonists commonly starts at about the time of the
peak acceleration and reaches its maximum at the peak velocity during the silent period
in the agonist.   In human and monkey subjects, this burst of activity varies in magnitude
with the peak velocity (LESTIENNE, 1974; SOECHTING et al., 1974).   While the silent
period in the agonist is primarily due to disfacilitation produced by the segmental actions
of muscle receptors following their unloading (ANGEL et al., 1965) and is also seen in the
cat, the burst of activity in the antagonist has been thought to reflect a transient excitatory
descending command forming part of the motor program (HALLET et al., 1975).   This
interpretation seems unlikely since the timed antagonist burst is not observed following
deafferentation (TERZUOLO et al., 1974).   Moreover, in the cat, this activity in the
antagonist is only present under anisometric conditions where limb displacement stretches
the antagonist muscle; it does not occur under isometric conditions (GHEZ and VICARIO,
in preparation).   Additionally, provided the 'set' of the animal is identical, this antagonist
activity is consistently greater when the limb is passively (and unexpectedly) displaced than
when the same velocity and acceleration are actively achieved by the animal (GHEZ and

VICARIO, in preparation).   These considerations strongly suggest that the burst of EMG activity in the antagonist during rapid limb movement represents a segmental stretch reflex upon which may be superimposed additional feedback actions of supraspinal centers receiving input from receptors sensitive to limb velocity (BURTON and ONODA, 1978; GHEZ and VICARIO, 1978a; EVARTS and TANJI, 1976).   When the descending excitatory drive is conveyed to the agonist, a concommitant inhibitory control appears to be exerted upon the antagonist (see also LAMARRE et al., 1978), but which may be insufficient to prevent the reflex when the velocity of stretch is high.   It is uncertain at present whether this inhibitory control includes both phasic and tonic components or whether the depth and duration of the inhibition can be modulated independently of the excitatory drive to the agonist.   Such an independent control could be especially important in the presence of high moments of inertia to facilitate the arrest of movement.

CONCLUDING REMARKS

An examination of tracking performance in the cat suggests that the processes controlling rapid limb movement can be considered to involve several distinct levels of control which operate to overcome constraints imposed by lower order processes.   In the first analysis, the animal's overall response can be considered as the expression of an input-output transformation whereby derivatives of display motion control the amplitude of both an initial pulsatile event and a terminal steady state.   The initial pulsatile component is required to overcome the constraints imposed by mechanical properties of the muscle and limb. Since the initial events are scaled from their onset to the final force required by randomly varying perturbations, they must represent the expression of central programs.   The gain of the underlying transfer function must be determined by higher order processes which enable the magnitude of the final output required to be estimated from the initial values of the derivatives of display motion, the properties of the peripheral plant and, in the case of limb displacement, the loads which will oppose movement.   This "resident" transfer function can be rescaled when either the display gain or the loading conditions are altered, but whether by different neural mechanisms remains to be investigated.   The establishment of such predictive behavior must be based upon information from the results of past responses and is an essential feature of "motor learning".   It is critical for accurate movements in an "evolving situation" (WELFORD, 1976) because of the long time which inevitably elapses between stimulus and feedback from the response.

The factors governing the duration of the initial pulsatile command are uncertain. While it is attractive to consider that the control policy aims to minimize flight time while preserving accuracy, motivational factors, over which we do not, as yet, have good control, must also be important.   BOUISSET and LESTIENNE (1974) have shown in humans that the kinematics of a movement of constant amplitude are critically dependent upon the instructions given to the subject.   From their figures it appears that when the instructions specified a higher velocity, the time to peak acceleration was reduced; it is legitimate to suppose that the subjects then programmed a shorter pulse of agonist activity.

It must be emphasized that the pulsatile nature of the initial output need not necessarily reflect any intermittency in the sampling of peripheral input (NAVAS and STARK, 1968). Indeed, the output pulse can, in the cat, be updated at all times by new sensory information even when it arrives during the course of the reaction time or the response itself (VICARIO et al., 1978; see also MEGAW, 1974).   The accuracy of such corrections is, however, limited by that of the transfer function in effect.   Thus, corrections may be ineffective in the case of unexpected loads (Fig. 8) which require a rescaling of the transfer function between input variables and the derivatives of the force output.

As regards the role of sensory events arising from afferents in the limb, consideration must be given to the fact that such inputs are necessary not only to provide information about the properties of the peripheral plant, but also about the initial position of the limb. While this may not be critical for the final position (BIZZI et al., 1976), it is critical for the accurate scaling of the early phasic events. This information could be incorporated in the motor program at a spinal level, perhaps using propriospinal neurons whose patterns of convergence have been elegantly described by Professor LUNDBERG (this volume) or at a higher level and/or after a reaction time. While the segmental actions of particular afferent systems may be important in the regulation of slow movements and in respiration (SEARS, 1973), in the case of rapid limb movements, we are more struck by the constraints which they seem to provide. It is within these constraints that the descending actions of central programs must operate. Thus, afferent input may, to paraphrase WEISS (1941), play more a constructive than a regulatory role. This could favor, during the acquisition of skill, the development of a pulse-height control policy, since the initial burst of neural activity will, as its action is exerted, be automatically terminated by the silent period. Since afferent input provides the information required to reset the gain of the input-output relations of rapid targeted movements, its role must certainly be constructive since it ultimately enables the purpose of such movements to be achieved.

ACKNOWLEDGEMENTS

The author is deeply indebted to D. VICARIO who collaborated in many of the experiments and to Ms. K. ARISSIAN, Ms. A. JEAN-MARIE and Ms. N. MARMOR for technical assistance.

REFERENCES

ANGEL, R. W., EPPLER, W. and IANNONE, A.: Silent period produced by unloading of muscle during voluntary contraction. *J. Physiol.*, *180*: 864–870 (1965)

BAHILL, A. T., CLARK, M. R. and STARK, L.: The main sequence, a tool for studying human eye movements, *Math. Biosci.*, *24*: 191–204 (1975)

BIZZI, E., POLIT, A. and MORASSO, P.: Mechanisms underlying achievement of final head position. *J. Neurophysiol.*, *39*: 435–444 (1976)

BOUISSET, S. and LESTIENNE, F.: The organization of a simple voluntary movement as analysed from its kinematic properties. *Brain Res.*, *71*: 451–457 (1974)

BUCK, L.: The boundary distance effects on overshooting. *J. Mot. Behavior*, *8*: 35–41 (1976)

BURKE, R. E. and RUDOMIN, P.: Spinal neurons and synapses. *In* BROOKHART, J. M. and MOUNTCASTLE, V. B. (eds): *Handbook of Physiology*, Section I. The Nervous System, Vol. I, pp. 877–944, American Physiological Society, Washington, D. C. (1977)

BURTON, J. and ONODA, N.: Dependence of the activity of interpositus and red nucleus neurons on sensory input data generated by movement. *Brain Res.*, *152*: 41-63 (1978)

EVARTS, E. V. and TANJI, J.: Reflex and intended responses in motor cortex pyramidal tract neurons of the monkey. *J. Neurophysiol.*, *39*: 1069–1080 (1976)

FITTS, P. M.: The information capacity of the human motor system in controlling the amplitude of a movement. *J. Exp. Psychol.*, *47*: 381–391 (1954)

FREUND, H. J. and BÜDINGEN, H. J.: The relationship between speed and amplitude of the fastest voluntary contractions of human arm muscles. *Exp. Brain Res.*, *31*: 1–12 (1978)

GHEZ, C. and VICARIO, D.: Discharge of red nucleus neurons during voluntary muscle contraction: activity patterns and correlations with isometric force. *J. Physiol. (Paris)*, *74*: 283-285 (1978a)

GHEZ, G. and VICARIO, D.: The control of rapid limb movement in the cat. I. Response latency. *Exp. Brain Res.*, *33*: 173-189 (1978b)

GHEZ, C. and VICARIO, D.: The control of rapid limb movement in the cat. II. Scaling of isometric force adjustments. *Exp. Brain Res.*, *33*: 191–202 (1978c)

GRANIT, R.: The functional role of the muscle spindles—facts and hypotheses. *Brain, 98*: 531–556 (1975)

HALLETT, M., SHAHANI, B. T. and YOUNG, R. R.: EMG analysis of stereotyped voluntary movements in man. *J. Neurol. Neurosurg. Psychiat., 38*: 1154–1162 (1975)

HEPP-REYMOND, M.-C. and WYSS, V. R.: Coding of static finger force in the primate motor cortex. *J. Physiol. (Paris), 74*: 287–291 (1978)

IKEDA, H. and WRIGHT, M.: Receptive field organization of 'sustained' and 'transient' retinal ganglion cells which subserve different functional roles. *J. Physiol. (Lond.), 227*: 769–800 (1972)

LAMARRE, Y., BIOULAC, B. and JACKS, B.: Activity of precentral neurones in conscious monkeys: effects of deafferentation and cerebellar ablation. *J. Physiol. (Paris), 74*: 253–264 (1978)

LESTIENNE, F.: Programme moteur et mechanismes de l'arret d'un movement monoarticulaire. These. Lille, France (1974)

MEGAW, E. D.: Possible modification to a rapid on-going manual response. *Brain Res., 71*: 425–441 (1974)

MERTON, P. A.: The silent period in a muscle of the human hand. *J. Physiol., 114*: 183–198 (1951)

NAVAS, F. and STARK, L.: Sampling or intermittency in hand control systems dynamics. *Biophys. J., 8*: 252–302 (1968)

PARTRIDGE, L. D.: Modification of neural output signals by muscles: a frequency response study. *J. Appl. Physiol., 20*: 150–156 (1965)

POULTON, E. C.: *Tracking Skill and Manual Control.* Academic Press, New York (1974)

ROBINSON, D. A.: The mechanics of human saccadic eye movement. *J. Physiol. (Lond.), 174*: 245–264 (1964)

ROBINSON, D. A.: Oculomotor unit behavior in the monkey. *J. Neurophysiol., 33*: 393–404 (1970)

SEARS, T. A.: Servo control of intercostal muscles. *In* DESMEDT, J. E. (ed.): *New Developments in Electromyography and Clinical Neurophysiology,* Vol. 3, pp. 404–417. Karger, Basel (1973)

SMITH, A. M., HEPP-REYMOND, M.-C. and WYSS, U. R.: Relation of activity in precentral cortical neurons to force and rate of force change during isometric contractions of finger muscles. *Exp. Brain Res., 23*: 315–332 (1975)

SOECHTING, J. F., RANISH, N. A., PALMINTERI, R. and TERZUOLO, C. A.: Changes in motor pattern following cerebellar and olivary lesions in the squirrel monkey. *Brain Res., 105*: 21–44 (1976)

TANJI, J. and KATO, M.: Recruitment of motor units in voluntary contraction of a finger muscle in man. *Exp. Neurol., 40*: 759–770 (1973)

TERZUOLO, C. A., SOECHTING, J. F. and RANISH, N. A.: Studies on the control of some simple motor tasks. V. Changes in motor output following dorsal root section in squirrel monkey. *Brain Res., 70*: 521–526 (1974)

VICARIO, D., BLUNK, T. and GHEZ, C.: Correction of ongoing motor output in the cat. *Soc. Neurosci. Abstracts, 8*: 977 (1978)

WEISS, P.: Does sensory control play a constructive role in the development of motor coordination? *Schweiz. Med, Wschr., 71*: 406–407 (1941)

WELFORD, A. T.: *Skilled Performance: Perceptual and Motor Skills.* Scott Foresman and Company, Glenview, Ill. (1976)

DISCUSSION PERIOD

BROOKS: Does the animal's accuracy go down as the displacement and velocity go up, and is the standard deviation of the error greater for higher velocities?

GHEZ: The accuracy of responses made by the cats to perturbations of randomly varied amplitudes was not dependent on their velocity *per se*.   Rather, as is also the case in human subjects performing a step tracking task with varied step sizes, accuracy is most heavily dependent on range effects, that is, the average value of preceding perturbations (POULTON, 1974) and boundary effects, that is, the difference between the maximal possible extent of display motion and that produced by the particular perturbation (BUCK, 1976). The latter effect results in a tendency towards undershooting for the largest perturbations. That both of these factors are important, underscores the role of predictive mechanisms in rapid movements.

Of course, movements of constant amplitude can be performed with different peak velocities and then, accuracy may decrease proportionally as velocity increases (FITTS, 1954).   With varied amplitudes of movement, the error will then increase as a function of the ratio between velocity and displacement.   Although this suggests an inverse relation between the duration of the initial pulsatile output and the error, we have not, as yet, studied this in the cat.

CONTROL OF INTENDED LIMB MOVEMENTS BY THE LATERAL AND INTERMEDIATE CEREBELLUM

Vernon B. BROOKS

Department of Physiology, University of Western Ontario
London, Ontario, Canada

INTRODUCTION

Control of a limb implies governance of all muscles that influence limb position, and the stiffness with which it is maintained or changed. The task of the nervous system is to adjust the timing and amount of force applied by these muscles according to the intentions of the individual and the circumstances in which they are to be carried out. Thus thought, mood and external conditions all influence posture and movements that are inextricably entwined. These are old thoughts (cf. Stetson and Bouman, 1935; Woodworth, 1899). How does the cerebellum participate in these controls? We will examine evidence about participation of spino- and neo-cerebellum, using these terms (not in the old lobular sense: cf. Brookhart, 1960; Dow and Moruzzi, 1958; Larsell and Jansen, 1967; Miller, 1926), to denote two rostro-caudally oriented strips (Chambers and Sprague, 1955): the *intermediate* part that primarily receives peripheral input from the ipsilateral limbs, and cerebral input from contralateral sensory and motor cortex by way of the pons and lateral reticular nucleus; and the *lateral* part that primarily receives cerebral input from contralateral association and sensorimotor cortex also by way of the brainstem (Allen et al., 1977, 1978; Bloedel, 1973; Brookhart, 1960; Evarts and Thach, 1969). Both cerebellar strips are also reached by projections from the inferior olives (cf. Bloedel, 1973; Oscarsson, 1973, 1976). Outputs from the intermediate and lateral parts travel through the anterior part (Courville and Cooper, 1970) of interpositus (IP) and dentate nuclei respectively (cf. Allen and Tsukahara, 1974; Allen et al., 1977; Bloedel, 1973; Brookhart, 1960; Eccles, 1969, 1973) reaching predominantly forelimb projections in contralateral cerebral motor areas 4 and premotor area 6, as opposed to more proximal projections for IP (Sasaki et al., 1976; Sasaki, 1977). Spinal projections are carried from dentate through the reticulospinal tract (Bantli and Bloedel, 1976), and from IP through the rubrospinal tract (cf. Allen and Tsukahara, 1974). The exact role of the short propriospinal system with convergent inputs is still unclear (Illert et al., 1977; Illert and Tanaka, 1978; cf. Lundberg in this Symposium). Electro-anatomical unit studies have revealed rostro-caudal gradient of hind- to forelimb projections in anesthetized monkey's nuclei (Allen et al., 1977, 1978). Dentate neurons receive input in decreasing order of prevalence from electrically stimulated premotor and supplementary motor cortex (area 6), frontal, motor and sensory cortex. IP neurons receive from motor and sensory cortex, peripheral nerves, pre- and supplementary motor cortex. The authors commented on the surprising lack, or great scarcity of inputs from parietal, temporal, prefrontal, insular, orbital and secondary visual cortex.

The subject of cerebellar limb control has its roots in analysis of clinical symptoms of cerebellar injuries, e. g. by Holmes (1917, 1939) and in the enormous development of cerebellar Physiology and Anatomy, variously summarized in Fulton and Dow (1937),

Dow and MORUZZI (1958), LARSELL and JANSEN (1967), BROOKHART (1960), ECCLES, ITO and SZENTAGOTHAI (1967), OSCARSSON (1976), ALLEN and TSUKAHARA (1974), LLINÁS (1969, 1975), THACH (1979) and many other works too numerous to cite.

Three questions will be considered: Does the cerebellum function at a cognitive level? How does evidence from cerebellar dysfunction fit with that obtained from unit recording in behaving animals? What common elements in the evidence can suggest at least one major mode of cerebellar limb control? These questions are treated together in the following Sections, that each conclude with a brief summary.

1. COGNITIVE FUNCTIONS?
2. MOVEMENT ONSET
3. MOVEMENT EXECUTION
4. MUSCLE TONE
5. MOTOR LEARNING
6. COMMON ELEMENTS

1. COGNITIVE FUNCTIONS?

To facilitate discussion, a diagram of sequential involvement of possible, functional connections, as drawn by ALLEN and TSUKAHARA (1974) is presented in Fig. 1 with its Legend. The "Idea" shown on the left [or the "Will" as ITO had it (ITO, 1970a, 1970b)] is some global process involving, at some stage, association areas of cerebral cortex. We shall consider movements from the selection of strategies, and getting set for an intended movement, to specifying movement directions and parameters, selection of muscles and details of their actions. When a movement begins is thus a matter of definition. All these processes take account of past experience, present circumstances, and future expectations. This holistic view sees 'hierarchies' of functions through a variety of distributed channels by multiple feedback and feedforward interactions, as has been reviewed elsewhere (BROOKS, 1979, and cf. MOUNTCASTLE in this Symposium).

The cerebellum cannot be considered in isolation from the rest of the sensorimotor apparatus, ranging from association cortex to spinal cord. Anatomical studies (JONES and POWELL, 1970; KUYPERS, 1960; PANDYA and KUYPERS, 1969) have shown that somatic, visual and auditory systems converge in the prefrontal and parieto-temporal association cortex. Successive convergences to prefrontal cortex were related to the psychological demonstration of loss of associative functions, including recent memory subsequent to lesions in these areas. "The significance of the double projection pattern—the one local and the other to the frontal lobe...may be... that in all [sensory] systems the frontal projection areas are more concerned with "praxic" functions of sensorimotor integration.... By contrast to the above, the local projections may have more to do with "gnostic" functions or the awareness of spatial and other relationships" (JONES and POWELL, 1970). Loss of higher levels of association between sensory input, its perception in the context of the situation, and appropriate motor output occurs in patients and monkeys after damage of association cortex, as has been reviewed particularly for the parietal cortex (MOUNTCASTLE, 1975). Visual guidance of finely controlled hand and finger movements depends critically on cortico-cortical connections between occipital and frontal cortex, which then projects back to area 6 (HAAXMA and KUYPERS, 1974; KUYPERS, 1960; PANDYA and KUYPERS, 1969). Subcortical integration of sensorimotor action has been considered on anatomical evidence (KEMP and POWELL, 1971) for parallel processing of information destined for motor cortex through basal ganglia in comparison to cerebellum

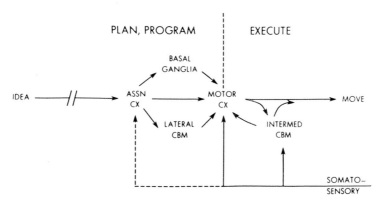

Fig. 1 A conceptual guide that will later be modified: ALLEN and TSUKAHARA's . . . "Scheme for proposed roles of several brain structures in movement. Thin dashed line represents a pathway of unknown importance . . . It is proposed that basal ganglia and cerebellar hemisphere are involved with association cortex in programming or volitional movements. At the time that the motor command descends to motoneurons, engaging the movement, the pars intermedia updates the intended movement, based on the motor command and somatosensory description of limb position and velocity on which the movement is to be superimposed. Follow-up correction can be performed by motor cortex when cerebellar hemisphere and pars intermedia do not effectively perform their functions . . .". (modified from ALLEN and TSUKAHARA, 1974)

(cf. ALLEN and TSUKAHARA, 1974; ALLEN et al., 1978; EVARTS and THACH, 1969). Both centers project to the VL complex of the thalamus that projects to motor cortex: the pallidum more rostrally than the cerebellar nuclei (STRICK, 1976a). Pathways from the substantia nigra to motor cortex are unknown (cf. STRICK, 1976a). Prefrontal as well as parietal cortex can communicate with motor cortex through cortico-cortical connections as well as subcortically through basal ganglia and lateral cerebellum (cf. EVARTS and THACH, 1969) (Fig. 1), "...but it is significant that there is an exceptionally small projection to each from the visual cortex" (KEMP and POWELL, 1971). There is however evidence for projections from the cat's (nonstriate) area 18 to rostral pontine nuclei whose visual properties resemble those of some in area 18. It is assumed that those pontine cells project to the cerebellum (GIBSON et al., 1978). Subcortical structures might thus handle information at 'higher' as well as 'lower' levels of integration although vision is of different importance for each (cf. ALLEN and TSUKAHARA, 1974; BUCHWALD et al., 1975). Visual information does not alleviate cerebellar symptoms (HOLMES, 1917, 1939; NASHNER, 1976; TERZUOLO and VIVIANI, 1974), but it assists Parkinsonian patients to walk (MARTIN, 1967), and to make arm movements (COOKE et al., 1978) much like monkeys with dysfunction of the globus pallidus (HORE et al., 1977). Lateral cerebellar visuomotor functions have been championed (STEIN, 1979) on the basis of 7 monkeys trained to track a visual target with a lever that could move sideways as well as up and down. Responses of 27 lateral Purkinje (P)-cells and of 42 dentate neurons were recorded to flashing or moving visual targets. Such responses were not observed with 64 intermediate P-cells and 42 IP-neurons, that responded only to somatic stimuli. Eye movements were not monitored.

At what cognitive level does the cerebellum fit in? It has been argued elsewhere (BROOKS, 1979) that selection of movement *strategies* is independent of neocerebellar action, because monkeys, made dysmetric by dentate dysfunction, chose a strategy appropriate to the constraints of their task (BROOKS et al., 1973a). To understand this, we need to know that monkeys, when in the set-up of Fig. 3, made two types of self-paced simple movements that are illustrated in Fig. 5, box 1, (and will be discussed in Section 3C). The type on the left was relatively independent of external cues for correct task performance

(BROOKS et al., 1973a) and oscillated at about 6 Hz (BROOKS et al., 1973b), while the one on the right depended on external cues, such as a tone or light when the handle entered the target area (BROOKS et al., 1973a), and oscillated at about 3 Hz (BROOKS et al., 1973b). Animals progressed from the '3 Hz'- to the '6 Hz'-type as their movement accuracy improved, and they regressed if the task was made more difficult (BROOKS et al., 1973a; BROOKS, 1979). (See Section 3C for equivalent data obtained with human subjects.) One animal, that was particularly well documented, worked successfully with '6 Hz'-movements as long as wide targets ensured success and hence reward. During cerebellar dysfunction, produced by ipsilateral dentate cooling, these movements became hypermetric but the wide targets still allowed successful task completion, and use of this movement strategy continued (Fig. 10 in BROOKS et al., 1973a). In contrast, two others that worked with narrower targets, changed during dentate cooling and the consequent hypermetria that deprived them of reward, to '3 Hz'-movements that they could bring to a halt in the targets in a few min as they 'compensated' (Fig. 7 in BROOKS et al., 1973a), like "...patients who have experienced the risk of overshooting the mark..." (HOLMES, 1939).

Another approach to assessing the level of complexity at which the cerebellum operates, is by *timing* cerebellar neural activities in relation to those in other brain parts (cf. EVARTS and THACH, 1969; EVARTS et al., 1972; THACH, 1972). For instance, in intended movements in trained monkeys, overt anticipatory discharge *does* occur during the interval of several sec between a learned instruction to prepare for, and the signal to execute, learned actions in prefrontal (FUSTER, 1973; KUBOTA et al., 1974) and parietal cortex (MOUNTCASTLE et al., 1975). The actions could for instance, be to point, after a delay, at a spot lit by a certain color or at a given intensity, or in a particular place. These discharges relate to the intended task for which the animal has been cued, rather than to the timing or sensory modality of instructional cues or the details of task execution. Some cells in supplementary (TANJI and TANIGUCHI, 1978b) and a few in motor cortex (SCHMIDT et al., 1975; TANJI and EVARTS, 1976; TANJI et al., 1978; THACH, 1978) also build up a discharge during the foreperiod before the animal has to either push or pull a lever with the contralateral wrist. The same is true for the basal ganglia (SOLTYSIK et al., 1975).

Precentral neurons are '*set*' for the intended movement about 0.3 sec after the correct instruction has been given, which may be several secs before the GO! signal. This was established with an instruction paradigm that permits separate correlation of cell firing in relation to direction of the required movement from that of direction of a perturbation serving as a GO! signal (EVARTS and TANJI, 1974, 1976; TANJI and EVARTS, 1976). The animals had to either push or pull with the wrist after the perturbation. *No overt* anticipatory discharge during the foreperiod of several *sec* with the same paradigm has been found in dentate or IP of 2 monkeys (STRICK, 1978). However, 46 dentate and 44 IP neurons discharged *within 70 msec* of movement onset. Over 50 % of the neurons in dentate but none in IP were "strongly" influenced by the animals' prior motor preparation", i. e. set. Similar results were obtained (THACH, 1978) with another paradigm that allowed correlation of neural discharge with wrist flexions or extensions against loads, or with holding in those positions until the next GO! signal was given. Neural discharge could be also related to the intended action since the 2 monkeys had to learn the sequences without being cued where to move after a hold. About one-third of dentate (18/62) and precentral (34/93) neurons discharged in relation to direction of the intended movement, in contrast to only 1/36 IP neurons.

These results, taken together, imply that the lateral cerebellum is important in events occurring just before (and after) movement onset (cf. Section 2), and the intermediate part mostly after onset (cf. Section 3). Hence, evidence from unit recording makes it unlikely that the cerebellum is involved in elaborating anticipatory 'set' for a learned task. Formation of such high-level, long-term functions might be better served by the areas linked through cortico-cortical connections, and perhaps even the posture-related basal ganglia that are known to discharge early enough (Buchwald et al., 1975; Denny-Brown and Yanagisawa, 1976; cf. Section 5 and Fig. 7B).

Discharge related to the direction of an intended movement is also evident in precentral activity of monkeys instructed to either push or pull a lever, and after a waiting period to respond according to the instruction to a push-or-pull perturbation (Evarts and Tanji, 1974, 1976; Tanji and Evarts, 1976). The 'set'-related discharge with regard to the intended direction occurs as the second of two 'early' precentral responses: it could be regarded as preparatory 'updating' of the movement. The first response occurs between 20–50 msec and the second, after an inhibition near 40 msec (cf. Evarts and Tanji, 1976), between 50–100 msec after the perturbation, i.e. just before its correction (Evarts and Tanji, 1976). Cerebellar involvement has been tested by cooling cerebellar nuclei and concomitant unit recording in motor cortex. Monkeys were trained to make self-paced elbow flexions and extensions by turning a handle in the horizontal plane, into mechanically undetectable, learned target zones, with the task area obstructed from view (see drawing in Fig. 3) (Meyer-Lohmann et al., 1975). The first precentral response to a perturbation is independent of the cerebellum, as it was neither affected in 41/46 precentral neurons by cooling the dentate nucleus in 2 monkeys (Meyer-Lohmann et al., 1975), nor by dentate and IP together for 47/58 precentral neurons in 2 other animals trained to hold the handle steady in a stationary target zone (Vilis et al., 1976). The second precentral response however, was depressed by nuclear cooling in 25/44 precentral neurons (Vilis et al., 1976), as were even later responses of 45/46 precentral neurons (Meyer-Lohmann et al., 1975). Fig. 2A (Conrad et al., 1975) defines the time relations of movement parameters, protagonist EMG, and precentral unit discharge. The second precentral response precedes 'intended', late, muscle activity. The paths and synaptic mechanisms upon alpha and gamma motoneurons to activate directional 'set' are unknown. Fig. 2B (Vilis et al., 1976) illustrates depression of the 2nd precentral response, for which some relevant cerebellar connections are drawn in Fig. 2C. How instructions for directional 'set' reach the cerebellum remains to be discovered: Fig. 2C suggests that it could result from various parts of the circuit. Set could have been stored in 'instructed' cerebellar P-cells, ready to act as a trigger upon receipt of appropriate combinations of inputs, as will be discussed in Sections 5 and 6.

Summary. The cerebellum does not appear to function at a high congitive level. Cerebellar dysfunction does not affect selection of movement strategies in monkeys or humans. "Anticipatory" set for a task delayed by several sec, is not conveyed from cerebellum to monkeys' motor cortex by overt cerebellar discharge. "Directional" set however, is expressed in discharge of dentate and precentral neurons just before correction of a perturbed posture or movement. This precentral discharge is diminished during cerebellar dysfunction.

2. MOVEMENT ONSET

Is the cerebellum involved in transmitting a command to Move!, and if so, from where and to what target? (cf. Evarts and Thach, 1969). The timing of precentral and cerebellar neural discharge in relation to movement implies a more important role for dentate than for IP. Impulses of most of a sample of 41 out of 50 dentate neurons, but only 17 out of 41 IP neurons, discharged before onset of prompt wrist flexions or extensions as tested in 4 monkeys (Thach, 1970a). In another 3 animals that exerted isometric force

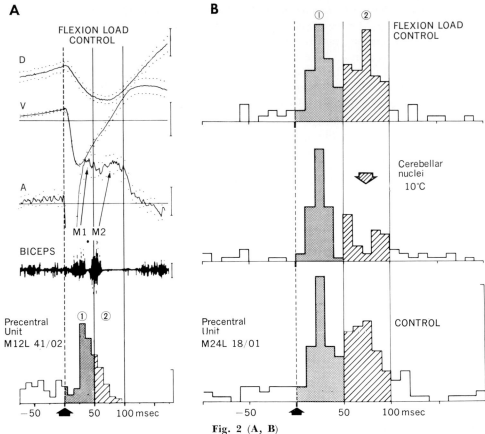

Fig. 2 (A, B)

A: Movement parameters, biceps EMG and activity of a precentral neuron to a perturbation that loaded elbow flexions of moderate speed, applied at time marked by upward arrow and dotted vertical line (Cebus monkey, see apparatus in Fig. 3). Computer generated averages ± SDs of 18 handle displacements (D), velocities (V), and acceleration (A), and histograms of precentral neuron (N) responses ① and ②. EMGs were obtained by photography of superimposed traces on a storage oscilloscope and were matched to the computer plots. Calibrations: time applies to all records, (D): 10 deg, (V): 200 deg/sec, (A): 5000 deg/sec², EMG: 2 mV, frequency of (N): 75 imp/sec. (from CONRAD et al., 1975).

B: Depression of second (directional set related) precentral response of a precentral neuron by cooling of cerebellar nuclei (dentate and IP). Normalized histograms are shown for first, response and another precentral neuron: dotted area ①; and for second response, cross-hatched ②, in response to a perturbation as in *A*. Same conventions and scales as in *A*. (Drawn on expanded time scale from VILIS et al., 1976).

about the wrist in response to a light signal (THACH, 1975), records from 256 dentate neurons and 225 precentral neurons yielded overlapping onset times, with the dentate slightly leading the precentral population in 2 animals. Median onset of discharge for the 3 animals was near 70 msec for dentate and 54 msec for motor cortex before force onset. Dentate discharge was sufficiently phasic so that it could have served as a trigger, once released from P-cell inhibition (THACH, 1972). In 2 other animals median onset times of discharge were compared for 93 precentral, 62 dentate and 36 IP neurons (THACH, 1978). All groups overlapped, but dentate led off, motor cortex followed by 15 msec, and IP by 26 msec.

HOLMES summarized in 1922 his observations (HOLMES, 1917, 1922b) that voluntary

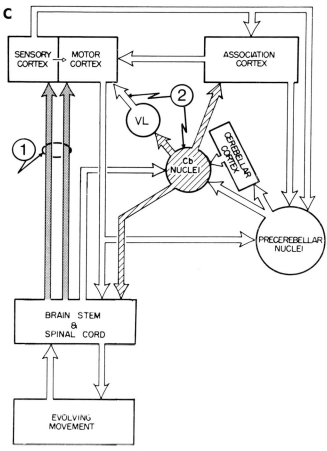

Fig. 2 (C)

C: Diagram of relevant functional connections. The first precentral response: ①, is thought to depend on thalamic route to sensorimotor cortex, not involving the cerebellum; while the second, set-related, precentral response: ②, depends on a route involving the dentate nucleus and VL of the thalamus. ("Cb nuclei" are marked because both dentate and interpositus were cooled in *B*). This diagram evolved in discussions with Drs. CONRAD, MEYER-LOHMANN, MATSUNAMI, WIESENDANGER, COOKE, HORE, and VILIS, 1975.

arm movements of patients with unilateral cerebellar injuries had a delayed onset with the ipsilateral arm by about 0.2 sec after the GO! command to move. Originally he believed that the cerebellum exerts a reinforcing or regulating influence on spinal motor mechanisms (HOLMES, 1917). However, by 1939, apparently under the influence of physiological discoveries made during the interim, he suggested that the delay may be at the cerebral rather than the spinal level, when he wrote that abnormalities in the rate and regularity of voluntary movement "are due to disorder in the cerebral mechanisms of voluntary movement, as a result of which there is a delay in initiating cortico-spinal innervation..." (HOLMES, 1939). HOLMES appears to have regarded the cerebellum not as a structure that details movement parameters for motor cortex, but rather as one which "...reinforces or tunes up the cerebral motor apparatus, including subcortical structures with motor functions, so that they respond promptly to volitional stimuli..." (HOLMES, 1939).

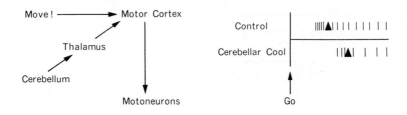

1. Cerebellar Nuclei Provide Background Excitation to Motor Cortex.

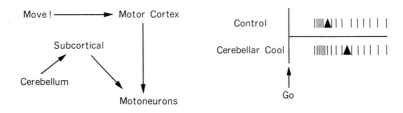

2. Cerebellar Nuclei Provide Background Excitation to Subcortical Structures.

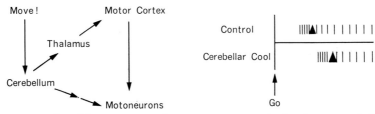

3. Cerebellar Nuclei Participate in Initiation of Movement.

Fig. 3 Dentate cooling delays onset of a learnt movement and related precentral discharge. *Left*: Three possible schemes for initiation of prompt arm movemenets. Pathways are drawn on the left, and on the right the expected time relations between discharge of a movement-related precentral neuron and movement onset (triangles). Control conditions above horizontal lines, and during cerebellar cooling below. Precentral discharge follows the visual GO! signal (vertical arrow). The three schemes predict three different discharge patterns during cerebellar nuclear cooling. Tonic precentral discharge levels would decrease in (1), but not in (2) and (3). Timing of discharge in relation to movement onset (triangles) differentiates between (2) and (3); precentral neural onset times would remain unchanged in (2) but would be delayed in (3). (from MEYER-LOHMANN et al., 1977).

Onset of arm movement of 2 monkeys trained to respond promptly were delayed by about 0.05–0.15 sec during dysfunction produced by brief, reversible cooling of the dentate nucleus (Fig. 3, MEYER-LOHMANN et al., 1977).   Delay of movement onset produced by dentate cooling has also been reported for baboons trained to a pointing task (TROUCHE et al., 1977); and prolonged reaction times have been seen after a dentate lesion in 1 monkey (THACH, 1975).   This reproduction of HOLMES' clinical observations could have been caused by withdrawal of tonic background support to motor cortex or to subcortical structures, as depicted in schemes 1 and 2 of Fig. 3.   Alternately, the cerebellum could be conveying a phasic Move! command, as in scheme 3.   Records from movement-related precentral neurons revealed that 42 out of 48 behaved as in scheme 3: their discharge remained tightly coupled to the movement and its protagonist muscles.   An

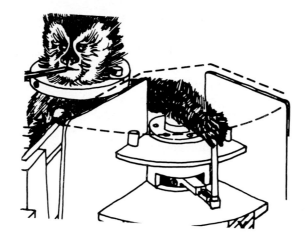

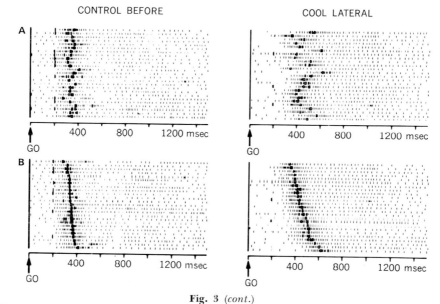

Fig. 3 *(cont.)*

Rasters next to scheme 3 correspond to scheme 3 and are typical of the majority, sampled by computer. *A*: discharge during 25 movements is plotted in raster format in successive lines one below the other with respect to the GO! signal (vertical arrow). *B*: same discharges as in *A* but ordered by increasing latency of movement onset (triangles). Vertical line at 0.2 sec is drawn to assist in recognition of delayed onset of precentral discharge and movement. (from MEYER-LOHMANN et al., 1977).

Inset drawing: Cebus monkey in experimental chair, with elbow supported on pivot of manipulandum, and hand grasping the handle, potentiometer and torque motor beneath. Juice reward tube in front of mouth; headholder and microdrive not shown. Opaque plate that blocks monkey's view of task area indicated by dotted lines.

example is provided in Fig. 3 to the right of scheme 3, where each raster dot represents an action potential of the neuron during a movement, and triangles mark the time of onset of these movements of moderate speed. Delay depended on extent of dentate cooling, but averaged about 0.1 sec. Similar data have been obtained recently for delay of antagonist muscles causing stop of corrected movements (VILIS and HORE, 1978). These results have been confirmed for monkeys with deafferented arms, before and after decerebellation (LAMARRE at al., 1978). All evidence indicates that delayed precentral discharge contributes to delayed movement onset.

The precentral discharge could be destined for actions that are only indirectly related to movement onset such as tonic disfacilitation of motor cortex, (scheme 1) but that was rarely seen (MEYER-LOHMANN et al., 1975, 1977). Tonic subcortical disfacilitation (scheme 2) may be involved, particularly when more extensive nuclear cooling slowed initial movement velocities, yielding a separate reproduction of that aspect of the clinical picture (HOLMES, 1917, 1922b, 1939; TERZUOLO and VIVIANI, 1974). If the motor command to Move! is sent from cerebellum to motor cortex over the VL pathway, then the divergence in that path (STRICK, 1976a) could disfacilitate many precentral neurons during dentate cooling, with a consequent delay in discharge onset. Cooling of the dentate may also prolong the computational time in the cerebellum of the command to Move! and thus delay its departure to motor cortex (NASHNER, 1976; PEW, 1974a, b; SEARS, 1974). Timing of such motor commands presumably depends on information available to the cerebellum about motor programs, for instance 'set' (Section 1), as well as about the current state of the body and of the external world, which is thought to be updated continuously between and during movements (ECCLES, 1967, 1969; ECCLES et al., 1972). Slight decreases in phasic discharge of precentral neurons observed during dentate cooling were the result of changes in discharge patterns in individual trials (MEYER-LOHMANN et al., 1977). This may support the notion that instructions from cerebellum to motor cortex arrive as patterned singnals (ECCLES, 1969; ECCLES et al., 1972), which is born out by the resemblance of discharge patterns of dentate and precentral neurons (THACH, 1978).

Some unresolved questions remain about pathways from cerebellum to spinal cord, and to motor cortex, with reference to participation in cerebellar movement generation. Dentate stimulation can produce stereotyped elbow flexions (SCHULTZ et al., 1976) and can potentiate some reflexes in monkeys deprived of sensorimotor and premotor cortex, presumably through the reticulo-spinal tract (BANTLI and BLOEDEL, 1976), which could be related to postural adjustments associated with movement preparation (ALLEN et al., 1978). Onset-times of discharge of movement-related neurons in the arm area of VL receiving dentate projections, also leave questions: of 160 units in 3 monkeys, (of which 142 were related to both ballistic and slow movements, i.e. less than 140 msec and more than 600 msec durations), VL-neuron onset preceded EMG onset in only 30/299 ballistic changes, and in only 10/115 slow changes. Pooled histogram displays however, can be deceiving: they suggest that all mean VL onsets preceded those of arm, shoulder, or trunk EMGs (STRICK, 1976b). Furthermore, lesions of the red nucleus, or thalamic nuclei VA/VL and VPL do not produce quite the same changes as cerebellar lesions in monkeys' elbow flexions (MILLER and BROOKS, 1977; RANISH and SOECHTING, 1976). These differences may be related to definition of the small volume of relevant thalamic tissue (STRICK, 1976a, b).

No matter how these problems will be resolved, the fastest pathway for generation of prompt arm movement appears to involve some sort of neocerebellar trigger function.

Summary. The cerebellum participates in onset of movements made by humans or monkeys by controlling the timing of supraspinal motor commands. Prompt movement onset after a GO! signal depends for monkeys on neocerebellar discharge to supraspinal motor centers, including motor cortex, beginning about 70 and 55 msec respectively before force onset. Dysfunction of the lateral cerebellum delays supraspinal motor commands in monkeys and delays movement onset by about 0.1–0.2 sec in monkeys and humans respectively.

3. MOVEMENT EXECUTION

HOLMES (1917, 1922a, b, c, d, 1939) set out the "fundamental" symptoms resulting from cerebellar lesions in humans as: generally decreased muscle tone and strength, abnormalities in the range, rate, regularity and force of voluntary movements, and delays in their onset and end. He regarded other signs as derived from those above, such as poor synchronicity and combinations of joints used in "compound" movements, and hence direction, and breakdown of rhythmic alternations. He urged that the total picture of disorganized posture and movements is explicable by defects of the constituent "simple" movements involving only one joint, namely errors in range, rate, force, and delays in starting and stopping. I follow this view, that the "coordinating" role of the cerebellum rests on simple functions concerning simple movements.

3A. Compound movements

Compound movements "involve change of posture at two or more joints". In "...cere-bellar ataxia...the affected limb decomposes the movements in time into its constituent parts, and this naturally leads to errors of direction. Delay in the initiation of one component relative to that of another, and excessive range of one element of the movement...are the chief causes...'". HOLMES (1939) also commented on loss of rhythm: "It is particularly in actions which require reversal of direction that...diversion of attention...increases the irregularities...indicating how dependent the rhythm of movement is on concentrated effort when cerebellar function is defective..." (HOLMES, 1939).

These symptoms have been reproduced in animals with cerebellar lesions (CARREA and METTLER, 1947) particularly with trained animals by the group at the Univ. of Pennsylvania. Recovery from ataxia to tremor has been described (GROWDON et al., 1967) as 5 monkeys were retrained after unilateral destruction of dentate and IP, to make goal-directed arm movements as well as hand and finger manipulations. Symptoms seemed to depend on the task context (cf. BROOKS, 1979), suggesting "...a single basic deficit following lateral cerebellar nuclear lesions in the monkey. This is the inability to control movements in goal directed behaviour. This basic deficit leads to an error, the voluntary correction of which results in ataxia, ataxic tremor and postural tremor...". Further experiments with another 4 such animals led to the conclusion that the primary deficit was "...a failure to start and stop movements with the proper timing" (LIU and CHAMBERS, 1971). Finally, 15 monkeys were trained to reach out and grasp a target object, and retraining of these animals was followed up to 1 year after bilateral lesions of dentate and IP interposed nuclei (GOLDBERGER and GROWDON, 1973). Data from accelerometers on the arm were correlated with motion pictures: "...Changes with time showed a progressive conversion of ataxic oscillations [3 5 Hz] to tremor [6–8 Hz] as reflex and locomotor performance improved. At any time, limb fixation combined with phasic movement initiated the oscillations, whereas a fixed position by itself could be maintained, or a phasic movement without a fixed end point performed without tremor or ataxia. Analysis...suggests...that the cerebellum provides a timing device for movement which matches limb fixation with phasic (usually distal) movement so that the limb fixation stops at the right moment for the phasic component to begin...". Reaching movement were re-studied more quantitatively recently (GILMAN et al., 1976), with 6 monkeys trained to reach, under direct vision, for a cube of apple placed before them in one out of 5 positions. Movement trajectories and velocities were computed from frames of movie film, taken from above. The animals could accomplish their task 10 days after removal of the entire cerebellum, despite dysmetria and a 3 Hz tremor originating at the shoulder. Movements deviated more however, from the previously linear path, and reached greater angular velocity.

Evidence for movement decomposition and delayed EMG termination and onset can be glimpsed in Fig. 6B (3 and 4) from an experiment with dentate cooling while a monkey performed an alternate-bar pressing task, outlined in Fig. 6A (HORVATH et al., 1970). Prolonged reaching times during dentate cooling in a pointing task carried out by baboons have also been noted (TROUCHE et al., 1977), and after cerebellectomy even in deafferented monkeys that have learned such a task (LAMARRE et al., 1978). Errors of rhythmic alternation have also been reproduced in monkeys by dentate cooling (HORVATH et al., 1970).

Records of cerebellar neural discharge during compound movements have by and large revealed relations to constituent simple parts of those movements. Monkeys were trained to pull a horizontal lever forward and hold it before releasing it and eating a reward. Unit records were made in intermediate cortex (HARVEY et al., 1977). Simple spike discharge (in response to mossy fiber input) of 173/183 task-related P-cells either increased or decreased during extensions or flexions, and in relation to their range or duration. Complex spikes (in response to climbing fiber input) also often changed in relation to some phase of the task, usually in opposite direction to that of the simple spikes. Only 9 P-cells gave complicated responses, of which 7 showed almost sinusoidal modulation of activity during successive phases of the task. Patterns of those 7 neurons resemble those recorded from 87 dentate neurons in 3 squirrel monkeys (ROBERTSON and GRIMM, 1975), trained to a compound sequential, button-pressing task. Most neurons gave some elevation of discharge at each button, but there was a suggestion that particular phases of the compound movement were specially effective. Discharge of all neurons increased somewhat on movement onset, and of some just prior to first button contact. Patterns of about one-third altered according to whether the 3-button panel was horizontal or tilted.

The evidence from animal experiments suggests that intent and circumstances are important in tasks that involve changes of position of several joints, action of many muscles, and contactual changes of the operant hand. This supports Holmes' view that explanations for cerebellar effects on compound movements are best sought by studying their constituent simple parts.

Summary. Compound movements depend for correctly timed sequencing of constituent simple movements on lateral and/or intermediate cerebellum. Their dysfunction causes movement decomposition and tremor in monkeys and in humans.

3B. Ballistic movements

Ballistic movements are voluntary, brief (about 0.15–0.2 sec), fast, and are launched without peripheral sensory guidance. Evidence for programming is presented in Fig. 4A (CONRAD and BROOKS, 1974) of the rhythm of such rapid, alternating arm movements, i. e. of the sequential timing of flexions and extensions. The traces are of handle position of a monkey, (representative of 3 so tested), using the same set-up as in Fig. 3, but in these trials the handle was slammed back and forth rapidly between two mechanical barriers, instead of being brought to an endpoint determined by voluntary arrest. Records of these movements, lasting about 0.15 sec between the usual positions of the stops, appear on the left. When the barriers were moved closer together unexpectedly, as shown in the subsequent records, the animal exerted protagonist and antagonist forces for the same durations as it has been used to, and thus maintained the learned rhythm. The upper part of Fig. 4B also illustrates that often protagonist muscle discharge ceased 10–40 msec before movement impact on the barrier, i. e. before feedback could cue it to cease. Other evidence from tests with normal and deafferented human subjects and monkeys supports the view that such rapid movements are preprogrammed (cf. BROOKS, 1979), but it is a

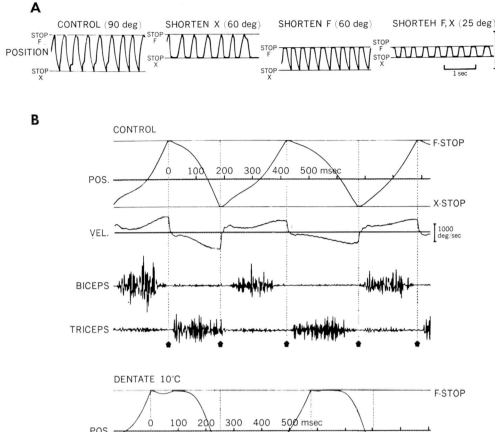

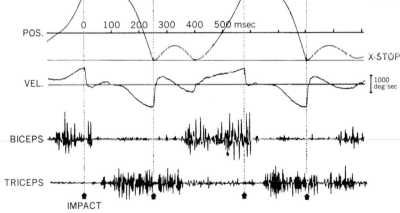

Fig. 4

A: Demonstration of programmed rhythmic ballistic movements. Rapid alternating arm movements of Cebus monkey (cf. Fig. 3) made after unexpected changes of positions of mechanical barriers ('stop') limiting movement range. Individual position traces shown between horizontal line sthat indicate barrier positions at Flexion (F) stop and Extension (X) stop. Time calibration: 1 sec.

B: Dentate cooling prolongs ballistic rhythm. Position, velocity and EMG during control (above) and cooling of dentate nucleus (below). Vertical broken lines and arrows indicate moment of impact on mechanical stops. Note prolongation of EMG by 0.1–0.2 sec. *A* and *B*: Position traces sampled by computer; velocity obtained by differentiating digitized position signal. *B*: tape recorded EMGs were matched to computer plots. (*A* and *B* from Conrad and Brooks, 1974).

matter of interpretation whether there is a controlled parameter such as movement duration (cf. KORNHUBER, 1971, 1974), or whether timing of muscles is controlled. There is now emerging evidence that monkeys' ballistic head (BIZZI et al., 1976, 1978) and arm (BIZZI and POLIT, 1979) movements are preprogrammed to reach the intended endpoint of the movement (not against a mechanical barrier as in Fig. 4) as governed by the expected length-tension curves of the pro- and antagonist muscles acting on the moved joint. This implies that 'initial' impulses (WOODWORTH, 1899) are generated and triggered centrally, for correct intensity and timing of the muscle actions involved, to achieve the programmed balance point.

Experiments with unit recording implicate the cerebello-cerebral circuit in rapid movements. 17 out of 71 hemispheric P-cells and 27 nuclear cells discharged in cadence with rapid flexions/extensions of the ipsilateral wrist, or pushing/pulling motions from the shoulder, as tested in 2 monkeys (THACH, 1968). Modulation of discharge frequency of simple spikes of 171 cells, and of 27 nuclear cells was established. During ballistic pronation/supination wrist movements of monkeys, 1/3 of 589 contralateral precentral neurons were solely related to these, as opposed to slower, movements; and these neurons emitted brief bursts which ceased prior to movement completion (FROMM and EVARTS 1977). That in itself does not prove them to be programmed 'command' neurons however, since they could be under the influence of residual fusimotor drive feedback (VALLBO, 1971), but the argument is strengthened because many large neurons in that sample (EVARTS and FROMM 1977) were unresponsive to sensory input from wrist perturbations.

Cerebellar participation in rhythmic rapid arm alternations has been tested with dentate cooling. The upper part of Fig. 4B (CONRAD and BROOKS, 1974) illustrates normal task execution on an expanded time scale. The lower part depicts performance during dentate cooling, when the protagonist muscle in each swing discharged for 0.1–0.2 sec longer than usual, instead of stopping before impact, and hence the animal pressed the handle against the mechanical barrier for that extra length of time. This is shown better in this record for the extensor: triceps, than for the flexor: biceps. Movement parameters as such remained unchanged: normal velocities and accelerations are evident. [It remains to repeat this experiment with self-terminated ballistic movements (cf. BIZZI and POLIT, 1979)]. The present results resemble human adiadochokinesis, first described by BABINSKI (1902), who blamed it on delayed braking of protagonist action by the antagonist. HOLMES (1917) described it thus: "...the slowness is due directly to delay at the turn and not to time lost in the movements themselves for there is rarely much difference in the rate of these and of those of the normal limb...". He also related cerebellar dysfunction and prolonged muscular effort for the case of equivalent hypermetria (HOLMES, 1939): "The movements, or rather the contractions of the muscles which effect it, may be continued for a fifth of second or more after the normal limb has come to rest...". Similar results have been obtained with 3 squirrel monkeys that had been trained to make a rapid forearm upward flexion when they could overcome a resistive force that was varied randomly (SOECHTING et al., 1976). After compensation for severe cerebellar symptoms during the first few weeks following lesions of all cerebellar nuclei on the side of the limb performing the task; peak velocity, acceleration and deceleration were unchanged, but agonist muscle action persisted for an abnormally long time. Unfortunately this 'release-and-let-go' paradigm does not produce simple ballistic movements (SOECHTING et al., 1976), but instead generates intended, isometric contractions against the restraint until release, when an "unloading reflex" (HANSEN and HOFFMANN, 1922) supervenes. Since its properties depend reactively on peripheral circumstances, SOECHTING et al., (1976) argued that such were also the properties of 'ballistic' movements. These are semantic points: in fact all results agree with those of others regarding unloading reflexes, and will be discussed at the end of Section 3C.

Summary. The cerebellum participates in rhythmic ballistic movements made by humans or monkeys, by controlling the relative timing of muscles moving the joint. Purkinje and nuclear cells can discharge in cadence with ballistic movements. Dysfunction of the lateral cerebellum prolongs protagonist muscle action, and delays antagonist action as well as movement return by about 0.1–0.2 sec in monkeys and in humans.

3C. Simple movements of moderate speed

Three fundamental cerebellar signs for simple voluntary movements: errors of range, rate and force, appeared as part of the syndrome discernible in compound movements of decerebellate monkeys, as described in Section 3A.   Errors in direction were taken up in Section 1.   Other fundamental signs, such as delay in starting simple movements were described in Section 2, and delay in stopping for ballistic movements in Section 3B. This now leads us to consider errors in range, rate and force.   Hypotonia will be next, in Section 4.

During the past decade there has been an intensive search for links between neural discharge in the sensorimotor system of trained animals with movements parameters, such as force, velocity, displacement, or duration (BROOKS and STONEY, 1971).   Some such correlations have been found, for instance for force particularly in motor cortex (cf. CONRAD et al., 1977; EVARTS et al., 1972).   Introduction of new task paradigms made it clear however, that many neurons discharge according to the intent of the animal as well as the circumstances (cf. BROOKS, 1979; EVARTS and THACH, 1969; EVARTS and TANJI, 1974; EVARTS and FROMM, 1977; FROMM and EVARTS, 1977; STRICK, 1978; THACH, 1978). Thus it is not surprising that no single, all-embracing, relation could be established for neurons in the sensorimotor system. *Different brain parts, such as sensory or motor cortex, cerebellum, or basal ganglia can no longer be regarded as candidates for separate control systems for specific parameters (Brooks and Stoney, 1971) or types of movements (Kornhuber, 1971, 1974).* The emerging view of sensorimotor control as interactive systems offers other new options to be studied (cf. BROOKS, 1979).   Different structures could, for instance, be regulators of gain (ITO, 1970, 1972, 1974; ROBINSON, 1976) or set-point (HOUK, 1978) of particular feedback servos, including an adaptive capability (Section 5).   Further options include functions as triggers (cf. BRAITENBERG, 1961, 1967; KORNHUBER, 1971, 1974), and more speculative engineering ideas such as differentiators, integrators etc.   It is most important however to keep in mind the properties of the anatomical connections that create preferential paths for information transfer, as well as the consequences of dysfunction.

IP neurons discharge overwhelmingly in relation to execution of ongoing, rather than to properties of intended, movements (STRICK, 1978; THACH, 1978) (cf. Section 1). Two parameters have been dissociated for correlation with wrist-turning (THACH, 1978): muscular patterns determined by load, and position of the wrist.   Dentate neuron discharge correlated (32/62) to muscle pattern and (14/62) to joint position, much as precentral neurons (34/93 and 25/93); whereas IP cells related mostly (30/36) to muscle patterns and the force exerted, only 5/36 related to joint position (cf. HARVEY et al., 1977, in Section 3A).

Monkeys were observed to make two kinds of simple elbow movements in our set-up, (Figs. 3 and 5, and description in Section 1): those that oscillated near '6 Hz' (left in box 1), and another type that oscillated near '3 Hz' (right).   The definition of frequency rests on whether the acceleration trace (A) crosses the zero-line.   Since oscillations could be of various amplitudes, the two types of movements differ mainly in the intensity of

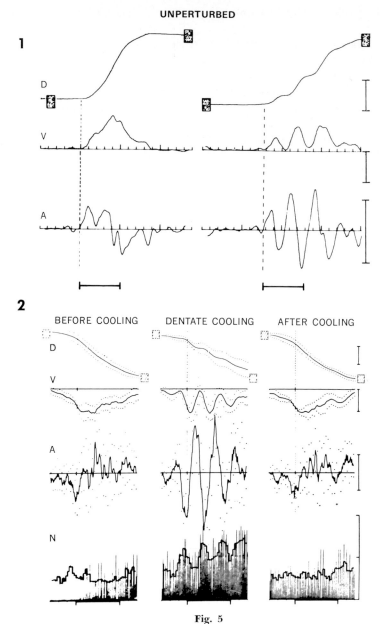

Fig. 5

1: Two types of simple movements of moderate speed. (Cebus monkey, see *Fig. 3*). Left and right columns: movements with oscillations at approx. 6 Hz and 3 Hz, respectively, made by the same animal. Target positions indicated on displacement (D) traces, sampled by computer. Velocity (V) and acceleration (A) obtained by differentiating digitized D signal. Calibrations for 1 and 2: time: 500 msec, (D): 25 deg, (V): 100 deg/sec, (A): 1000 deg/sec², (N): 100/sec. (from BROOKS et al., 1973b)

2: Dentate cooling causes animal to decrease oscillation frequency from '6 Hz' to '3 Hz'. Averages (± SD: dots) of about 20 elbow extensions. Sample at 10°C 3 min after first control, second control 5 min after end of cooling. (D) and (V) traces sampled by computer. (A) obtained by differentiating digitized (V) signal. (N): Normalized histograms of discharge of a precentral unit during those movements. (from MEYER-LOHMANN et al., 1975)

PERTURBED

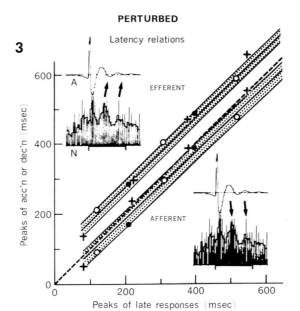

3 Latency relations

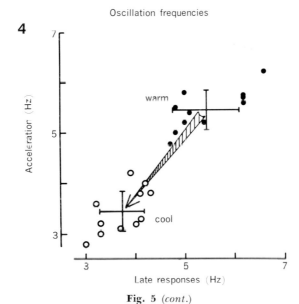

Oscillation frequencies

Fig. 5 *(cont.)*

3: Tightly coupled timing of late precentral responses to arm perturbations and of movement oscillations. Regression lines: (± SDs) for 18 neurons plotted in relation to peaks of (A) oscillations. (D) and (V) as in *2*. Insets: traces of (A) and histograms of discharge of another precentral neuron (N) (time marker: 500 msec). Arrows indicate "efferent" lead time from cortex to limb, and "afferent" lag time from limb to cortex. (from CONRAD et al., 1975)

4: Dentate cooling slows oscillations of movements and of late precentral responses from '6 Hz' '3 Hz'. Points (± SDs) for 11 precentral neurons, as in *3*. (from MEYER-LOHMANN et al., 1975) cyclic force application (BROOKS et al., 1973b), but they coexist as shown by power spectral density analysis that revealed peaks at 3–5 Hz and 5–7 Hz (COOKE and THOMAS, 1976). This indicates that the two types may be a continuum with 2 peaks, for which '3 Hz' and '6 Hz' are convenient names.

Oscillations at these frequencies also predominate in such analyses of feedback-guided and predictive muscle force, respectively, applied about the elbow joint by normal human subjects to steady a vibrating rod ("action tonic stretch reflex": NEILSON and LANCE, 1978). The most striking, and unique, change paralleling hypotonia in 10 patients with cerebellar dysfunctions, was loss of EMG phase lead in relation to external forces that had to be overcome (NEILSON and LANCE, 1978; cf. Section 6). The predominant peaks in the power spectrum also disappeared. In contrast, during dentate cooling with 2 monkeys (COOKE and THOMAS, 1976), the relative power of the 6 Hz peak declined and that near 3 Hz increased. Peak accelerations of oscillations increased in our samples, (BROOKS et al., 1973a; MEYER-LOHMANN et al., 1975) and so did their peak velocities in an earlier sample (BROOKS et al., 1973a), which was stressed then since it fits well with HOLMES' description of movements unopposed by any load (HOLMES, 1922a, 1939). This view had to be modified however, when it was realized that speed and accuracy are traded off in monkeys' movements just as they are in humans, depending on their set for conditions of the task (cf. BROOKS, 1979). It may therefore be more useful to search for basic cerebellar deficiencies by considering the apparent need to change movement rhythms to compensate for errors of range (cf. Section 1). Fig. 5 (box 2) illustrates quick compensation during dentate cooling for errors of range (D) and rate (V), but reveals residual larger variabilities and slowed cyclic applications of force in extensions, as reflected in the acceleration trace (A). HOLMES (1939) recognized that "...an...important...disorder in all movements, but particularly those executed slowly and deliberately, is a lack of uniformity in their velocity...The instability of a limb and the irregular tremor which develops in it... are evidently due to defective postural fixation and to voluntary corrections of its deviations...". Originally we (BROOKS et al., 1973a) like others (GOLDBERGER and GROWDON, 1973; GROWDON et al., 1967; LIU and CHAMBERS, 1971) thought that this also applied to monkeys, but we now also have to take into account the servo-properties of tremor (VILIS and HORE, 1977) (cf. Section 6).

The changes of movement oscillations that occur in min during repeated nuclear cooling (cf. Fig. 5), correspond closely to those observed during weeks of recovery from lesions of dentate and IP (cf. Section 2). Lesions cause degeneration, and hence lasting effects on many structures: 'diaschesis' (Monakow, 1914). The advantage of the cooling method, begun in 1910 (Trendelenburg) is that local dysfunctions can be produced reversibly, so that the results can be compared quickly to normal function before permanent re-organization of brain parts takes place.

Histograms of the discharge of a precentral neuron (N) during the movement in Fig. 5 illustrate unchanged tight coupling to movement oscillations during dentate cooling (representative of 10 so tested). Better insight into timing could be gained by examining responses to perturbations (load or unload) that changed in the same way as self-paced movements during dentate cooling. The insets in box 3, illustrate damped oscillations of accleration (A) and discharge of a precentral neuron (N) that occurred late after the first and second precentral responses, illustrated in Fig. 2B. [Unlike the second 'early' response, 'late' precentral responses do not reflect directional set since they always reacted 'reflexly' to perturbations, i. e. in the same direction sense as the first 'early' response, as tested with 111 neurons (CONRAD et al., 1975). The first response need not be reconsidered since it does not involve the cerebellum (Fig. 2C)]. Timing of peaks of late responses of a larger sample is plotted in box 3 of Fig. 5 in relation to acceleration oscillations. Average "efferent" lead-time between late precentral responses and these oscillations was of the same order (70–80 msec) as that between the first precentral response and the acceleration peak arising from the spinal stretch reflex (cf. Fig. 2A). Conversely, average "afferent" lagtime from limb to motor cortex (above 20 msec) was of the same order as the first precentral response after the initial displacement (cf. Fig. 5, in CONRAD et al., 1977), and furthermore varied with their time evolution (Fig. 6 in CONRAD et al., 1975, and Fig. 6 in MEYER-LOHMANN et al., 1975). Analogy of timing suggests that both first and late precentral responses involve interaction of periphery and motor cortex (MEYER-LOHMANN et al., 1975). During dentate cooling, with much (VILIS and HORE, 1976) or with only little (MEYER-LOHMANN et al., 1975) involvement of IP, during moving (MEYER-LOHMANN et al., 1975) or holding (VILIS and HORE, 1976), movement oscillations (and discharge bursts of 64 precentral neurons: MEYER-LOHMANN et al., 1975), slowed from their normal values of 5–8 Hz to 3–4 Hz (box 4 in Fig. 5: MEYER-LOHMANN et al., 1975). Frequency reduction amounted to a delay of about 0.15 sec, and EMG records in 14 cases showed equivalent changes (cf. Fig. 9 in MEYER-LOHMANN et al., 1975).

The results imply that rhythms of movements and those of their spinal and supraspinal commands, normally depend on the lateral cerebellum: timing is the critical factor (cf. MARSDEN et al., 1977). Rhythms might be slowed during cerebellar dysfunction because of time-consuming precentral interaction with peripheral events, as has been suggested (ALLEN and TSUKAHARA, 1974; ITO, 1970; MEYER-LOHMANN et al., 1975; MURPHY et al., 1975b; VILIS et al., 1976; VILIS and HORE, 1977; see Fig. 2C). Other alternatives how central delay could be prolonged will be discussed in Section 6. Compensation for errors of range accomplished by '3 Hz' movements indicates parallel processing in distributed systems (cf. MURPHY et al., 1974), presumably involving association cortex for reorganization. The monkeys did not recover their original capacity, but now succeeded with a degraded performance through use of the '3 Hz' strategy (cf. Section 1). During dysfunction of the lateral cerebellum, errors of timing of force thus remain uncompensated. The relative lack of effects by cooling IP (neither exaggerated oscillations, nor hypermetria; UNO et al., 1973) suggests that sensory feedback for overtrained movements can be carried by paths paralleling those of the intermediate cerebellum, for instance the medial lemniscal one (MURPHY et al., 1975a) (see Fig. 2B). Onset-timing of self-initiated movements appears to fit into ongoing oscillations, since their rhythm cohered across at least 8 such movements, tested in 2 monkeys (COOKE and THOMAS, 1976). This result does not conflict with demonstration of oscillation-reset by perturbations tested in 2 other monkeys (VILIS and HORE, 1977), as the neural command sequences may be different.

Cyclic force applications, timed by the cerebellum, might therefore time onset of voluntary movements: the slowing of oscillations in ordinary and in perturbed movements (Meyer-Lohmann et al., 1975; Vilis and Hore 1977) and of movement onset (Section 2) (Meyer-Lohmann et al., 1975) as well as of termination (Conrad and Brooks, 1974) (Section 3B) during dentate dysfunction are of the same order: about 0.1–0.2 sec. The emphasis on timing does not imply that the cerebellum is regarded as a clock with a 0.1 sec period (e.g. Braitenberg, 1961, 1967), but rather that deranged timing is an adventitious sign of released dysfunction. This dysfunction, common to all investigated situations, amounts to application of force that is scaled and timed less than optimally, but still matched as well as possible to the properties of the task and the moved limb (cf. Section 6).

Very similar results to ours were obtained when monkeys' elbows were unloaded (SOECHTING et al., 1976) while the animals applied set-dependent force for rapid upward flexions until they could overcome a restraint. Description of these results has been held over from Section 3B for comparison to our data; and to emphasize that their human subjects and presumably also monkeys, did indeed try to make ballistic movements, but that onset was commingled with an "unloading reflex". SOECHTING et al. (1976) observed, exactly as we had done, pauses in agonist EMG with corresponding bursts in antagonist EMG near peak acceleration and velocity. Timing of the pauses was tightly coupled to the time evolution of these movements parameters (cf. Figs. 6 in CONRAD et al., 1975; MEYER-LOHMANN et al., 1975). After uni- or bilateral lesions of monkeys' cerebellar nuclei, the (more prominent) pause at peak velocity was absent, leading to cocontraction (cf. Fig. 9 in MEYER-LOHMANN et al., 1975) and slowed adjustments. EMG reductions were no longer accurately timed, but fluctuated from 10 msec prior to, to 15 msec after, peak velocity. Furthermore, adaptability was lost: there was degradation of the usually detailed relation between EMG pauses and the kinematic movement variables, whose evoluion in time and intensity were manipulated by changing the inertial load or resitive force of the lever moved by the upswinging arm. Ordinarily the "duty cycle of the [cerebellar] automatic system" (TERZUOLO et al., 1973a; TERZUOLO and VIVIANI, 1974) in human normal volunteers was thought to last to peak acceleration or velocity, which coincided with a pause of agonist muscle discharge and an antagonist burst. It was only after this first "unintentional deceleration", about 0.1 sec after movement onset, that 7 normal human subjects (under similar circumstances, in which they had to overcome the maximal tension that each was able to exert), could initiate voluntary accelerations or decelerations of "ballistically" initiated upward elbow flexions (TERZUOLO and VIVIANI, 1974). Tests were made with 3 patients that had undergone surgical partial removal of a cerebellar hemisphere. The outstanding characteristics of their movements were cocontraction, slowed adjustments, and the absence of the "unintentional deceleration", as well as of "structured" EMG patterns, i.e. the silent period pauses described above.

Summary. The cerebellum participates in simple movements by preparation and guidance, as indicated by discharge of lateral cerebellar neurons shortly before onset and thereafter, and that of intermediate cerebellum more after onset. Some neurons in dentate, but none in IP, discharge in relation to the intended next movement. All IP, and some dentate neurons, discharge in relation to muscle action with regard to movement execution. Error of range, rate, and force involve prolongation of muscle action up to 0.1–0.2 sec. This is the most "fundamental"sign that could account for the change to slower movement oscillations at about 3 Hz, observed initially after cerebellar dysfunction in monkeys and humans.

4. MUSCLE TONE

Hypotonia, i. e. decreased maintained resistance to passive muscle stretch can be a long-lasting consequence of acute lateral cerebellar lesions in man (HOLMES, 1917, 1922a, 1939). The condition was first reproduced in cats and dogs by LUCIANI (1891, 1915), who considered it the main symptom of decerebellation (cf. Dow and MORUZZI, 1958; MILLER, 1977). It appears most clearly if other release phenomena are avoided by restricting the lesion to the neocerebellum (BREMER, 1935). Monkeys, baboons (BOTTERELL and FULTON, 1938a, b, c) and chimpanzees (BOTTERELL and FULTON, 1937) are (said to be progressively more severely and longer) hypotonic after dentate, rather than IP lesions (cf. BROOKHART, 1960; Dow and MORUZZI, 1958; GILMAN, 1969; GRANIT, 1970). No systematic tests were made, but hypotonia was reported to have lasted as long as ataxia: on average about one month (cf. Section 3A). Pendular tendon reflexes were first related to atonia by Andre THOMAS (1897, 1911). We have not studied muscle tone in clinical fashion during cooling of cerebellar nuclei, because Cebus monkeys withdraw their arm violently when passive manipulation is attempted.

Evidence that hypotonia can be caused by depressed function of muscle spindles was produced by cooling of intermediate cerebellar cortex of decerebrate cats, which reduced spindle responses to maintained extension of the soleus to passive levels, although alpha motoneuron activity increased (GRANIT et al., 1965). This work was extended to the demonstration of deficient function of gastrocnemius primary spindle afferents in monkeys decerebellated 5–6 days previously. Thresholds were raised and static and dynamic sensitivities were depressed paralleling the degree of hypotonia. Responses of muscle spindle secondary afferents, however were normal at short muscle lengths (GILMAN and MacDONALD, 1967; GILMAN and VAN DER MEULEN, 1965). Reduction of spindle sensitivity to graded static stretches of gastrocnemius, and to a variety of natural, external inputs after total cerebellectomy in decerebrate cats, was supplemented by establishing low baseline rates of gamma motoneuron fibers (GILMAN and EBEL, 1970) (reviewed in the clinical perspective: GILMAN, 1969, 1972). The cerebellum was therefore thought to regulate gamma bias on spindle output (GILMAN and VAN DER MEULEN, 1965), implying "that, in the recently decerebellate animal, alpha anterior horn cells having synaptic connection with spindle receptors innervated by afferent fibers of high conduction velocity receive a falsely low indication of static muscle length" (GILMAN and MacDONALD, 1967). In addition there is cerebellar control over the dynamic gamma system because dynamic stretch-sensitivity in the cat is abolished by interfering stimulation of the anterior lobe (JANSEN and MATTHEWS, 1962) or by cerebellectomy (GLASER and HIGGINS, 1966).

GRANIT (1970) concluded in his overview "...that the cerebellum controls a neural switch directing excitation into the alpha or gamma route. Alternatively this may be thought of as a neuronal link governed by the Purkinje cells. In the normal animal fusimotor activity would then rise and fall with the level of activity of these cells. Destruction of the link in cerebellar disease could explain well known symptoms such as dysmetria and adiodochokinesis. There would then be no organized gamma activity to enable the spindles to measure, and by their messages to control muscle length and change...". This statement was made with regard to ongoing feedback in active movements, but it can also be applied to preparatory 'updating' of preprogrammed movements (cf. ALLEN and TSUKAHARA, 1974; ECCLES, 1967, 1969; ECCLES et al., 1972; and Sections 1 and 6), that would also function most efficiently with alpha-gamma coactivation (cf. GRANIT et al., 1955; GRANIT, 1970; PHILLIPS and PORTER, 1977). Programming of precentral neurons innervating gamma motoneurons has been mooted (FROMM and EVARTS, 1977), including a route through the lateral cerebellum (HORVATH et al., 1970; MEYER-LOHMANN, 1975, and cf. PHILLIPS and PORTER, 1977), but so far without direct evidence.

Granit (1970) viewed alpha-gamma uncoupling as a basic deficit that could explain the signs of cerebellar dysfunction. I agree, and in addition I propose that such uncoupling is fundamentally caused by loss of adaptive capability in central connections of the cerebellum.

Clinical assessments of hypotonia are subjective. Quantitative measurements of the "action tonic stretch reflex" by NEILON and LANCE (1978) (Section 3C), revealed loss of predominant oscillation frequencies, and loss of phase lead at higher (predictive) frequencies, near 5 Hz. Application of this method is still vitiated however, by the dependence of tone in active movements on attitude or 'set'. We are thus returned to the problems considered in Section 1 e.g. Fig. 2. HOLMES (1939) in review allowed... "that in long-standing disease of the cerebellum...the muscles regain through the activities of other parts of the nervous system some capacity to fix attitudes and to resist stretch so that hypotonia is not so easily recognized on clinical examination, *but the more complex function of adapting tone to changing posture during movement remains defective and contributes to the disturbances included in the term ataxia...*" (my italics). *This is illustrated, in a way, in Figs. 2–6 for monkeys. Clinical hypotonia thus should probably be removed from the list of "fundamental" defects, and instead should be considered another sign of loss of cellebellar adaptability (cf. Section 5 and 6).*

Summary. Hypotonia can be is a consequence of acute dysfunction of the lateral

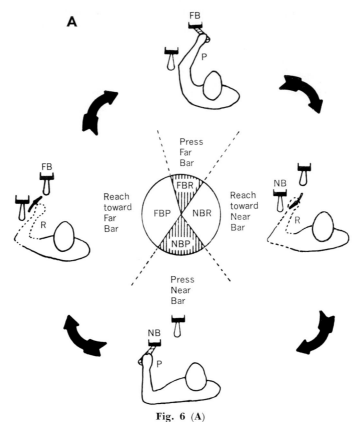

Fig. 6 (A)

A: Task cycle for an alternate bar pressing task, requiring compound movements. Task is divided into sequential phases (arrows) of pressing the far bar (**FBP**), shown at the top, reaching toward the near bar (**NBR**), pressing the near (**NBP**), and reaching toward the far bar (**FBR**). Cebus monkey learned bar positions without visual guidance because a horizontal plate was inserted between the head and the task area for arm movements. Relative times for each phase are indicated by relative widths of circle sectors. Total cycle time was about 1.5 sec.

cerebellum in monkeys and humans, said to be caused in monkeys by depression of gamma motoneurons. It is argued that hypotonia may be fundamentally a consequence of loss of cerebellar adaptability.

5. MOTOR LEARNING

HOLMES (1939) doubted that the cerebellum has a 'cognitive' learning function because intelligent patients comprehend their difficulties. He also commented (HOLMES, 1939) that ..."It is a striking feature of acute cerebellar injury that its symptoms gradually decrease in intensity and may in time disappear. This fact...has been explained by compensation by intact parts of the cerebellum and by other parts the nervous system. But even in the acute stages of disease the disturbances may be...reduced by training and by concentrated effort...".

The ability to adjust to the unexpected is compromised: 4 patients with cerebellar signs have been described who could not adapt their 'long-loop' (120 msec) stretch reflexes (in the gastrocnemius) to unexpected, postural adjustments (cf. Fig. 2). whereas 5/12 normal humans could do so within 3–5 trials, by adjusting gain (NASHNER, 1976).

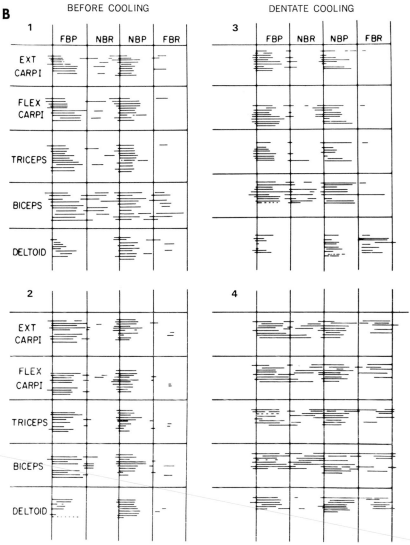

Fig. 6 (B)

B: Improved EMG coordination during motor learning (boxes 1, 2), and its reversal during dentate cooling (boxes 3, 4). Standardized displays of EMG activity (rows) and task cycle phases (columns). Each horizontal line represents duration of EMG in relation to standardized phase of task, regardless of real times, (cf. *A*.) 1: Early training with bars in a new position. 2: Improvement 2 min later. 3: A few min later while denate temperature fell from 27°C to 23°C. 4: A few min later yet, when temperature was 21°C to 19°C. (*A* and *B* from HORVATH et al., 1970)

Degradation of learned, skilled limb movements during brief, reversible dysfunction of neocerebellar output was demonstrated by cooling the dentate nucleus in a monkey trained to make reaching movements with the arm in executing an alternate bar-pressing task (HORVATH et al., 1970) as explained schematically in Fig. 6A. Smooth task execution was disturbed more by cooling if either bar was placed in a position that was difficult to reach: e.g., requiring shoulder retraction (extension) and extreme elbow flexion, or shoulder flexion and full elbow extension. When a new combination of bar positions was presented, the monkey learned the task during the first few trials with longer and more variable reaching and pressing times than those in a well-rehearsed situation. Within a few minutes, however, the original speed and reliability were regained; and well-synchronized patterns for shoulder, arm and wrist muscles evolved for that bar arrangement (Fig. 6B: 1 and 2). Thus, as 'skill' developed, muscular coordination improved and movement times became shorter. These learned improvements were reversed by dentate cooling, producing EMG patterns characteristic of performance before training (Fig. 6B: 3 and 4). We described this decomposition of compound movements as unlearning: "The changes in performance during cooling tended to resemble the changes in performance which occurred when positions of the bars were altered so that the monkey had to learn a new situation. Both task modification and cooling were followed by... disruption in timing patterns of movements,...and disruption of patterned EMG activity" (HORVATH et al., 1970). This seemed far-fetched at the time, and unfortunately was not pursued further, except to note and stress that compensation after reversible or permanent cerebeller lesions became unstable or was even lost when task conditions changed (BROOKS et al., 1973a).

Two theories for motor learning were advanced independently in 1968/9. ITO (1970a) proposed that the cerebellum might function as an adaptive feedforward control mechanism for movements, by replacing guidance through long peripheral-cerebral feedback loops with a "short-cut, side-loop" through the cerebellum, acting as a "dummy". ..."Voluntary movement would be performed in the way programmed in the cerebellum without referring to its actual end effect. This seems to be the case with learned, skilled movements" (ITO, 1970a). "Adequate performance of this feedforward system is secured only when the model in the neocerebellum is a faithful miniature of the combination of spinal motor system, the external world and the sensory pathways. Various input pathways into the cerebellum in addition to those from the motor area may serve for adjusting characteristics of the internal model from time to time, just as it is an adaptive control system (ITO, 1970b). Cerebellar syndromes such as dysmetria, intention tremor may be understandable...as the results from loss or impairment of the internal model in the neocerebellum. The cerebrum then has to perform an action by the aid of a large loop passing through the external world, just as in the stage before the patient learned that action" (ITO, 1970b). Fig. 7A (ROBINSON, 1976) depicts a simplified version of ITO's scheme for the vestibulo-ocular reflex (VOR) which was ITO's original model as tested in rabbits (ITO et al., 1974). Changes were reported of the VOR when visual dysmetria was produced in 17 cats by wearing reversing prisms (ROBINSON, 1976), or in rabbits by sustained head rotation combined with visual stimulation (ITO et al., 1974). VOR gain nearly doubled in 3 monkeys after they had worn 2 × magnifying spectacles for a few days, and returned towards normal when they were removed. By the same token, normal gains were reduced to 0.7 when 0.5 × spectacles were used (MILES and FULLER, 1974). Eye movements were adapted in all these cases to stabilize the image on the retina during motion, but only if there was an intact cerebellum, not after its removal.

How learning of skill could be accomplished was first proposed by MARR (1969), by suggesting "...that each olivary cell corresponds to a 'piece of output' which it is necessary to have under control during movements. This could be a movement of a limb or of a digit—and will be called an 'elemental movement'. Each olivary cell is thought to be driven by an instruction [from the cerebral cortex] for that movement to take place. During learning, the cerebrum organizes the movement, and in so doing, causes the appropriate olivary cells to fire in a particular sequence. This causes the P-cells to learn the *contexts* within which their corresponding elemental movements are required, so that next time such a context occurs the mossy fiber activity stimulates the Purkinje

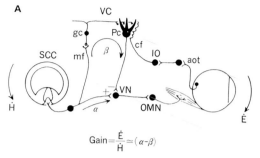

$$\text{Gain} = \frac{\dot{E}}{\dot{H}} \approx (\alpha - \beta)$$

Fig. 7A An example of a learning theory: Automatic gain control as proposed by Ito (ref. 1970b) (Diagram and Legend from ROBINSON, 1976) for the continuous adjustment of the vestibuloocular reflex. The gain of the reflex is eye velocity, E, divided by head velocity, H. The main reflex path of gain α is paralleled by a wide branch through the vestibulo-cerebellum, VC, of gain β so that total gain is proportional to $\alpha - \beta$. The theory hypothesizes that the gain β can be altered (adaptively) by visual information arriving on climbing fibers (cf) (after error detection in the inferior olive, IO). Dysmetria produced by a disorder of any of the main pathway components is detected by the retina which readjusts until the gain is restored to its normal value. SCC, semicircular canals; VN, vestibular nucleus; OMN, oculomotor nucleus; mf, mossy fibers; gc, granule cells; Pc, Purkinje cells; aot, accessory optic tract; IO, inferior olive.

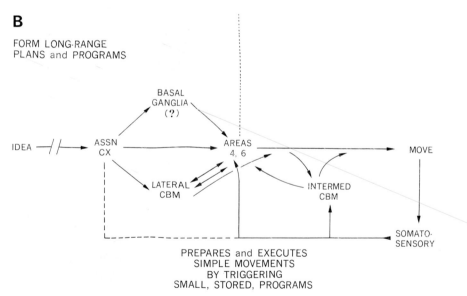

Fig. 7B Proposed roles of several brain structures in movement. It is proposed that association cortex, and perhaps also basal ganglia, are involved in forming 'longrange' plans and programs for volitional movements. The lateral and intermediate parts of the cerebellum store and trigger small programs that prepare and execute simple movements. (see text, Section 6)

cell, which evokes the relevant elemental movement...that are probably small movements..." (MARR, 1969). [Unbeknown to most physiologists, the notion of synaptic learning had been put forward for the cerebellume earlier by BRINDLEY (1964), following HEBB's suggestion (1949) of leaning by synaptic change; and MARR's theory was paralled by a similar, but independent one by ALBUS (1971) who proposed heterosynaptic depression rather than facilitation "...by the climbing fibre teacher..."] ROBINSON (1976) commented that Marr's.... "...theory casts the inferior olive into a very complicated role: it would have to detect dysmetria. That is, it would have to compare the result of the actual reflex behavior (reafference) with what was wanted (derived from efference copy) and use the difference to modify the contributions of the cerebellar cortical path in successive trials until dysmetria was eliminated" (Robinson, 1976). The olive is well suited for this role as a 'comparator', because it receives peripheral and central inputs, critically also those from association cortex (Oscarsson, 1976). Ito incorporated this idea (Ito, 1970b) and added a "teaching line" from the periphery through inferior olive to cerebellum, so that "...the cerebellum could be informed of the results of its performance..." for optimum compensation (Ito, 1972, 1974). Marr's theory was revised in 1970 extending its versatility (Bloomfield and Marr, 1970) and its speed (Gilbert, 1974) so that movement "...corrections can eventually be run by the cerebellar P-cells, without reference to the cerebrum. If a number of similar mossy fiber inputs have been learned and later an unlearned input is presented which is near enough to those which have been learned, then the P-cell may treat the new input as if it had been learned...". Furthermore the theory was extended to neo- and archicortex (Marr, 1971a, b), indicating that the proposed type of learning could occur at many levels. I certainly do not think that only the cerebellar cortex 'learns': this must be a distributed function (cf. Section 6). The evolution of learning theories, and of their speed and versatility, has been reviewed recently (Eccles, 1977). Ito's forthcoming book (1979) is unfortunately not yet available.

Lesions of the inferior olive should and do (Carrea et al., 1947) mimic those of the cerebellum, particularly when tested in the appropriate task context (cf. Brooks, 1979). Ito et al. (1977) have shown that stimulation of the cells of origin of the climbing fibers (in the contralateral inferior olive) could depress the VOR in acute experiments with rabbits, and that this was abolished by destruction of the ipsilateral flocculus. Destruction of the caudal part of the inferior olive in chronically maintained rabbits (Ito and Miyashita, 1975) abolished, or delayed, the visual modification of the horizontal VOR. Procedural problems still plague some of these experiments: the gains of some rabbits' VOR were low, and showed little plasticity as discussed in a recent symposium (Baker and Berthoz, 1977) and those of monkeys actually decreased (Miles and Braitman, 1978). There is by no means universal agreement on a 'learning' role for the olivocerebellar circuit however, with accent on Purkinje-cells (cf. Llinás, in this Symposium). Turning to limb movements, symptoms of cerebellectomy have been reproduced in 2 squirrel monkeys after lesion of the inferior olive contralateral to the operant arm (confirmed histologically for 1 animal) (Soechting et al., 1976). The animals exhibited for weeks ataxia of the head and trunk, dysmetria and oscillations in the course of some movements, and greater movement variability. When tested later, their unloading reflexes were affected as they had been by cerebellar nuclear lesions (cf. Section 3C).

Information about error between intended and actual eye movements (retinal slip) needed for vestibulo-ocular adjustments, is known to ascend towards the olive in the accessory optic tract (cf. Ito, 1972), but olivary error detection remains yet to be proved for limb movements. Such function requires climbing fiber discharge to have low thresholds for changes of detail about movements. This fits the exceedingly fine projections into microzones, recently discovered by electrical stimulation experiments (Oscarsson, 1976) and by radioautographic histological techniques (Courville, 1975). It finds its counterpart by analysis of such discharge giving remarkably detailed information about various parameters of passive joint movements in anesthetized or decerebrate cats (Rubia and Kolb, 1978; Rushmer et al., 1976), but not in awake monkeys (Bauswein et al., 1978). Presumably error-detection is signalled only in intact, conscious animals: in them climbing fibers discharge more consistently only when there may be uncertainty about a level of skilled execution, such as refining pressing-movements (HARVEY et al., 1977), or turning-movements into mechanically undetectable target zones (THACH, 1970b); but not when the task is stereotyped and over-learnt (THACH, 1968). An early attack on this problem (MANO, 1974) had failed, perhaps because the task was too complex for cerebellar processing (cf. Section 1): monkeys were trained to make selective alternate reaching hand movements to push a number of buttons for reward in complicated sequences. Only 4/21 analyzed P-cells showed correlation of climbing fiber discharge to selective task performance.

That climbing fibers do indeed dicharge during adaptation of *simple* limb movements to a new situation has been shown by GILBERT and THACH (1977), who found that P-cells could respond to climbing fiber input in time-locked manner during adaptation of 3 monkeys' wrist movements opposing a new load situation, until the animals learned to make smooth, skilled, movements in that situation within 20–50 trials. This was true for 14 out of 20 transient-related and 5 out of 8 load-related cells. Responses of these cells to parallel (mossy) fiber input, moreover, remained altered thereafter. *If that turns out to be a causal consequence of 'newness', then we could imagine that the cerebellum triggers off immediately usable instructions for adjustments, e.g. of thresholds for peripheral events or limb compliances, to achieve desired timing for muscle forces. The number of trials required for adaptation seems small in all experiments where this has been tested (e.g. also Evarts and Tanji, 1974, 1976 and Fig. 6).*

Summary. The cerebellum may participate in motor learning, but, according to clinical evidence, at a non-cognitive level dealing with motor skill. Cerebellar patients cannot quickly adapt the gain of set-dependent long-loop reflex responses to sudden, unexpected postural changes. Climbing fibers discharge Purkinje cells in time-locked cadence while a new simple motor task is learned by monkeys, and destruction of their cells of origin in the inferior olive degrades adaptability of the vestibulo-ocular reflex in rabbits, cats and monkeys. The mechanisms in motor learning may be of the olivo-cerebellar kind proposed by MARR, and ITO, or ALBUS.

6. COMMON ELEMENTS

Facts. What common elements about cerebellar functions and dysfunctions have emerged in this survey? Observations of human patients and of monkeys with experimental cerebellar lesions show equivalent problems, that in all cases fit like corollary evidence with the properties of cerebellar and precentral neural discharge. The lateral cerebellum does not act cognitively (Section 1), but it participates in imparting 'directional set', as witnessed by special discharge shortly before movement onset and before corrections for perturbed positions; while equivalent precentral discharge is depressed by nuclear dysfunction (Section 1, Fig. 2). This causes us to abandon the notion of cerebellar 'long-term planning' implied in Fig. 1, and to substitute the term 'preparation' in Fig. 7B. The cerebellum has no special role in the production of complicated events like compound movements as such, but instead it sequences constituent simple movements of appropriate force in appropriate time order (Section 3A). The 'updating' function of intermediate cerebellum is retained in Fig. 7B together with the term 'executes'. These two functions overlap with 'preparation' for movements of moderate speed.

The cerebellum exerts many of its effects by governing precentral cortex, whose discharge remains tightly coupled in time to the movement during all conditions of cerebellar performance. Discharge of lateral cerebellum, followed by precentral cortex, triggers movement onset. Both are delayed about 0.1–0.2 sec by lateral cerebellar dysfunction (Section 2, Fig. 3). Ballistic movements are preceded by discharge of lateral cerebellar and precentral neurons. Lateral cerebellar dysfunction prolongs protagonist muscle action during rhythmic ballistic alternations, and thus delays that of the antagonist and hence movement return, by 0.1–0.2 sec (Section 3B, Fig.4). The same delays occur during lateral cerebellar dysfunction in simple movements of moderate speed when monkeys use a strategy of slowed movement oscillations matched by equally prolonged precentral discharge (Section 3C, Fig. 5).

Why should the common element of lateral cerebellar dysfunction for these diverse phenomena, revealed by our experiments, be a delay of about 0.1–0.2 sec? It could be coincidence, or because these phenomena also share a common element, of which the most obvious would be that during cerebellar dysfunction, movements of moderate speed are governed by long and slower loops between periphery and cortex. This view has been taken by most authors (ECCLES, 1967, 1969, 1972; GRANIT, 1970; ITO, 1970b; MEYER-LOHMANN et al., 1975; ROBINSON, 1976, also cf. ALLEN and TSUKAHARA, 1974; PHILLIPS and PORTER, 1977) (Section 3B).

Speculations. Other interpretations can be entertained. Onset of movements of moderate speed was described as being 'triggered', a term that is also applicable to ballistic movements which may be programmed according to length-tension properties of muscles (BIZZI and POLIT, 1979). The implication here is that an array of lateral cerebellar P-cells 'triggers' on coincident arrival of appropriate inputs, mostly from areas 6 and 4, but also from other cortical areas (Section 1), the combination having been learnt previously with the help of the inferior olive (Section 5). P-cell discharge inhibits dentate neurons, that give however post-inhibitory bursts (ECCLES, 1967; THACH, 1972) destined mostly for areas 6 and 4, via VL, that may constitute a Move! command (THACH, 1972) (Figs. 2C, 3 and 7B). These bursts of appropriate combinations of lateral cerebellar neurons may constitute a triggered program forwarded to their targets, including the cortical neurons, where they in turn trigger off stored programs, that compose movements out of muscles. *Fig. 2C is meant to suggest a distributed system: the same argument about lodging program outputs in target cells could be made right around the circle of presumably adaptive neural structures, as well as other circuits. Such feedforward functions do not imply a 'top-down' hierarchy of programs (cf. Brooks, 1979).* Lateral P-cells are assumed to be poised well before movement onset, although they do not discharge at that time, as a result of asynchronous previous learning from integratively functioning brain parts, but they do not act until called upon to prepare the learnt movement (cf. Section 1). Intermediate P-cells and IP-neurons would deal analagously with area 4. Thus initiation of intended movements of all speeds may be programmed (EVARTS and TANJI, 1976; HOUK, 1978), perhaps according to muscle properties for length-tension and force-velocity. *It could be a crucial cerebellar function to smoothly fit intended movements into ongoing spinal and suraspinal servo-control, according to intent as well as peripheral circumstances (cf. Houk, 1978, also Brooks, 1979).*

The inscription beneath Fig. 7B assigns the same 'trigger' function to lateral and intermediate cerebellum. Their programs are thought to be small because simple elbow movements oscillate rapidly and because cerebellar neurons discharge continuously and even more rapidly (cf. ECCLES, 1967, 1969, 1972, 1973). This view transforms the 'updating' function to also include an 'adaptive' mode. The '6 Hz' oscillations of normal monkeys' elbow movements, [that depend on limb properties (cf. VILLS and HORE, 1976), but little on external guidance (BROOKS, 1976)], might set an upper time limit on updating (ALLEN and TSUKAHARA, 1974) of programs for ongoing movements of moderate speed, and thus perhaps also timing onset of the next movement (Section 3B). The deliberate change, in a new situation, to a new strategy (Section 1) using slower oscillations near '3 Hz' may be adequate for the cerebral system to gather peripheral information for movement guidance, when 'predictive' cerebellar capability fails (cf. Section 3C). During this delay of 0.1–0.2 sec, cerebellar computation could be more effectively updated to eliminate inappropriate responses (cf. NASHNER, 1976; PEW, 1974a, b; PHILLIPS and PORTER, 1977), and programs could be 'repaired' to guide movements once more (cf. ROBINSON, 1976). Both might occur in adaptation of postural reflexes (NASHNER, 1976) or of skill in correcting arm perturbations (cf. BROOKS, 1979; HOUK, 1978) of humans and monkeys.

When the adaptive capacity of the lateral cerebellum is impaired by dysfunction however, signs of inappropriate responses remain in monkey's simple elbow movements: muscular actions are prolonged or delayed by about 0.1–0.2 sec. This could be due to slower operation of extracerebellar loops, as pointed out above. In addition moreover, the original programs as learned previously by the cerebral cortex from the normal cerebellum, might be still capable of being triggered by extra-cerebellar inputs; but degraded preparatory updating would now yield degraded responses to commands that were timed and scaled for normal activation (Section 4). *Accuracy of intended movements during cerebellar dysfunction could be determined by the balance of these two processes: slower long-loop feedback guidance and inappropriate feedforward commands.*

These are many suppositions, of which each has been championed by some investigators. Their speculative juxtaposition will be justified if it leads to experimental tests. We need to link programmed movements, the "inverse" relationship between speed and accuracy, and the most "fundamental" consequence of lateral cerebellar dysfunction: delayed sequencing of neural instructions for muscular actions by about 0.1 sec.

ABSTRACT

Evidence is reviewed on function and dysfunction of lateral and intermediate cerebellum in the control of intended limb movements of humans and animals. The main fundamental sign of dysfunction is that actions of precentral neurons and of muscles are delayed or prolonged by about 0.1 sec. The possibility is raised that these degraded functions might arise 1) during loss of cerebellar adaptive capability, because inappropriate movements are initiated upon loss of preparatory updating according to programs learnt when muscles were engaged normally; and 2) by slower, peripheral feedback guidance including long loops through cerebral cortex.

ACKNOWLEDGEMENTS

The author wishes to express his appreciation for research support in past years to the Medical Research Council of Canada; the U. S. Public Health Service; and the Richard and Jean Ivey Fund, London, Canada. Figures are reproduced by permission of the Int. J. Neurol., Elsevier Publishing Co., Plenum Publishing Corp., and the American Physiological Society.

REFERENCES

ALBUS, J. S.: A theory of cerebellar function. *Math. Biosci., 10*: 25–61 (1971)

ALLEN, G. I. and TSUKAHARA, N.: Cerebrocerebellar communication systems. *Physiol. Rev., 54*: 957–1006 (1974)

ALLEN, G. I., GILBERT, P. F. C., MARINI, R., SCHULTZ, W. and YIN, T. C. T.: Integration of cerebral and peripheral inputs by interpositus neurons in monkey. *Exp. Brain Res., 27*: 81–99 (1977)

ALLEN, G. I., GILBERT, P. F. C. and YIN, T. C. T.: Convergence of cerebral inputs onto dentate neurons in monkey. *Exp. Brain Res.*, *32*: 151–170 (1978)

ANDRÉ-THOMAS.: *Le Cervelet*: *Etude Anatomique, Clinique, et Physiologique.* G. Steinheil, Paris (1897)

ANDRÉ-THOMAS.: *La Fonction Cérébelleuse.* Doin et Fils, Paris (1911)

BABINSKI, J.: Sur le role du cervelet dans les actes volitionnels necessitants une succession rapide de mouvements. (Diadococinésie). *Rev. neurol.*, *10*: 1013–1015 (1902)

BAKER, R. and BERTHOZ, A. (eds.): *Control of Gaze by Brain Stem Neurons, Developments in Neuroscience.* Elsevier/North Holland Biomedical Press, Amsterdam, 1 (1977)

BANTLI, H. and BLOEDEL, J. R.: Characteristics of the output from the dentate nucleus to spinal neurons via pathways which do not involve the primary sensorimotor cortex. *Exp. Brain Res.*, *25*: 199–220 (1976)

BAUSWEIN, E., KOLB, F. P. and RUBIA, F. J.: Responses of cerebellar units in the awake rhesus monkey during active and passive movements. *Pflügers Arch.*, *373*: 73 (1978)

BIZZI, C. and POLIT, A.: Characteristics of the motor program underlying visually evoked movements. *In* TALBOTT, R. E. and HUMPHREY, R. (eds.): "*Posture and Movement*: *Perspectives for Integrating Sensory and Motor Research on the Mammalian Nervous System*". Raven Press, New York, 1979. (in press)

BIZZI, E., POLIT, A. and MORASSO, P.: Mechanisms underlying achievement of final head position. *J. Neurophysiol.*, *39*: 435–444 (1976)

BIZZI, E., DEV, P., MORASSO, P. and POLIT, A.: The effect of load disturbances during centrally initiated movements. *J. Neurophysiol.*, *41*: 542–556 (1978)

BLOEDEL, J. R.: Cerebellar afferent systems: A Review. *Prog. Neurobiol.*, *2*: 3–68 (1973)

BLOOMFIELD, S. and MARR, D.: How the cerebellum may be used. *Nature*, *227*: 1224–1228 (1970)

BOTTERELL, E. H. and FULTON, J. F.: Functional localization in the cerebellum of primates. (I. Unilateral section of the peduncles). *J. Comp. Neurol.*, *69*: 31–46, (1938a)

BOTTERELL, E. H. and FULTON, J. F.: Functional localization in the cerebellum of primates. (II. Lesions of midline structures [vermis] and deep nuclei). *J. Comp. Neurol.*, *69*: 47–62 (1938b)

BOTTERELL, E. H. and FULTON, J. F.: Functional localization in the cerebellum of primates. (III. Lesions of hemispheres [neocerebellum]). *J. Comp. Neurol.*, *69*: 63–87 (1938c)

BOTTERELL, E. H. and FULTON, J. F.: Functional localization in the cerebellum of primates. (IV. "Hypotonia" and "ataxia" following lesions of the cerebellum in the chimpanzee). 1938. Unpublished, but cited in FULTON, J. F. and DOW, R. S.: The cerebellum: a summary of functional localization. *Yale J. Biol. Med.*, *10*: 89–119 (1937)

BRAITENBERG, V.: Functional interpretation of cerebellar histology. *Nature, 190*: 539–540 (1961)

BRAITENBERG, V.: Is the cerebellar cortex a biological clock in the millisecond range? *Prog. Brain Res.*, *25*: 334–346 (1967)

BREMER, F.: Le Cervelet: *In* ROBER, G. H. and BINET, L. (eds.): *Traité de Physiologie Normale et Pathologique.* pp. 39–134, Masson, Paris, Vol. 10, Pt. 1, (1935)

BRINDLEY, G.S.: The use made by the cerebellum of the information that it receives from sense organs. *IBRO Bull.*, *3*: 80 (1964) (Abstract)

BROOKHART, J. M.: The cerebellum. *In*: *Handbook of Physiology.* Sect. I, Vol. 2, 1245–1280, Am. Physiol. Soc., Washington, D. C., (1960)

BROOKS, V. B. and STONEY, S. D. Jr.: Motor mechanisms: the role of the pyramidal system in motor control. *Ann. Rev. Physiol.*, *33*: 337–392 (1971)

BROOKS, V. B., KOZLOVSKAYA, I. B., ATKIN, A., HORVATH, F. E. and UNO, M.: Effects of cooling the dentate nucleus on tracking-task performance in monkeys. *J. Neurophysiol.*, *36*: 974–995, (1973a)

BROOKS, V. B., COOKE, J. D. and THOMAS, J. S.: The continuity of movements. *In* STEIN, R. B., PEARSON, K. G., SMITH, R. S. and REDFORD, J. B. (eds.): *Control of Posture and Locomotion.* pp. 257–272, Plenum Press, New York, (1973b)

BROOKS, V. B.: Motor programs revisited. *In* TALBOTT, R. E. and HUMPHREY, D. R. (eds.): *Posture and Movement*: *Perspectives for Integrating Sensory and Motor Research on the Mammalian Nervous System.* pp. 13–49, Raven Press, New York (1979)

BUCHWALD, N. A., HULL, C. D., LEVINE, M. S. and VILLABLANCA, J.: The basal ganglia and the regulation of response and cognitive sets. *In* BRAZIER, M. A. B. (ed.): *Growth and Development of the Brain* pp. 171–189, Raven Press, New York, (1975)

CARREA, R. M. E. and METTLER, F. A.: Physiologic consequences following extensive removals of the cerebellar cortex and deep cerebellar nuclei and effect of secondary cerebral ablations in the primate. *J. Comp. Neurol.*, *87*: 169–288 (1947)

CARREA, R. M. E., REISSIG, M. and METTLER, F. A.: The climbing fibers of the simian and feline cerebellum. Experimental inquiry into their origin by lesions of the inferior olives and deep cerebellar nuclei. *J. Comp. Neurol.*, *87*: 321–365 (1947)

CHAMBERS, W. W. and SPRAGUE, J. M.: Functional localization in the cerebellum. II. Somatotopic organization in cortex and nuclei. *Archi. Neurol. Psychiat. (Chicago)*, *74*: 653–680 (1955)

CONRAD, B. and BROOKS, V. B.: Effects of dentate cooling on rapid alternating arm movements. *J. Neurophysiol.*, *37*: 792–804 (1974)

CONRAD, B., MEYER-LOHMANN, J., MATSUNAMI, K. and BROOKS, V. B.: Precentral unit activity following torque pulse injections into elbow movements. *Brain Res.*, *94*: 219–236 (1975)

CONRAD, B., WIESENDANGER, M., MATSUNAMI, K. and BROOKS, V. B.: Precentral unit activity related to control of arm movements. *Exp. Brain Res.*, *29*: 85–95 (1977)

COOKE, J. D. and THOMAS, J. S.: Forearm oscillation during cooling of the dentate nucleus in the monkey. *Can. J. Physiol. Pharmacol.*, *54*: 430–436 (1976)

COOKE, J. D., BROWN, J. D. and BROOKS, V. B.: Increased dependence on Visual Information for Movement Control in Patients with Parkinson's Disease. *Can. J. Neurol. Sciences, 5*: 413–415 (1978)

COURVILLE, J. and COOPER, C. W.: The cerebellar nuclei of Macaca mulatta: a morphological study. *J. Comp. Neurol.*, *140*: 241–254 (1970)

COURVILLE, J.: Distribution of olivocerebellar fibers demonstrated by a radioautographic tracing method. *Brain Res.*, *95*: 253–263 (1975)

DENNY-BROWN, D. and YANAGISAWA, N.: The role of the basal ganglia in the initiation of movement. *In* YAHR, M. D. (ed.): *The Basal Ganglia.* pp. 115–149, Raven Press, New York, (1976)

DOW, R. S. and MORUZZI, G.: *The Physiology and Pathology of the Cerebellum.* The University of Minnesota Press, Minneapolis (1958)

ECCLES, J. C., ITO, M. and SZENTAGOTHAI, J.: *The Cerebellum as a Neuronal Machine.* Springer Verlag, New York (1967)

ECCLES, J. C.: Circuits in the cerebellar control of movement. *Proc. Nat. Acad. Sci. U. S. A.*, *58*: 336–343 (1967)

ECCLES, J. C.: The dynamic loop hypothesis of movement control. *In* LEIBOVIC, K. N. (ed.): *Information Processing in the Nervous System.* Springer Verlag, Heidelberg, (1969)

ECCLES, J. C., SABAH, N. H., SCHMIDT, R. F. and TABORIKOVA, H.: Mode of operation of the cerebellum in the dynamic loop control of movement. *Brain Res.*, *40*: 73–80 (1972)

ECCLES, J. C.: Review lecture: the cerebellum as a computer: patterns in space and time. *J. Physiol. (London)*, *229*: 1–32 (1973)

ECCLES, J. C.: An instruction-selection theory of learning in the cerebellar cortex. *Brain Res.*, *127*: 327–352 (1977)

EVARTS, E. V. and THACH, W. T.: Motor mechanisms of the CNS: cerebro-cerebellar interrelations. *Ann. Rev. Physiol.*, *31*: 451–498 (1969)

EVARTS, E. V., BIZZI, E., BURKE, R. E., DeLONG, M. and THACH, W. T. (eds.): *Central Control of Movement.* Neurosci. Res, Symp. Summaries, *6*: 1–170 (1972)

EVARTS, E. V. and TANJI, I.: Gating of motor cortex reflexes by prior instruction. *Brain Res.*, *71*: 479–494 (1974)

EVARTS, E. V. and TANJI, J.: Reflex and intended responses in motor cortex pyramidal tract neurons of monkey. *J. Neurophysiol.*, *39*: 1069–1080 (1976)

EVARTS, E. V. and FROMM, C.: Sensory responses in motor cortex neurons during precise motor control. *Neurosci. Letters, 5*: 267–272 (1977)

FROMM, C. and EVARTS, E. V.: Relation of motor cortex neurons to precisely controlled and ballistic movements. *Neurosci. Letters, 5*: 259–265 (1977)

FULTON, J. F. and DOW, R. S.: The cerebellum: a summary of functional localization. *Yale J. Biol. Med.*, *10*: 89–119 (1937)

FUSTER, J. M.: Unit activity in prefrontal cortex during delayed response performance: neuronal correlates of transient memory. *J. Neurophysiol.*, *34*: 61–78 (1973)

GIBSON, A., BAKER, J., MOWER, G. and GLICKSTEIN, M.: Corticopontine cells in area 18 of the cat. *J. Neurophysiol.*, *41*: 484–495 (1978)

GILBERT, P. F. C.: A theory of memory that explains the function and structure of the cerebellum. *Brain Res.*, *70*: 1–18 (1974)

GILBERT, P. F. C. and THACH, W. T.: Purkinje cell activity during motor learning. *Brain Res.*, *128*: 309–328 (1977)

GILMAN, S.: The mechanism of cerebellar hypotonia. An experimental study in the monkey. *Brain*, *92*: 621–638 (1969)

GILMAN, S.: The nature of cerebellar dyssynergia. *In* WILLIAMS, D. (ed.): *Modern Trends in Neurology.* pp. 60–79, Butterworths, London, (1972)

GILMAN, S. and EBEL, H. C.: Fusimotor neuron responses to natural stimuli as a function of prestimulus fusiomotor activity in decerebellate cats. *Brain Res.*, *21*: 367–384 (1970)

GILMAN, S. and MACDONALD, W. I.: Relation of afferent fiber conduction velocity to reactivity of muscle spindle receptors after cerebellectomy. *J. Neurophysiol.*, *30*: 1513–1522 (1967)

GILMAN, S. and VAN DER MEULEN, J. P.: Recovery of muscle spindle activity after cerebellar ablation. *J. Neurophysiol.*, *28*: 943–957 (1965)

GILMAN, S., CARR, D. and HOLLENBERG, J.: Kinematic effects of deafferentation and cerebellar ablation. *Brain*, *99*: 311–330 (1976)

GLASER, G. H. and HIGGINS, D. C.: Motor stability, stretch responses and the cerebellum. *In* GRANIT, R. (ed.): *Muscular Afferents and Motor Control. Nobel Symposium I.* pp. 121–138, Almquist and Wiksell, Stockholm, (1966)

GOLDBERGER, M. E. and GROWDON, J. H.: Pattern of recovery following cerebellar deep nuclear lesions in monkeys. *Exp. Neurol.*, *39*: 307–322 (1973)

GRANIT, R., HOLMGREN, B. and MERTON, P. A.: The two routes for excitation of muscle and their subservience to the cerebellum. *J. Physiol. (London)*, *130*: 213–224 (1955)

GRANIT, R.: The Basis of Motor Control; Integrating the Activity of Muscles, Alpha and Gamma Motoneurons and Their Leading Control Systems. Academic Press, New York, (1970)

GROWDON, J. H., CHAMBERS, H. W. and LIU, C. N.: An experimental study of cerebellar dyskinesia in the rhesus monkey. *Brain*, *90*: 603–632 (1967)

HAAXMA, R. and KUYPERS, H.: Role of occipito-frontal cortico-cortical connections in visual guidance of relatively independent hand and finger movements in rhesus monkeys. *Brain Res.*, *71*: 361–366 (1974)

HANSEN, K. and HOFFMANN, P.: Weitere Untersuchungen uber die Bedeutung der Eigenreflexe fur unsere Bewegungen. I. Anspannungs und Entspannungsreflexe. *Z. Biol.*, *75*: 293–304 (1922)

HARVEY, R. J., PORTER, R. and RAWSON, J. A.: Activity related to the performance of a learned motor task in Purkinje cells of the intermediate zone of the monkey cerebellum. *J. Physiol. (London)*, *271*: 515–536 (1977)

HEBB, D. O.: "*The Organization of Behaviour; A Neurophysiological Theory*". Wiley, New York (1949)

HOLMES, G.: The symptoms of acute cerebellar injuries due to gunshot injuries. *Brain*, *40*: 461–535 (1917)

HOLMES, G.: Clinical symptoms of cerebellar disease and their interpretation. The Croonian lectures I. *Lancet*, *1*: 1177–1182 (1922a)

HOLMES, G.: Clinical symptoms of cerebellar disease and their interpretation. The Croonian lectures II. *Lancet*, *1*: 1231–1237 (1922b)

HOLMES, G.: Clinical symptoms of cerebellar disease and their interpretation. The Croonian lectures III. *Lancet*, *2*: 59–65 (1922c)

HOLMES, G.: Clinical symptoms of cerebellar disease and their interpretation. The Croonian lectures IV. *Lancet*, *2*: 111–115 (1922d)

HOLMES, G.: The cerebellum of man. (The Hughlings Jackson memorial lecture). *Brain*, *62*: 1–30 (1939)

HORE, J., MEYER-LOHMANN, J. and BROOKS, V. B.: Basal ganglia cooling disables learned arm movements of monkeys in the absence of visual guidance. *Science*, *195*: 584–586 (1977)

HORVATH, F. E., ATKIN, A., KOZLOVSKAYA, I., FULLER, D. R. G. and BROOKS, V. B.: Effects of cooling the dentate nucleus on alternating bar-pressing performance in monkey. *Int. J. Neurol.*, *7*: 252–270 (1970)

HOUK, J. C.: Participation of reflex mechanisms and reaction-time processes in the compensatory adjustments to mechanical disturbances. *In* DESMEDT, J. E. (ed.): *Cerebral Motor Control in Man: Long Loop Mechanisms.* Vol. 4, *Prog. Clin. Neurophysiol.* pp. 193–215, Karger, Basel (1978)

ILLERT, M., LUNDBERG, A. and TANAKA, R.: Integration in descending motor pathways controlling the forelimb in the cat. 3. Convergence on propriospinal neurons transmitting disynaptic excitation from the corticospinal tract and other descending tracts. *Exp. Brain Res., 29*: 323–346 (1977)

ILLERT, M. and TANAKA, R.: Integration in descending motor pathways controlling the forelimb in the cat. 4. Corticospinal inhibition of forelimb motoneurones mediated by short propriospinal neurones. *Exp. Brain Res., 31*: 131–141 (1978)

ITO, M.: The cerebello-vestibular interaction in cat's vestibular nuclei neurones. *In* GRAYBIEL, A. (ed.): *Proc. 4th Symposium on the Role of the Vestibular Organs in Space Exploration.* Pensacola-1968 National Research Council, Florida, NASA SP-187 (1970a)

ITO, M.: Neurophysiological aspects of the cerebellar motor control system. *Int. J. Neurol., 7*: 162–176 (1970b)

ITO, M.: Neural design of the cerebellar motor control system. *Brain Res., 40*: 81–84 (1972)

ITO, M., SHIIDA, T., YAGI, N. and YAMAMOTO, M.: The cerebellar modification of rabbit's horizontal vestibulo-ocular reflex induced by sustained head rotation combined with visual stimulation. *Proc. Japan Acad., 50*: 85–89 (1974)

ITO, M.: The control mechanisms of cerebellar motor systems. *In* SCHMITT, F. O. and WORDEN, F. G. (eds.): The Neurosciences, Third Study Program. pp. 293–303, MIT Press, Cambridge, (1974)

ITO, M.: *The Cerebellum and Neural Control.* Raven Press, New York, (1979 in press)

ITO, M. and MIYASHITA, Y.: The effects of chronic destruction of the interior olive upon visual modification of the horizontal vestibulo-ocular reflex of rabbits. *Proc. Japan Soc., 51*: 716–720 (1975)

ITO, M., NISIMARU, N. and YAMAMOTO, M.: Specific patterns of neuronal connexions involved in the control of the rabbit's vestibulo-ocular reflexes by the cerebellar flocculus. *J. Physiol. (London), 265*: 833–854 (1977)

JANSEN, J. K. S. and MATTHEWS, P. B. C.: The central control of the dynamic response of muscle spindle receptors. *J. Physiol. (London), 161*: 357–378 (1962)

JONES, E. G. and POWELL, T. P. S.: An anatomical study of converging sensory pathways within the cerebral cortex of the monkey. *Brain, 93*: 793–820 (1970)

KEMP, J. M. and POWELL, J. P. S.: The connexions of the striatum and globus pallidus: synthesis and speculation. *Philos. Trans. R. Soc. Lond. (Biol.), 262*: 441–457 (1971)

KORNHUBER, H. H.: Motor functions of cerebellum and basal ganglia: the cerebellocortical saccadic (ballistic) clock, the cerebello-nuclear hold regulator, and the basal ganglia ramp (voluntary speed smooth movement) generator. *Kybernetic, 8*: 157–162 (1971)

KORNHUBER, H. H.: Cerebellar cortex, cerebellum and basal ganglia. An introduction to their motor function. *In* SCHMITT, F. O. and WORDEN, F. G. (eds.): *The Neurosciences, Third Study Program.* pp. 267–280, MIT Press, Cambridge, (1974)

KUBOTA, K., IWAMOTO, T. and SUZUKI, H.: Visuokinetic activities of primate prefrontal neurons during delayed-response performance. *J. Neurophysiol., 37*: 1197–1212 (1974)

KUYPERS, H. G. J. M.: Central cortical projections to motor and somatosensory cell groups. *Brain, 83*: 161–184 (1960)

LAMARRE, Y., BIOULAC, B., and JACKS, B.: Activity of precentral neurones in concious monkeys: Effects of deafferentation and cerebellar ablation. *J. Physiol. (Paris), 74*: 253–264 (1978)

LARSELL, O. and JANSEN, J. (eds.): *The Comparative Anatomy and Histology of the Cerebellum.* Vol. 3. The Human Cerebellum, Cerebellar Connections, and Cerebellar Cortex. University of Minnesota Press, Minneapolis (1967)

LLINAS, R. (ed.): *Neurobiology of Cerebellar Evolution and Development.* American Medical Association, Chicago (1969)

LLINAS, R.: The cerebellar cortex. *In* TOWER, D. B. (ed.): *The Nervous System.* 1, pp. 235–244, Raven Press, New York (1975)

LIU, C. N. and CHAMBERS, W. W.: A study of cerebellar dyskinesia in the bilaterally deafferented forelimbs of the monkey (Macaca Mulatta and Macaca speciosa). *Acta Neurobiol. Exp., 31*: 263–289 (1971)

LUCIANI, L.: Il Cervelletto: Nuovi Studi di Fisiologia Normale e Patologica. Le Monnier, Firenze (1891)

LUCIANI, L.: *Muscular and Nervous System* (Vol. 3 of "Human Physiology"). Macmillan, London (1915)

LUNDBERG, A.: Control of spinal mechanisms from the brain. *In* TOWER, D.B. (ed.): *The Nervous System.* 1, pp. 253–265, Raven Press, New York (1975)

MANO, N.: Simple and complex spike activities of the cerebellar Purkinje cell in relation to selective alternate movement in intact monkey. *Brain Res., 70*: 381–393 (1974)

MARR, D.: A theory of cerebellar cortex. *J. Physiol. (London), 202*: 437–470 (1969)

MARR, D.: A theory of cerebral neocortex. *Proc. Roy. Soc. London (Biol.), 262*: 23–81 (1971a)

MARR, D.: Simple memory: a theory for archicortex. *Philos. Trans. R. Soc. Lond. (Biol.), 262*: 23–81 (1971b)

MARSDEN, C. D., MERTON, P. A., MORTON, H. B., HALLETT, M., ADAM, J. and RUSHTON, D. N.: Disorders of movement in cerebellar disease in man. *In* ROSE, F.(ed.): *The Physiological Aspect of Clinical Neurology.* pp. 179–199, Blackwells, Oxford, (1977)

MARTIN, J. P.: *The Basal Ganglia and Posture.* Pitman Medical, London (1967)

MATTHEWS, P. B. C.: *Mammalian Muscle Receptors and Their Central Actions.* Edward Arnold Ltd., London (1972)

MEYER-LOHMANN, J., CONRAD, B., MATSUNAMI, K. tnd BROOKS, V. B.: Effects of dentate cooling on precentral unit activity following torque pulse injections into elbow movements. *Brain Res., 94*: 237–251 (1975)

MEYER-LOHMANN, J., HORE, J. and BROOKS, V. B.: Cerebellar participation in generation of prompt arm movements. *J. Neurophysiol., 38*: 871–908 (1977)

MILES, F. A. and BRAITMAN, D. J.: Effect of prolonged optical reversal of vision on the vestibular reflex: Some neurophysiological observations. *Abstracts, 8th Ann. Meet. Soc. Neurosci., 4*: 167 (1978)

MILES, F. A. and FULLER, J. H.: Adaptive plasticity in the vestibulo-ocular responses of the rhesus monkey. *Brain Res., 80*: 512–516 (1974)

MILLER, A. D. and BROOKS, V. B.: Effects of cooling ventral lateral thalamus (VL) and sensori-motor cortex on long-loop reflexes in monkeys. *Abstracts, 7th Ann. Meet. Soc. Neurosci., 3*: 274 (1977)

MILLER, F. R.: The physiology of the cerebellum. *Physiol. Rev., 6*: 124–159 (1926)

MONAKOW, V. C.: *Die Lokalisation im Grosshirn (und der Abbau der Funktion durch kortikale Herde).* J. F. Bergmann, Wiesbaden (1914)

MOUNTCASTLE, V. B., LYNCH, J. C., GEORGOPOULOS, A., SAKATA, H. and ACUNA, C.: Posterior parietal association cortex of the monkey: command functions for operations within extrapersonal space. *J. Neurophysiol., 38*: 871–908 (1975)

MOUNTCASTLE, V. B.: The world around us: neural command functions for selective attention. Schmitt lecture. *Neurosci. Res. Program Bull., 14*, Suppl.: 1–41 (1975)

MURPHY, J. T., WONG, Y. C. and KWAN, H. C.: Distributed feedback systems for muscle control. *Brain Res., 71*: 495–506 (1977)

MURPHY, J. T., WONG, Y. C. and KWAN, H. C.: Afferent-efferent linkages in motor cortex for single forelimb muscles. *J. Neurophysiol., 38*: 990–1014 (1975a)

MURPHY, J. T., KWAN, H. C., MacKAY, W. A. and WONG, Y. C.: Physiological basis of cerebellar dysme'ria. *Can. J. Neurol. Sci., 2*: 279–284 (1975b)

NASHNER, L. M.: Adapting reflexes controlling the human posture. *Exp. Brain Res., 26*: 59–72 (1976)

NEILSON, P. D. and LANCE, J. W.: Reflex transmission characteristics during voluntary in normal man and patients with movement disorders. *In* DESMEDT, J. E. (ed): *"Cerebral Motor Control in Man: Long Loop Mechanism".* Prog. clin Neurophysiol., Karger Basel, *4*: 263–299 (1978).

OSCARSSON, O.: Functional organization of spinocerebellar paths. *In* IGGO, A. (ed.): *Handbook of Sensory Physiology,* Vol. II, Somatosensory System. pp. 339–380, Springer Verlag, Heidelberg, (1973)

OSCARSSON, O.: Spatial distribution of climbing and mossy fibre inputs into the cerebellar cortex. *In* CREUTZFELDT, O. (ed.): Afferent and Intrinsic Organization of Laminated Structures in the Brain. *Exp. Brain Res.,* Suppl. *1*: 36–42 (1976)

PANDYA, D. N. and KUYPERS, H. G. J. M.: Cortico-cortical connections in the rhesus monkey. *Brain Res., 13*: 13–36 (1969)

PARTRIDGE, L. D.: Muscle properties: a problem for the motor physiologist. *In* TALBOTT, R. E. and HUMPHREY, D. R. (eds.): *Posture and Movement: Perspecitves for Integrating Sensory and Motor Research on the Mammalian Nervous System.* Raven Press, New York (1979 in press)

PEW, R. W.: Human perceptual-motor performance. *In* KANTOWITZ, B. (ed.): *Human Information Processing: Tutorials in Performance and Cognition.* pp. 21–39, Lawrence Erlbaum Associates, Potomac, Md., (1974a)

PEW, R. W.: Levels of analysis in motor control. *Brain Res., 71*: 393–400 (1974b)

PHILLIPS, C. G. and PORTER, R.: *Corticospinal Neurones: Their Role in Movement.* Academic Press, New York (1977)

RANISH, N. A. and SOECHTING, J. F.: Studies on the control of some simple motor tasks. Effects of thalamic and red nuclei lesions. *Brain Res., 102*: 339–345 (1976)

ROBERTSON, L. and GRIMM, R.: Responses of primate dentate neurons to different trajectories of the limb. *Exp. Brain Res., 23*: 447–462 (1975)

ROBINSON, D. A.: Adaptive gain control of vestibuloocular reflex by the cerebellum. *J. Neurophysiol., 39*: 954–969 (1976)

RUBIA, F. J. and KOLB, F. P.: Responses of cerebellar units to a passive movement in the decerebrate cat. *Exp. Brain Res., 31*: 387–401 (1978)

RUSHMER, D. S., ROBERTS, W. J. and AUGTER, G. K.: Climbing fiber responses of cerebellar Purkinje cells to passive movement of the cat forepaw. *Brain Res., 106*: 1–20 (1976)

SASAKI, K., KAWAGUCHI, S., OKA, H., SAKAI, M. and MIZUON, N.: Electrophysiological studies on the cerebellocerebral projections in monkeys. *Exp. Brain Res., 24*: 495–507 (1976)

SASAKI, K.: The cerebro-cerebellar interconnections. *Proc. Intern. Union Physiol. Sci., 12*: 619 (1977)

SCHMIDT, E. M., JOST, R. G. and DAVIS, K. K.: Cortical cell discharge patterns in anticipation of a trained movement. *Brain Res., 75*: 309–311 (1975)

SCHULTZ, W., MONTGOMERY, E. B. Jr, and MARINI, R.: Stereotyped flexion of forelimb and hindlimb to microstimulation of dentate nucleus in Cebus monkeys. *Brain Res., 107*: 151–155 (1976)

SEARS, T. A.: The afferent regulation of learnt movements. *Brain Res., 71*: 465–473 (1974)

SOECHTING, J., RANISH, N., PALMINTERI, R. and TERZUOLO, C.: Changes in a motor pattern following cerebellar and olivary lesions in the squirrel monkey. *Brain Res., 105*: 21–44 (1976)

SOLTYSIK, S., HULL, C. D., BUCHWALD, N. A. and FEKETE, T.: Single unit activity in basal ganglia of monkeys during performance of a delayed response task. *Electroencephalogr. Clin. Neurophysiol., 39*: 65–78 (1975)

STEIN, J.: Neural mechanisms in visually controlled arm movements. *In* CHIVERS, D. J. and HERBERT, J. (eds.): *Recent Advances in Primatology: Behaviour.* Academic Press, London (1979 in press)

STETSON, R. H. and BOUMAN, H. D.: The coordination of simple skilled movements. *Arch. Neerland. Physiol., 20*: 179–254 (1935)

STRICK, P. L.: Anatomical analysis of ventrolateral thalamic input to the primate motor cortex. *J. Neurophysiol., 39*: 1020–1031 (1976a)

STRICK. P. L.: Activity of ventrolateral thalamic neurons during arm movement. *J. Neurophysiol. 39*: 1032–1044 (1976b)

STRICK, P. L.: Cerebellar involvement in 'volitional' muscle responses to load changes. *In* DESMEDT, J. (ed.): *Prog. Clin. Neurophysiol.* Vol. 4, pp. 85–93 (1978)

TANJI, J. and EVARTS, E. V.: Anticipatory activity of motor cortex neurons in relation to direction of an intended movement. *J. Neurophysiol., 39*: 1062–1068 (1976)

TANJI, J. and TANIGUCHI, J.: Does the supplementary motor area play a part in modifying motor cortex reflexes? *In* MASSION, J., PAILLARD, J., and WIESENDANGER, M. (eds.): *Pyramidal Microconnexions and Motor Control. J. Physiol.* (Paris), *74*: 317–318 (1978)

TANJI, J., TANIGCHI J., and FUKUSHIMA, Y.: Relation of slowly conducting pyramidal tract neurons to specific aspects of forearm movement. *In* MASSION, J., PAILLARD, J. and WIESENDANGER, M. (eds.): *Pyramidal Micro-connexions and Motor Control. J. Physiol.* (Paris). *74*: 293–296 (1978)

TERZUOLO, C. A., SOECHTING, J. F. and VIVIANI, P.: Studies on the control of some simple motor tasks. II. On the cerebellar control of movements in relation to the formulation of intentional commands. *Brain Res., 58*: 217–222 (1973a)

TERZUOLO, C. A., SOECHTING, J. and PALMINTERI, R.: Studies on the control of some simple motor tasks. III. Comparison of the EMG pattern during ballistically initiated movements in man and squirrel monkey. *Brain Res., 62*: 242–246 (1973b)

TERZUOLO, C. A. and VIVIANI, P.: Parameters of motion and EMG activities during some simple motor tasks in normal subjects and cerebellar patients. *In* COOPER, I. S.. RIKLAN, M. and SNIDER, R. S. (eds.): *The Cerebellum, Epilepsy, and Behavior.* pp. 173–215, Plenum Press, New York, (1974)

THACH, W. T.: Discharge of Purkinje and cerebellar nuclear neurons during rapidly alternating arm movement in the monkey. *J. Neurophysiol., 31*: 785–797 (1968)

THACH, W. T.: Discharge of cerebellar neurons related to two maintained postures and two prompt movements. I. Nuclear cell output. *J. Neurophysiol., 33*: 527–536 (1970a)

TACH, W. T.: Discharge of cerebellar neurons related to two maintained postures and two prompt movements. II. Purkinje cell output and input. *J. Neurophysiol. 33*: 537–547 (1970b)

THACH, W. T.: Cerebellar output; properties, synthesis and uses. *Brain Res., 40*: 89–97 (1972)

THACH, W. T.: Timing of activity in cerebellar dentate nucleus and cerebral motor cortex during prompt volitional movement. *Brain Res., 88*: 233–241 (1975)

THACH, W. T.: Correlation of neural discharge with pattern and force of muscular activity, joint position, and direction of the intended movement in motor cortex and cerebellum. *J. Neurophysiol., 41*: 654–676 (1978)

THACH, W. T.: The cerebellum. *In* MOUNTCASTLE, V. B. (ed.): *Medical Physiology.* 14th ed. C. V. Mosby, St. Louis, MO. (1979 in press)

TRENDELENBURG, W.: Untersuchungen über reizlose vorübergehende Ausschaltung am Zentralnervensystem. III. Die Extremitatenregion der Grosshirnrinde. *Pflügers Arch. ges. Physiol., 137*: 515–544 (1911)

TROUCHE, E., BEAUBATON, D. and GRANGETTO, A.: Reaction time and movement time during cooling of dentate nucleus in monkeys performing a visuomotor pointing task. *Proc. Intern. Union Physiol. Sci., 13*: 764 (1977)

UNO, M., KOZLOVSKAYA, I. B. and BROOKS, V. B.: Effects of cooling the interposed nuclei on tracking-task performance in monkeys. *J. Neurophysiol., 36*: 996–1003 (1973)

VALLBO, A. B.: Muscle spindle response at the onset of isometric voluntary contractions in man. Time difference between fusimotor and skeletomotor effects. *J. Physiol. (London), 218*: 405–431 (1971)

VILIS, T., HORE, J., MEYER-LOHMANN, J. and BROOKS, V. B.: Dual nature of the precentral responses to limb perturbations regealed by cerebellar cooling. *Brain Res., 117*: 336–340 (1976)

VILIS, T. and HORE, J.: Effects of changes in mechanical state of limb on cerebellar intention tremor. *J. Neurophysiol., 40*: 1214–1224 (1977)

VILIS, T. and HORE, J.: A possible explanation of cerebellar tremor. *Abstracts, 8th Ann. Meet. Soc. Neurosci., 4*: 69 (1978)

WELFORD, A. T.: On sequencing of action. *Brain Res., 71*: 381–392 (1974)

WOODWORTH, R. S.: Tht Accuracy of Voluntary Movement. *Psychol. Monograph*, Suppl. 13. pp. 1–114, Macmillan, New York, (1899)

DISCUSSION PERIOD

AMASSIAN: I wonder if measuring the isotherms is quite as fundamental as measuring the firing rates of the neurons. There is a very real possibility that the roof nuclei may show a mixture of depression of firing rates by direct postsynaptic action and also a change in the efficacy of the inhibitory Purkinje cell and the excitatory inputs. As you know, elsewhere in the nervous system, remarkable paradoxes occur in which much bigger outputs occur as a result of cooling. Now, have you substituted a microelectrode for the thermistor in the nucleus dentatus and shown what the firing rates do under these cooling conditions?

BROOKS: No. We have not done it that way. But, we have measured the changes of temperature across histologically identified structures, with reference to a thermocouple on the cooling probe sheath. And we know from other work, particularly that of Professor Chandler BROOKS, who is here, that you first have an 'exaltation', excitability and firing rates go up. Per ANDERSSEN has shown that the cadence of neural discharge changes even with only one or two degrees of cooling. These changes are so subtle that they might disturb the temporal sequence that Professor MOUNTCASTLE was talking about. And then you get to this oversimplification that we all use, namely that synaptic block occurs around 20°, and fiber conduction block around 15° to 10°. One must look at the time course however, because you have to cool fibers for quite a long time before they block at that temperature, not just in a minute under the conditions of spatial distribution that we use. The most important point though, is to establish, by isotherms, what structures *other* than the "target" have been cooled, particularly in a crowded space like the thalamus.

MOUNTCASTLE: It is true that in human material the set of symptoms and signs you describe in cerebellar disease can be dissociated. There are many patients with those signs but with little or no hypotonia. That would favor your alternative hypothesis wouldn't it?

BROOKS: I think it might very well. And I have stressed that we cannot measure hypotonia quantitatively. Perhaps at some future time, we will find out if hypotonia means loss of adaptive capability.